Ethical Issues in Cardiovascular Medicine

This book provides an exploration of the ethics of cardiology practice. It provides a variety of frameworks for analyzing ethical issues that arise in cardiovascular medicine.

Cardiovascular medicine—the diagnosis and treatment of congenital and acquired diseases of the heart, major arteries, and veins—has seen rapid change in diagnosis, treatment, and the organization of practice in the last half of the twentieth and the beginning of the twenty-first century. The complexity of these developments has resulted in increasing subspecialization, and many practitioners are challenged to stay abreast with the latest developments in cardiology. These changes also bring with them various ethical challenges. The chapters in this volume are divided by five broad areas of practice: beginning-of-life; end-of-life; allocation of expensive or scarce resources; professionalism; and research. The case-based approach presented across the volume provides a perspective that will allow readers to reason through current and future ethical issues as they arise in this rapidly changing field.

Ethical Issues in Cardiovascular Medicine will be of interest to researchers working in bioethics, clinical ethics, and the philosophy of medicine, as well as practicing physicians, nurses, and students who work in cardiovascular medicine.

David M. Zientek is Clinical Assistant Professor at the Department of Internal Medicine, University of Texas at Austin Dell Medical School, USA. He has practiced general and interventional cardiology for 29 years and served as co-chair of the Ascension Seton Medical Center ethics committee for 17 years and a member of the American College of Cardiology Ethics and Disciplinary committee for 6 years.

Mark J. Cherry is the Dr. Patricia A. Hayes Professor in Applied Ethics and Professor of Philosophy, St. Edwards University, USA. He is Editor of *The Journal of Medicine and Philosophy*, Senior Editor of *Christian Bioethics*, and Editor-in-Chief of *HealthCare Ethics Committee (HEC) Forum*. He is the author of *Kidney for Sale by Owner: Human Organs, Transplantation, and the Market* (2005/2015) and *Sex, Family and the Culture Wars* (2016).

Routledge Annals of Bioethics

Series Editors:

Mark J. Cherry
St. Edward's University, USA

Ana Smith Iltis
Wake Forest University, USA

Ethical Issues in Cardiovascular Medicine

Edited by David M. Zientek
and Mark J. Cherry

Routledge
Taylor & Francis Group

NEW YORK AND LONDON

First published 2022
by Routledge
605 Third Avenue, New York, NY 10158

and by Routledge
2 Park Square, Milton Park, Abingdon, Oxon, OX14 4RN

Routledge is an imprint of the Taylor & Francis Group, an informa business

Library of Congress Cataloging-in-Publication Data
Names: Zientek, David M., editor. | Cherry, Mark J., editor.
Title: Ethical issues in cardiovascular medicine / edited by David M. Zientek and Mark J. Cherry.
Description: New York, NY : Taylor & Francis, 2022. | Series: Routledge annals of bioethics | Includes bibliographical references and index.
Subjects: LCSH: Cardiovascular system--Diseases. | Heart--Diseases. | Cardiology--Moral and ethical aspects.
Classification: LCC RC667 .E84 2022 (print) | LCC RC667 (ebook) | DDC 174.2/961--dc23
LC record available at https://lccn.loc.gov/2021032734
LC ebook record available at https://lccn.loc.gov/2021032735

ISBN: 978-1-032-13998-2 (hbk)
ISBN: 978-1-032-14631-7 (pbk)
ISBN: 978-1-003-24027-3 (ebk)

DOI: 10.4324/9781003240273

Typeset in Bembo
by SPi Technologies India Pvt Ltd (Straive)

Contents

Notes on Contributors

Dawn Allain is Director, Genetic Counseling Graduate Program and Associate Professor in the Division of Human Genetics, Department of Internal Medicine, The Ohio State University, USA

Emily E. Anderson is Associate Professor at the Neiswanger Institute for Bioethics, Stritch School of Medicine, Loyola University Chicago, USA

Teresa Lynne Caples is Adjunct Faculty at the Graduate School of Nursing and Master of Public Health Program, University of West Florida, USA

Alexandra Charrow is Attending Dermatologist at Brigham and Women's Hospital and Instructor of Medicine at Harvard University Medical School, USA

Sara Cherny is Cardiovascular Genetic Counselor at Ann & Robert H. Lurie Children's Hospital of Chicago and Assistant Professor of Pediatrics at Northwestern University Feinberg School of Medicine, USA

Mark J. Cherry is the Dr. Patricia A. Hayes Professor in Applied Ethics and Professor of Philosophy, St. Edwards University, USA

Angela Clark is Associate Professor Emeritus at The University of Texas at Austin School of Nursing

Dalia M. Feltman is Clinical Associate Professor at University of Chicago Pritzker School of Medicine, Neonatologist at NorthShore University HealthSystem Evanston Hospital, USA

Mark A. Hoffman is Partner at Ross Feller Casey, LLP, USA

Ana S. Iltis is Director of the Center for Bioethics, Health and Society and Professor of Philosophy at Wake Forest University, USA

Pamela Jordi is an Obstetrician and Gynecologist at Clinic Sofia OBGYN, USA

James N. Kirkpatrick is Professor of Medicine and Bioethics and Humanities, Section Chief, Cardiac Imaging, Division of Cardiology, and Director of Echocardiography at University of Washington Medical Center, USA

Douglas E. Lemley is a retired physician and bioethicist in Greensboro, North Carolina, USA

Daniel D. Matlock is Head of the Division of Geriatrics, Director of the Colorado Program for Patient Centered Decisions, and Associate Professor of Medicine at the University of Colorado School of Medicine, USA

Kayhan Parsi is Professor of Bioethics and Director of the Graduate Program at the Neiswanger Institute for Bioethics, Loyola University Chicago Stritch School of Medicine, USA

Behzad Pavri is Professor in the Department of Medicine and Director of the Cardiac Electrophysiology Fellowship Program at Thomas Jefferson University, USA

Joy Penticuff is Professor Emeritus at The University of Texas at Austin School of Nursing, USA

James Smith, Jr. is Professor in the School of Medicine, Creighton University, USA

Keith M. Swetz is Professor of Medicine at the University of Alabama School of Medicine and Medical Director of UAB Medicine's Supportive Care Clinic, USA

Sara E. Wordingham is Assistant Professor of Medicine, Mayo Clinic College of Medicine, USA

David M. Zientek is Clinical Assistant Professor at the Department of Internal Medicine, University of Texas at Austin Dell Medical School, USA

Acknowledgments

The development of this volume benefited through the kind efforts of many friends and colleagues. Its origin was a realization on the part of the editors of the need more fully to explore the significant bioethical issues that arise in cardiovascular medicine. Our goal was to produce a volume punctuated with case studies and theoretical analysis that would speak to practicing physicians, nurses, bioethicists, and other cardiovascular caregivers, while also being useful for medical students or residents as they complete their training. We are deeply thankful to the contributors, who recast their essays several times to craft the final versions that appear herein.

David Zientek wishes to recognize his partners at Ascension Texas Cardiovascular for allowing him time from a busy clinical practice to pursue his interest in bioethics, and the many colleagues whose thoughtful questions provided many of the issues addressed in these chapters, in particular Mary Beth Cishek, David Kessler and George Rodgers. I am indebted to the faculty at the Neiswanger Institute for Bioethics and Healthcare Leadership for their assistance with the initial outline for this volume, especially Nanette Elster, Kayhan Parsi, and Mark Kuczewski. Finally, the completion of this project would not have been possible without the loving encouragement and patience of my wife, Colleen, and daughters, Emily, Sarah, and Kate.

Mark J. Cherry wishes to recognize the ongoing generosity of St. Edward's University, the School of Arts and Humanities, and the Philosophy Department, especially Sharon Nell, Peter Wake and Jack Musselman. Each has been instrumental, though in quite diverse ways, to the success of this project. As with all of my projects, this volume would not exist without the constant support, kindness, and love of my wife, Mollie.

David Zientek
Mark J. Cherry
June, 2021

Cardiovascular Ethics

An Introduction

David M. Zientek

I Introduction

Cardiology, and more broadly cardiovascular medicine, the diagnosis and treatment of congenital and acquired diseases of the heart, major arteries, and veins, has seen rapid change in diagnosis, treatment, and the organization of practice in the last half of the twentieth and the beginning of the twenty first century (Braunwald 2003; Mehta and Khan 2002). These changes bring with them various ethical challenges. Evolution in the practice of cardiology has been particularly influenced by large-scale clinical trials. For example, the Framingham Heart Study, begun in 1948, recruited and prospectively followed a cohort of 5,209 men and women from Framingham, Massachusetts without symptoms of cardiovascular disease and first demonstrated that hypertension, smoking, and elevated cholesterol were risk factors for the development of disease (Braunwald 2003; Kannel, Dawber, Kagan, Revotskie and Stokes 1961; Mehta and Khan 2002). These findings provided a basis for the development of multiple diagnostic and therapeutic strategies for primary (before the development of clinical disease) and secondary (after the development of clinical disease) prevention and treatment of cardiovascular disease. In order to detect small, but significant benefits of various diagnostic and therapeutic modalities, many studies have recruited hundreds or thousands of patients. The size of these studies often preclude a single academic center from conducting the research, resulting in many studies being conducted at multiple sites with widespread involvement of non-academic clinical cardiologists and pharmaceutical or device companies in research.[1] While research has led to many pharmaceutical and lifestyle modifications to treat heart disease, when compared to other medical subspecialties, cardiology is uniquely dependent on technology. In particular, recent decades have seen the development of devices implanted in patients such as pacemakers and defibrillators to regulate the heart rhythm, ventricular assist devices to support the failing heart, and intracoronary stents for the treatment of myocardial infarction and chronic coronary artery disease (Braunwald 2003; Klaidman 2000; Mehta and Khan 2002; Patel, Kalra, Doshi, Bajaj, Arora, and Arora 2018). The rapid pace of new research coupled with the increasing complexity has resulted in difficulty mastering the entire field, leading to the development of multiple subspecialties

DOI: 10.4324/9781003240273-1

within cardiology.[2] Despite such advances, cardiovascular disease remains the leading non-infectious cause of death worldwide with 17.9 million deaths versus 9.0 million for the second cause, cancer. As a result, advances in medical care and changes in practice have a significant global impact on individual and community health, the cost and distribution of healthcare, and health policy (World Health Organization 2020).

While large clinical trials and the resulting changes in diagnostic and therapeutic approaches have had a major impact on the clinical practice of cardiology, the specialty has also evolved in the larger context of medicine and society in general. The United States continues to have a complex system of paying for healthcare with federal programs such as Medicare and Medicaid, a variety of private insurance programs, and a significant proportion of uninsured patients. Changes in the way cardiologists are reimbursed and new requirements for documentation have had a profound impact on the way cardiology is practiced. For example, 90% of cardiologists were in independent private practice groups in 2007, but by 2013 only 29% remained in independent practice. A major reason for this shift to practices integrated with large hospital and health systems was a change in Medicare reimbursement: there was a significant decrease in payment for several types of imaging studies when performed in a physician office, but no change in reimbursement if the study was performed in a hospital facility (Jaskie and Rodgers 2014). At the same time, federal mandates requiring adoption of costly electronic medical records and new forms of reimbursement based on achieving certain quality measures (requiring significant time and manpower to document) were other forces that made independent private practice difficult financially to sustain (Jaskie and Rodgers 2014). Similarly, uncertainty in the availability of outside research funding and institutional pressure to increase financially lucrative clinical work has forced many academic physicians to change from a more research-based, to a more clinically-oriented practice with an ever-more significant increase in research being performed in the private practice setting, funded by pharmaceutical and device companies (Fanari and Weiss 2015). In addition to changes in reimbursement, and reporting requirements, the practice of cardiology has been influenced by efforts to improve quality and reduce error. Since the publication of the Institute of Medicine's Study *To Err is Human* demonstrating that a significant number of patients die each year from medical errors, there has been an increased focus on evaluating systems, rather than individual practitioners as a major factor in these errors (Kohn, Corrigan, and Donaldson 1999). One aspect of this system level focus has been a cultural change emphasizing the importance of teamwork among all healthcare providers, including nurses, aides, therapists, and others in reporting and helping prevent errors and harm to patients, rather than viewing the physician alone as the "captain of the ship."[3]

Over the same time frame, as cardiology has developed into a broad and complex field and practice has been shaped by financial and other pressures outside the scientific realm, the field of bioethics has also gained increasing prominence (Jonsen 1998). Much of the interest in bioethics has arisen from the forces shaping medicine in general and cardiology in particular. As medicine has become more complex with the ability to extend life, though at times at the expense of significant complications or poor quality of life for patients, physicians, theologians, philosophers, lawyers, and others began to ask if there were legitimate limits to the use of advanced medical interventions, how those limits could be defined, and whether treatment could be stopped once initiated (Jonsen 1998). Revelations of the use of prisoners for research in Nazi Germany during the Nuremburg trials and later instances of researchers exposing patients to unnecessary risk, such as the Tuskegee study in the United States, led to new policies to regulate clinical research and emphasized the importance of informed consent both for research and clinical treatment (Weindling 2004; Jones 2008). As the cost of healthcare has increased with resources in some instances remaining limited, such as the availability of human organs for transplant, there has been interest in how fairly to distribute expensive or scarce resources (Jonsen 2007, Persad, Wertheimer, and Emanuel 2009). Finally, changes in the way practice is structured by different forms of reimbursement, and how healthcare organizations ensure quality while minimizing unintended harm to patients has stimulated the study of conflicts of interest, and organizational structures best suited to provide quality care.[4] Case-based and topic-focused, this book provides an exploration of ethical issues in five broad areas of cardiology practice: beginning-of-life, end-of-life, allocation of expensive or scarce resources, professionalism, and research. The discussions in the book will be useful to practitioners, ethicists, and students. Together, they provide a variety of frameworks for analyzing ethical issues that arise in cardiovascular medicine. Here, I begin with an overview of the evolution of cardiology as a medical specialty and subsequently consider the ethical implications of the evolving practice.

II An Overview of Cardiovascular Advances in the Twentieth and Twenty-first Centuries

While much was known about the anatomy and function of the heart prior to the twentieth century, a number of developments in the past 120 years have led to the practice of cardiology as we know it today. In a review of the history and future of cardiology in 2003, Eugene Braunwald identified the use of a string galvanometer by Willem Einthoven in the early 1900s, to record the first standardized electrocardiograms measuring the electrical activity of the heart, as giving birth to modern cardiology (Braunwald 2003; Mehta and Khan 2002). Within ten years, patterns on the electrocardiogram were found to correlate with structural abnormalities of the heart, arrhythmias and ischemic changes revolutionizing the diagnosis of heart disease. The electrocardiogram also serves as the basis for stress testing for the diagnosis and risk assessment of those with coronary artery disease and arrhythmias.

Advances in understanding the electrical activation of the heart and arrhythmias has led to the development of electrophysiology as a subspecialty within cardiology. Major advances in this field have included the ability to correct abnormal rhythms with an external shock, with the first external defibrillation of a human in 1956 by Paul Zoll (Zoll, Paul, Linenthal, Norman, and Gibson 1956). This led to the development of coronary care units in the 1960s where patients with life-threatening arrhythmias, one of the leading causes of death post-myocardial infarction, could be treated successfully with the defibrillator (Mehta and Khan 2002). The first implantation of an internal pacemaker to regulate the electrical activation of the heart was reported in 1959 in Switzerland by Rune Elmqvist and Ake Senning (Elmqvist and Senning 1960). More recently, Michel Mirowski working at Sinai Hospital in Baltimore developed an implantable electrical defibrillator allowing conversion of ventricular arrhythmias in ambulatory patients with the first implantation in 1980 (Mirowski et al. 1980). While implantable defibrillators are life-saving, converting lethal arrhythmias back to a normal rhythm, the shocks delivered within the chest can be extremely painful and psychologically traumatic. These devices have since been modified to allow resynchronizing the activation of the ventricles of the heart, significantly improving symptoms in a subset of heart failure patients.

While some researchers advanced our understanding about the electrical activity of the heart, others were studying the blood supply to, and the mechanical structure of, the heart. In 1929, a German surgeon, Werner Forssman, hoping to find a means of injecting drugs for cardiac resuscitation, performed what is considered the first cardiac catheterization on himself by inserting a catheter into the vein of his left arm and confirming its position in the right atrium by radiography (Forssmann 1974). Subsequently, in the 1940s, Andre Cournand and Dickinson Richards used cardiac catheterization to measure cardiac output and pressures in the right side of the heart (Cournand, Riley, Breed, Baldwin, Richards, Lester, and Jones 1945). Building on these techniques, in 1958 Mason Sones performed the first coronary angiograms allowing detailed evaluation of coronary artery anatomy and the natural history of coronary artery disease (Sones and Shirey 1962).

Cardiac catheterization and angiography paved the way for cardiovascular surgery and later percutaneous revascularization of the heart. In 1953, surgeon John Gibbon performed the first surgery using a heart-lung machine to repair an atrial septal defect. He had worked closely with engineers at IBM to develop the device to oxygenate and pump blood outside the body allowing protection of other organs during surgery (Gibbon 1954; Klaidman 2000). Interestingly, in this early collaboration between clinicians and industry, IBM foreswore any future profits from the invention (Comroe 1983; Klaidman 2000). The heart-lung machine allowed the development of coronary artery bypass surgery with the first internal mammary artery to coronary artery anastomosis performed in 1964 by Vasilii Kolessov, and the first use of saphenous vein grafts by Rene Favaloro in 1967 (Favaloro 1971; Kolessov 1967). Further, the heart-lung machine expanded the ability to repair congenital heart defects and perform repair and replacement of cardiac valves. Andreas Gruentzig performed the first coronary artery angioplasty, using a balloon catheter to dilate an obstructed coronary artery in 1977 (Gruentzig, Myler, Hanna, and Turina 1977). This last development has led to the field of interventional cardiology with the development of coronary artery stents as a less invasive treatment for coronary artery disease versus bypass grafting in certain patients, and, increasingly less invasive, percutaneous treatment of structural and valvular heart disease.

The improved ability to treat coronary artery, congenital and valvular heart disease has allowed many patients to live significantly longer lives, but has also led to an increasing prevalence of chronic problems such as congestive heart failure (Chair, Yu, Ng, Wang, Cheng, Wong, and Sit 2016). Patients who, in the past, may have died suddenly from a myocardial infarction, often now survive, but with significant damage to their heart (cardiomyopathy), leading to heart failure. Here, again, there have been significant advances in the past century. While newer medical regimens have significantly altered the course of the disease, cardiomyopathy remains a significant cause of mortality and morbidity with over 58,000 deaths in the United States alone (Chair, Yu, Ng, Wang, Cheng, Wong, and Sit 2016). Cardiac transplantation, first successfully reported in 1967 by Christiaan Barnard in South Africa, is still considered the treatment of choice for end-stage cardiomyopathy (Kittleson and Kobashigawa 2017; Sliwa and Zilla 2017). However, the limited pool of available donor hearts has led to the search for alternatives such as the left ventricular assist device, with the first successful implantation by Dr. Louis De Bakey in 1966 (Chair, Yu, Ng, Wang, Cheng, Wong, and Sit 2016). These devices were originally used as a temporary "bridge" to support patients awaiting transplantation, but with improved technology, and reductions in the size of the devices, they are now often used as permanent therapy for patients who are not candidates for transplantation, albeit with significant impacts on lifestyle and the potential for significant complications (Pinney, Anyanwu, Lala, Teuteberg, Uriel, and Mehra 2017).

In addition to electrocardiography, other techniques for noninvasive evaluation of the heart have grown exponentially. A notable step in noninvasive imaging occurred in the early 1950s when Inge Edler, a cardiologist, and Helmuth Hertz, a physicist, in Sweden adapted a sonar, developed to detect submarines during World War II, to obtain ultrasound images of the heart, giving rise to the field of echocardiography to image cardiac structures and motion (Edler and Hertz 1954). Interest in noninvasive imaging over the years has extended to the use of nuclear isotopes in imaging, magnetic resonance imaging (MRI) and computed tomography (CT) of the heart, all with their distinct strengths, weaknesses, and indications for diagnosing cardiac disease.

Along with technological advances, preventive cardiology and drug therapy have rapidly advanced. The Framingham Study is often credited with introducing the idea of risk factors for developing cardiovascular disease, such as hypertension, hyperlipidemia, and smoking, and emphasized the importance of correcting these risk factors (Kannel, Dawber, Kagan, Revotskie, and Stokes 1961). The identification of these factors provided targets for drug development, including the development of beta blockers and angiotensin-converting enzyme inhibitors for hypertension and systolic heart failure, thrombolytic agents, antiplatelet and anticoagulant drugs for coronary artery disease, valvular disease and atrial fibrillation, and statins (3-hydroxy-3-methylglutaryl coenzyme A reductase inhibitors) for hyperlipidemia. These medications and others have revolutionized the treatment of both risk factors and established cardiovascular disease.

More recently, genetics has assumed a growing role in the study of cardiovascular disorders. A genetic component has been identified for many cardiovascular diseases, including various arrhythmias such as long QT syndrome, hypertrophic and dilated cardiomyopathies, and aortic aneurysms in patients with the Marfan syndrome among others (Ahmad, McNally, Ackerman, Baty, Day, Kullo, Madueme, Maron, Martinez, Salberg, Taylor and Wilcox 2019). Currently, most genetic testing is applied to patients, or family members of patients, to determine their risk for developing clinical disease, or prenatal testing to assess for congenital disease or risk for transmission of disease to a patient's children. Yet, despite the hope for personalized medicine based on genetic testing, since the completion of the human genome project there has not yet been a significant impact on mortality, and genetic testing is typically not a part of day-to-day practice (Emmert-Streib, Dehmer, and Yli-Harja 2017; Shah 2020).

III Implications of the Rapid Advances in Cardiovascular Diagnostics and Therapeutics

This review of recent history demonstrates the broad trends in cardiovascular medicine and provides a starting point to discuss the ethical challenges of today's practice. The first notable trend is the rapid progress in diagnostic and therapeutic options cardiologists are able to offer patients. Several seminal developments in the first half of the previous century, such as electrocardiography, echocardiography, and cardiac catheterization, have provided a platform for the explosive development of new and increasingly complex modalities in the last half of the century. This pace of growth has several implications. First, the pace of development of new knowledge and techniques and the resulting complexity of practice strains the ability of many cardiologists to keep pace with the nuanced indications and potential complications of interventions. This complexity has resulted in increasing subspecialization within cardiology. Cardiologists may specialize, for example, in interventional cardiology, electrophysiology, or noninvasive imaging. Such subspecialization has the benefit of producing cardiologists who are highly focused on a particular modality and are subsequently well-trained at performing and interpreting highly complex procedures and studies. However, they will be challenged to stay abreast with the latest developments in other areas of cardiology, and may be less likely to be in a position to coordinate an overall plan for the patient's care. Braunwald has noted, "…one may ask: where is the conductor—the physician who oversees and integrates the care of the cardiac patient?" (Braunwald 2003). As chronic cardiac disease becomes more prevalent, an elderly patient may present with coronary artery disease, congestive heart failure and significant arrhythmias as well as dementia. Based on the ejection fraction, a measure of the heart pumping function, prophylactic implantable cardioverter–defibrillators can be considered. The electrophysiologist may be asked to consult on the patient and recommend an implantable defibrillator based purely on the ejection fraction, the interventional cardiologist may find significant lesions on angiography amenable to intracoronary stenting or coronary bypass surgery. Yet these interventions may not be a good use of resources, or what the patient would want, given a very poor overall prognosis. While each of the cardiac issues may have several options for treatment, it remains important to look at the "big picture" and consider what should be done in the patient's best interest according to his or her wishes and goals, rather than blindly doing what can be done for each individual problem.

Second, is the difficulty of obtaining informed consent. It has become increasingly challenging and yet essential to provide patients with adequate information prior to pursuing many of the more complex interventions currently available. While the cardiologist may conscientiously spend time explaining the indications and the nature of the procedure prior to placing a ventricular assist device in a patient with advanced heart failure, it may be difficult for the patient fully to understand or envision the implications for their lifestyle of having to live with an external battery source, including the requirements to have a backup battery available and the ability to deal with device malfunctions until they are actually in that position. It is important before proceeding with implantation that the patient fully understands the potential for disabling stroke, bleeding, or infection related to the device and discusses with the cardiac team what he or she would want done with the device should those complications occur. Similarly, implantable defibrillators are very effective at treating lethal arrhythmias by delivering a shock to convert the rhythm back to a normal one. Yet these shocks can be both physically and psychologically traumatic for patients. Death from ventricular arrhythmias is typically sudden and painless. In the patient with advanced heart failure, it is essential to discuss that this life-saving device may, at the end of life, cause repeated shocks if arrhythmias become more frequent and thus the patient may exchange a sudden, painless death for a prolonged painful course. This is a difficult conversation for the physician to have, and it is important to carefully balance the discussion such that the patient is not unduly frightened of having this life-saving device placed, while at the same time recognizing the possibility that the defibrillator and shocks may become burdensome at the end of life.

A third trend related to the complexity of ethical issues in cardiology is the increasing reliance on devices permanently implanted in the patient. Often these are life-sustaining, as with pacemakers for patients with extremely slow heart rates or ventricular assist devices for patients with severe heart failure. As patients approach the end of life, and the treatments become increasingly burdensome relative to their benefits, both patients and medical staff struggle with how to manage these devices. Often deactivating or removing a device "feels" different than, for example, forgoing cardiopulmonary resuscitation, both because of the life-sustaining nature and the fact that the device is now "part of the body." Physicians and patients may struggle with worries that deactivating a device is equivalent to assisted suicide or euthanasia.

The first two parts of this book, on beginning of life and end of life, deal extensively with these types of questions arising from the rapid pace of progress. In the first part, the authors discuss ethical issues relating to cardiac illness at the beginning of life. Common to these discussions are the importance of clinicians being familiar with recent advances in diagnosis and therapy and implications of these advances for assessing the benefits and burdens of treatment and diagnostic decisions. This awareness is fundamental to the clinician's ability to engage patients or surrogates in shared decision-making.

In the first chapter Sara Cherny and Dawn Allain discuss the ethical challenges in counseling families about genetic testing prior to or during pregnancy (Cherny and Allain 2022). They note the increasing number of cardiac diseases that have been correlated with genetic mutations or variants, but recognize that rarely does a single gene invariably lead to clinical disease. Genes associated with cardiac disease may have variable penetrance, meaning the gene may or may not cause clinical disease, or may manifest the disease to different degrees even in the same family. In addition, the likelihood of a genetic variant causing disease is dependent on interactions with other genes and environmental factors, and while some may cause disease in childhood, many predispose to illness in adult patients. These facts complicate advising patients or families about the benefits of genetic testing and counselors must be able to clearly explain the uncertainties associated with genetic testing and discuss the implications of knowledge of genetic variants given this uncertainty. The authors note that while genetic counselors generally focus on respecting a client's autonomy and attempt to provide "nondirective" counseling there are significant limitations to this approach. In the case they discuss, a family requests testing for a future pregnancy after having a child with a cardiomyopathy requiring transplantation. While testing of the parents and offspring may identify the gene associated with the cardiomyopathy, other genes may be identified that may put a future child at risk for cardiac disease late in life. The question arises whether testing for an adult onset gene should be offered to the parents either as part of preimplantation evaluation during *in vitro* fertilization, or evaluation of an already established pregnancy, given that the parents may destroy the embryo or terminate a pregnancy based on this knowledge. If the parents do not terminate a pregnancy, ethical dilemmas arise about how the knowledge of this variant will be provided to the child and how it will impact the child's own medical decision-making. The authors point out that there is a general consensus in professional genetics societies against testing for adult onset conditions, but that it will be the role of the individual counselor to decide whether and how to present these options to parents. Similarly, the counselor must elicit and respect the views of parents who may, for religious, moral, or personal reasons, see pregnancy termination, or *in vitro* fertilization, as ethically inappropriate and include discussion of all genetic testing and reproductive options.

In the second chapter, Pamela Jordi and James Smith discuss the ethical issues that arise in advising patients with cardiovascular disease about their risks for pregnancy (Jordi and Smith 2022). In this chapter, the authors discuss two scenarios that often raise ethical issues during pregnancy because of the high risk of maternal and fetal mortality. In the first, peripartum cardiomyopathy (PPCM) patients develop cardiac failure in late pregnancy or early after delivery. These patients have a significant risk of recurrent failure, even if the heart completely recovers normal function after an initial episode. As a result, patients are typically advised to avoid pregnancy. The authors present the case of a patient with a history of PPCM who wishes to have another child, and presents requesting infertility treatment after failing to conceive. Here, the clinician is not only advising the patient of the risk of pregnancy, but must consider if, in his or her opinion, the risk of helping the patient become pregnant is unacceptably high. The authors argue that in such circumstances it is acceptable for a provider to refuse to participate in the fertility treatments and may offer referral for a second opinion. The second type of case regards patients with pulmonary hypertension, elevated pressures in the circulation between the right and left sides of the heart that may occur in isolation or as a result of acquired or congenital heart disease. Here, the patient presents with an already established pregnancy. The traditional recommendation is for termination of pregnancy; however, there has been significant improvement in treatment, though mortality with pregnancy remains high. Given that a successful outcome of the pregnancy is possible, the authors argue for careful counseling of the patient about the anticipated risks and potential outcomes of continuing the pregnancy, and the option of termination. Should the patient decide to continue pregnancy after informed consent, the clinician should provide optimal care to provide the best chance for a good outcome.

In the final chapter on beginning of life issues, Dalia Feltman presents a discussion of treatment decision-making for newborns with severe congenital cardiac defects (Feltman 2022). Two congenital defects are discussed in this essay: hypoplastic left heart syndrome and trisomy 18 with a ventricular septal defect (a hole between the two ventricles of the heart). Neither condition is curable, and in the past there would have been a consensus for providing only comfort measures and hospice care to these patients; however, significant improvements in treatment have improved survival and quality of life for both. Treatment of hypoplastic left heart has advanced to the degree that patients have been able to deliver healthy babies of their own, and notably the patient's self-reported quality of life is higher than their parents' perception. Comparatively, survival remains much worse with trisomy 18; however, a small fraction may live beyond ten years and parents report significant interaction of these children with family members. There is significant variation between clinicians' views of the appropriateness of aggressive intervention versus comfort measures and their opinions about patient quality of life. Feltman documents that most authors argue that given that there is no clear "best interests" analysis for these patients, comfort care and intensive care can both be ethical decisions requiring careful shared decision-making with parents in light of their goals and values.

The next part of the book addresses issues surrounding cardiovascular illness near the end of life. The complexity in determining prognosis and in managing symptoms for patients with advanced heart failure and other severe cardiac disease is outlined in the initial chapter of this portion. Sara Wordingham and Keith Swetz present the typical course of these patients with intermittent, and progressively worsening, exacerbations followed by stable periods (Wordingham and Swetz 2022). This pattern of illness makes accurate assessment of prognosis difficult. While medical therapy and interventions, such as implantable defibrillators and ventricular assist devices, have significantly impacted the course of disease, mortality and morbidity remains high. The choice of optimal therapy may vary with the stage of disease and severity of co-morbidities, along with the patients' goals and values. While patients value conversations about long-term prognosis and treatment options, the authors note that clinicians are often uncomfortable discussing these topics. The chapter concludes that shared decision-making with regard to therapeutic options and resuscitation is essential despite prognostic uncertainty, and they argue for a significant role for palliative care specialists on the team caring for these patients to aid with symptom management and discussion of goals.

In Chapter 5, Keith Swetz, Sara Wordingham, Daniel Matlock, and David Zientek review potential dilemmas surrounding deactivation of implantable electronic and circulatory devices at the end of life (Swetz, Wordingham, Matlock, and Zientek 2022). The authors briefly review ethical and legal opinion in the United States with the current consensus being that patients or appropriate surrogates have the right to refuse or remove life-sustaining treatment that has become burdensome. While courts have not upheld a constitutional right to physician assistance in dying, individual states are allowed to legalize this assistance. Many clinicians, however, continue to see a distinction between allowing a patient to die and killing a patient by actively introducing a new pathology. As the indications for both implantable electronic devices, such as pacemakers and defibrillators, and mechanical circulatory support devices, such as left ventricular assist implants, have grown, patients are reaching the end of life with these life-sustaining devices in their bodies. Many healthcare providers have raised concerns about whether it is ethical to deactivate or remove these devices since they may replace bodily functions and to some degree become part of the body. Building on the work of Pellegrino and Sulmasy, the authors argue that the appropriateness of deactivating these devices at the end of life can be evaluated in much the same way as withdrawing a ventilator or dialysis (Pellegrino 2000; Sulmasy 2008). They argue for the importance of informing both physicians and patients that deactivation of devices when they become burdensome is an option.

Along with the complexity of diagnostic and therapeutic technology comes a significant increase in the cost of cardiac care. Healthcare providers struggle with how these costly and, at times, scarce resources can be justly distributed within resource-rich countries and more resource-poor parts of the world. Some may question if the few extra months of life with a ventricular assist device justifies the cost when Medicare and other insurance covers them, rather than investing in treatments, such as vaccines or optimal control of blood pressure that may have a larger impact on overall mortality in the population. If Medicare and other insurance programs cover these expensive treatments, clinicians and hospital administrators must struggle with how to approach patients who are good candidates for a device but lack insurance coverage or personal resources to cover the cost. Similarly, the healthcare provider may find it difficult repeatedly to provide costly treatments to poorly compliant patients, such as the ongoing intravenous drug user who may require repeated surgery to replace a heart valve infected as a result of the drug use. Another consideration is whether it is legitimate for wealthy Western countries to send used, but still functional, technology, or expired but still active medications to poorer nations, where such treatments would otherwise be unavailable. Some have argued that justice demands working toward global equity in access to, and clinical outcomes from, these devices and to offer older, previously used, or past expiration date medications does not advance this goal (Farmer and Bukhman 2012).

The next part of this volume addresses questions regarding how to best distribute costly and scarce resources. In the first chapter in this section, Behzad Pavri addresses ethical issues arising from global healthcare disparities (Pavri 2022). He considers the appropriateness of sterilizing and reusing implanted devices such as pacemakers and defibrillators in patients in resource-poor nations, who otherwise would not have any access to these life-saving devices. He argues that while some have seen this practice as similar to providing substandard medications, these devices are the same as those offered to patients in wealthy countries, albeit with shorter battery life due to prior use. Given data that there is not a significant increase in infection rates among recipients of resterilized devices, he argues that it is preferable to offer to reuse these devices in patients, who would otherwise have a high mortality, rather than to wait for an ideal global distribution of resources that would allow them to receive new devices. He also considers whether it is preferable to offer these devices via charitable means, or a commercial approach offering discounted or subsidized pricing with the author arguing for a continued charitable approach.

In Chapter 7, Kayhan Parsi and David Zientek review the ethics of allocating scarce or costly resources to patients using left ventricular assist devices (LVADs) as a case study (Zientek and Parsi 2022). The authors briefly consider several philosophical approaches to a just distribution of healthcare, finding that there is no clear consensus in the United States. As a result, decisions by government and insurance companies about what therapies will be compensated are often unpredictable, and this fact, along with the reality that some patients have no insurance coverage at all, often places the onus for deciding how to distribute scarce resources on regional or local healthcare systems. Given the overlap in patients who are candidates for heart transplantation and LVADs, existing methods for allocating donor hearts to patients with advanced heart failure are used as a basis for determining appropriate candidates for LVAD placement. The authors propose that the patient's prognosis and psychosocial situation may be ethically relevant to these decisions, and if there are more candidates than available resources, some form of lottery may be required. In addition, they propose circumstances in which charitable LVADs may be considered with the proviso that the institution may have a transparent set of criteria for deactivating the device or requiring the patient to provide material support for ongoing care in situations where prognosis has significantly worsened or patients are not compliant with required treatment.

The final chapter in this section considers ethical dilemmas faced by clinicians in providing costly treatment to patients who are noncompliant with medical recommendations, such as those continuing to use intravenous drugs after replacement of an infected heart valve (Charrow and Kirkpatrick 2022). Here, the ethical dilemma faced by clinicians is their obligation to treat an individual who presents with an infected prosthetic valve versus their obligation to avoid wasting society's resources when the patient's ongoing drug use makes it highly likely that a new valve may again become infected. The authors discuss the possible harm that may occur if physicians are responsible for bedside rationing in terms of patient trust and the potential inequities in rationing based on the biases of the individual physician. Ultimately, they argue for administrative gatekeeping whereby the specialist participates at the hospital system level in setting policy related to rationing, but remains able to advocate for their individual patients. In determining if an individual patient should be referred for a costly treatment, Alexandra Charrow and James Kirkpatrick argue that understanding the different conceptions of futility and the nuances of applying the concept to a particular case may be the most appropriate means of decision-making. Declaring a particular treatment futile may necessitate the assistance of ethics consultants and specialists in treating addiction.

As costs have increased, and the complexity of care has resulted in reorganization of cardiovascular practice with a focus on preventing error, medical societies have begun to publish guidelines for the utilization of medical technology. In addition, there has been attention to the importance of collaboration between physicians and other members of the care team along with concerns about conflicts of interest with different models of practice. As evidence has grown of significant geographic variations in the frequency of using cardiovascular procedures, payers have increasingly used a variety of methods, such as requiring prior authorization before procedures to contain costs and improve the quality and consistency of care. Beginning in 2005, the American College of Cardiology and other subspecialty groups have published "appropriate use criteria" (Hendel, Lindsay, Allen, Brindis, Patel, White, Winchester, and Wolk 2018). These guidelines provide recommendations that categorize a diagnostic or therapeutic procedure as "appropriate care", "may be appropriate care", or "rarely appropriate care" (Hendel, Lindsay, Allen, Brindis, Patel, White, Winchester, and Wolk 2018, p. 940). These recommendations carry significant weight on how physicians practice and how insurers reimburse for these procedures. As a consequence, concerns have been raised about physicians following the guidelines prescriptively rather than considering the nuances of a particular patient's situation, and there is concern that the writers of the guidelines (often clinicians and researchers with close ties to the pharmaceutical or medical device industry) may have conflicts of interest, either financial or professional, that may influence the recommendations (Hendel, Lindsay, Allen, Brindis, Patel, White, Winchester, and Wolk 2018). At the same time, changes in reimbursement, and efforts to improve quality of care while reducing cost, have led to alterations in the way clinical practice and research is organized, and the way physicians interact with patients and other caregivers to enhance quality of care. Conflicts of interest are again a significant concern when physicians are pressured by financial or other incentives to alter the care of patients.[5] Also, the importance of cooperation among caregivers and a team approach has been seen as essential to improving safety and quality of care (Vitalsmarts 2005).

Professionalism, conflict of interest, quality and teamwork are all themes addressed by authors in Part IV. The first chapter of this section addresses conflicts of interest faced by clinicians in routine practice (Zientek 2022a). David Zientek provides a brief definition of conflicts of interest and argues that the ways in which physician practices are organized, the methods for compensating members, and marketing of the practice all have the potential to induce physicians, or the institutions they work for, to act against a patient's best interests. The different forms that conflicts of interest may take in various practice settings are discussed and a variety of methods for preventing or minimizing these conflicts are reviewed: these include prohibition of particularly egregious ones, disclosure, or management utilizing professional codes of ethics and guidelines or consultation with outside experts. These methods are then applied to a case illustrating many of the situations that may be faced by the practitioner.

Chapter 10, by Mark Hoffman and James Kirkpatrick, considers conflicts of interest in a different setting (Hoffman and Kirkpatrick 2022). As cardiology has become more dependent on technology and pharmaceuticals, there has been an increasingly close relationship between practitioners and specialty societies on the one hand, and the manufacturers of devices and medications on the other. The authors argue that at the root of conflicts of interest is the expectation that physicians will place the interests of their patients above their own. Since professional organizations represent and advance the goals of physicians, these organizations should reflect the obligations of individual practitioners. These organizations increasingly promulgate clinical practice guidelines with the goal of improving quality of care and providing evidence-based recommendations for diagnosis and treatment of cardiac conditions. Such guidelines strongly influence clinicians' treatment of patients and are often referenced as the standard of care by insurers determining reimbursement and in legal proceedings. When professional societies or the members of their guideline-writing committees have close relationships with industry, there is concern that these relationships may influence the final document and undermine trust in the objective and impartial nature of these recommendations. As a consequence, the authors argue for strong rules for disclosing potential conflicts, and for limiting participation of those with strong industry ties in the guideline writing process.

In the next chapter, Zientek turns to efforts to enhance the quality of care with a consideration of the appropriate professional response of caregivers and institutions when patients suffer unanticipated harm from diagnostic or therapeutic interventions (Zientek 2022b). He distinguishes three types of unintended harm: medical error, malpractice, and complication and their moral implications. The chapter notes the importance of all members of the care team being alert for actual and potential harms to patients and the ability of all members to report these issues. He argues that, in all instances, there should be transparent disclosure to the patient or surrogates of unintended harm with an investigation of the underlying cause of the event and a plan put in place to change institutional systems or policies if appropriate to prevent future events when error or malpractice occurs. In the case of a complication, when all procedures were appropriately followed and the event not preventable, an expression of sympathy for the harm suffered is appropriate. However, in instances where investigation confirms a medical error or malpractice as a cause of harm, justice requires a formal apology, often with some form of compensation to the patient or their appropriate surrogates.

In the final chapter of this section, Joy Penticuff and Angela Clark consider ethical challenges cardiovascular nurses face in clinical practice (Penticuff and Clark 2022). Bedside nurses spend significantly more time with individual patients than many other members of the care team, and subsequently may be more in tune with patient suffering. They are often more aware if the patient or surrogates do not fully understand the clinical situation or feel that their wishes are not being followed. The structural hierarchy in large hospitals with cardiac programs often places the nurse in a situation where they may have a limited voice in responding to these patient issues as a result of the power imbalance between them and physicians and administration. Moral distress occurs when the nurse feels he or she cannot respond in an ethically appropriate manner to care dilemmas, and the harm this distress causes individual caregivers, and institutional quality of care are reviewed. The authors identify structural features of healthcare institutions that contribute to moral distress and discuss a case study demonstrating methods for improving communication and collaboration among the care team to address these issues. Finally, the authors demonstrate how the American Nurses Association Code of Ethics applies to the case.

We began with the observation that research has been a driving force for the changes in cardiovascular practice. The increasing complexity of technology and medical therapy requires a multidisciplinary approach among clinicians, engineers, pharmaceutical companies, and the medical device industry to advance cardiovascular care. While this collaboration has been beneficial in delivering new therapy to patients, as new discoveries of medications and technology accelerate and the economic impact of these on the practice of cardiology has increased, there has been an increased volume of basic and clinical research and pressure to publish these studies. Increased competition to be the first to bring new technology to practice, increased pressure to publish studies to burnish one's academic credentials, and the retraction of several studies due to irregularities in the research have led a group of cardiology journal editors to publish guidelines for improving the ethics of the conduct and publication of studies (HEART Group 2008; Kolata 2018).

The final part of this volume addresses ethical issues surrounding research in cardiovascular medicine. In Chapter 13, Ana Iltis and Douglas Lemley provide a broad overview of ethical issues in clinical research (Iltis and Lemley 2022). The essay begins with a brief historical overview of events leading to the development of current concepts of ethical human subjects research. While the Nuremberg Code remains important, it is noted that the United States did not adopt significant protections for clinical research until the Belmont report was published in 1979 in the wake of revelations of misconduct by researchers in the United States Public Health Service Syphilis Study. Three principles from the report undergird the regulation of research in the United States: respect for persons, beneficence, and justice. The chapter then provides an overview of ethical principles and controversies in a number of areas. These include discussions of the role of institutional review boards in the review and oversight of research, and the importance of designing studies in such a way that significant questions are answered and patients are not subjected to risks in a poorly designed study. The importance of informed consent and selecting patient populations to avoid victimizing vulnerable populations for high-risk interventions or denying those populations the opportunity to participate in studies likely to have significant benefit is also considered. Other topics, such as subsequent research on samples collected in the initial study, continuing access to study drugs or devices after the completion of the protocol, treatment of conditions unrelated to the research, conflicts of interest and the involvement of community members in research, are also discussed.

In the final chapter, ethical issues arising when cardiovascular research protocols are terminated before the planned completion of the trial are considered by Lynne Caples and Emily Anderson (Caples and Anderson 2022). The authors note that there has been an increase in the frequency of terminating randomized controlled trials before completion of the protocol. They review a variety of reasons for stopping trials, some of which they find ethically appropriate, while others may be ethically inappropriate after careful analysis. For example, trials that are stopped because interim analysis clearly demonstrates the intervention to be harmful, or non-beneficial are typically ethically appropriate. Similarly, if concomitant studies published while the trial is underway clearly answer the questions being addressed in the study, it may be appropriate to end the study rather than deprive patients in a placebo arm of a now proven treatment. The essay finds termination of studies for an apparent benefit more complex. At times a benefit is so clear, particularly for a novel treatment, it is appropriate to end a study and make the intervention widely available. However, the authors present examples where an optimistic interim analysis is not borne out in the final data, or a delayed harmful effect may arise after longer follow-up. Even more problematic are studies terminated for commercial reasons. For example, terminating a study early when it becomes clear the medication will be unlikely to generate a profit or because the pharmaceutical company wishes to rush a promising and likely profitable drug to market when there are still important scientific questions to be answered would be ethically inappropriate. A significant concern raised in this chapter is the frequent failure to explain to patients or in the literature why a study was terminated or even the failure to report that data at all. The authors offer guidelines for determining if it is ethically appropriate to terminate a study and for publication of these studies.

While it is not possible to address all the ethical dilemmas that may arise in research and the practice of clinical cardiovascular medicine, the case-based approach presented in this volume will provide readers, including cardiovascular specialists, students, and members of ethics committees, a perspective that will allow them to reason through current and future ethical issues as they arise in this rapidly changing field. In summary, as one of the contributors to this volume has noted:

> Cardiovascular care is increasingly complicated and requires striking balances between quality of life and longevity, high-tech interventions and supportive care, an unexpected but mercifully sudden death and a prolonged but predictable disease course. The modern cardiovascular specialist must understand and explain each of these spectra considering the individual patient's wishes and best interests, the maleficence of side-effects, and the impact of therapeutic interventions in the larger social context.

This nuanced approach requires skill in the "art" of medicine.

(Kirkpatrick, Fields, and Ferrari 2010)

Not only cardiologists, but also cardiothoracic and vascular surgeons, cardiac nurses and technicians, physical and occupational therapists, hospital ethicists, and, of course, our patients and their families, deal with these ethical dilemmas on a regular basis. It is with these issues that the authors of the following chapters will engage.

Notes

1 For example the GISSI trial, one of the early studies showing the benefit of clot lysis for the treatment of myocardial infarction enrolled 11,712 patients (Rovelli, De Vita, Feruglio, Lotto, Selvini, Tognoni, and GISSI Investigators 1987). For further insight into the evolution of industry involvement and the expansion of research in the private practice setting see, e.g., Klaidman (2000) and Fanari and Weiss (2015).

2 For example, the American College of Cardiology publishes separate research journals in cardiovascular interventions, heart failure, clinical electrophysiology, basic to translational science, cardiovascular imaging, and cardio-oncology, in addition to the Journal of the American College of Cardiology. American College of Cardiology (2020).

3 See, e.g., Vitalsmarts. Silence Kills: The Seven Crucial Conversations for Healthcare (2005).

4 See, for example: Zientek (2003), Moore (2003), Allman (2003), Stout and Warner (2003), and Spece (2003).

5 For insight on the impact of concerns about conflicts of interest on practice and research see: Zientek (2003), DuBois (2011), Bierut, Cruz-Flores, Hodges, et al. (2011), Anderson and Kraus (2011), and Wynia and Crigger (2011).

References

Ahmad, F., E.M. McNally, M.J. Ackerman, L.C. Baty, S.M. Day, I.J. Kullo, P.C. Madueme, M.S. Maron, M.W. Martinez, L. Salberg, M.R. Taylor, and J.E. Wilcox. 2019. Establishment of specialized clinical cardiovascular genetics programs: Recognizing the need and meeting standards: A scientific statement from the American Heart Association. *Circulation: Genomic and Precision Medicine* 12: 286–305.

Allman, R.L. 2003. The relationship between physicians and the pharmaceutical industry: Ethical problems with the every-day conflict of interest. *Healthcare Ethics Committee (HEC) Forum* 15(2): 155–170.

American College of Cardiology. 2020. *Jacc Journals*. Available at: www.acc.org.

Anderson, E.E., and E.M. Kraus. 2011. Re-examining empirical data on conflicts of interest through the lens of personal narratives. *Narrative Inquiry in Bioethics* 1(2): 91–99.

Bierut, L.J., S. Cruz-Flores, L.E. Hodges, A.A. Mikulec, G.K. Nagaldinne, E.L. Bakanas, J.F. Peppin, J.S. Perlmutter, W.H. Seitz Jr., E. Diao, A.N. Sofair, and D.M. Zientek. 2011. Personal narratives: Conflicting interests in medicine. *Narrative Inquiry in Bioethics* 1(2): 67–90.

Braunwald, E. 2003. Cardiology: The past, the present, and the future. *Journal of the American College of Cardiology* 42(12): 2031–2041.

Caples, L., and E.E. Anderson. 2022. Early termination of cardiovascular research protocols. In: *Ethical issues in cardiovascular medicine*, D.M. Zientek and M.J. Cherry (eds). New York: Routledge.

Chair, S.Y., D.S.F. Yu, T.M. Ng, Q. Wang, H.Y. Cheng, E.M.L. Wong, and J.W.H. Sit. 2016. Evolvement of left ventricular assist device: The implications on heart failure management. *Journal of Geriatric Cardiology* 13: 425–430.

Charrow, A., and J.N. Kirkpatrick. 2022. The cardio-ethics of endocarditis. In: *Ethical issues in cardiovascular medicine*, D.M. Zientek and M.J. Cherry (eds). New York: Routledge.

Cherny, S., and D. Allain. 2022. Ethical issues in reproductive testing for cardiovascular disease. In: *Ethical issues in cardiovascular medicine*, D.M. Zientek and M.J. Cherry (eds). New York: Routledge.

Comroe, J.H. 1983. *Exploring the heart*. New York: W.W. Norton.

Cournand, A., R.L. Riley, A.S. Breed, E.D. Baldwin, D.W. Richards Jr., M.S. Lester, and M. Jones. 1945. Measurement of cardiac output in man using the technique of catheterization of the right auricle or ventricle. *The Journal of Clinical Investigation* 24(1): 106–116.

DuBois, J.M. (2011). Conflicting interest in medicine: Stories by physicians on how financing affects their work. *Narrative Inquiry in Bioethics* 1(2): 65–66.

Edler, I., and C.H. Hertz. 1954. Use of ultrasonic reflectoscope for the continuous recording of movements of heart walls. *Kungl. Fysiografiska Sallskapets i Lund Forhandlingar* 24: 1–19.

Elmqvist, R., and A. Senning. 1960. *Implantable pacemaker for the heart*. In: *Medical electronics: Proceedings of the second international conference on medical electronics, Paris, June 1959*, Smyth, C.N. (ed). London: Ilife and Sons.

Emmert-Streib, F., M. Dehmer, and O. Yli-Harja. 2017. Lessons from the human genome project: Modesty, honesty, and realism. *Frontiers in Genetics* 8: 184.

Fanari, Z., and S.A. Weiss. 2015. Academic versus private cardiology. *Journal of the American College of Cardiology* 65(3): 303–305.

Farmer, P., and G. Bukhman. 2012. Reuse of medical devices and global health equity. *Annals of Internal Medicine* 157(8): 591–592.

Favaloro, R.G., D.B. Effler, C. Cheanvechai, R.A. Quint, and F.M. Sones, Jr. 1971. Acute coronary insufficiency (impending acute myocardial infarction and myocardial infarction): Surgical treatment by the saphenous vein graft technique. *American Journal of Cardiology* 28: 598–607.

Feltman, D. 2022. Severe congenital anomalies in the fetus or infant: "Best-interests" decisions for ambiguous outcomes. In: *Ethical issues in cardiovascular medicine*, D.M. Zientek and M.J. Cherry (eds). New York: Routledge.

Forssmann, W. 1974. *Experiments on myself. Memoirs of a surgeon in Germany*. New York: St. Martin's Press.

Gibbon, J.H., Jr. 1954. Application of a mechanical heart and lung apparatus to cardiac surgery. *Minnesota Medicine* 37: 171–175.

Gruentzig, A.R., R.K. Myler, E.S. Hanna, and M.I. Turina. 1977. Coronary transluminal angioplasty (abstr). *Circulation* 84: 55–56.

HEART Group. (2008). A statement on ethics from the HEART group. *Journal of the American College of Cardiology* 51(18): 1821–1823.

Hendel, R.C., B.D. Lindsay, J.M. Allen, R.G. Brindis, M.R. Patel, L. White, D.E. Winchester, and M.J. Wolk. 2018. *Journal of the American College of Cardiology* 71(8): 935–948.

Hoffman, M.A., and J.N. Kirkpatrick. 2022. Ethical challenges for cardiology societies: Conflicts of interest and clinical practice guidelines. In: *Ethical issues in cardiovascular medicine*, D.M. Zientek and M.J. Cherry (eds). New York: Routledge.

Iltis, A.S. and D. Lemley. 2022. Ethics in cardiovascular research. In: *Ethical issues in cardiovascular medicine*, D.M. Zientek and M.J. Cherry (eds). New York: Routledge.

Jaskie, S. and G. Rodgers. 2014. Current trends in U.S. cardiology practice. *Trends in Cardiovascular Medicine* 24(8): 350–359.

Jones, J.H. 2008. The Tuskegee syphilis experiment. In: *The Oxford textbook of clinical research ethics* (pp. 86–96), Emanuel, E.J., Grady, C., Crouch, R.A., Lie, R.K., Miller, F.G., and Wendler, D. (eds). New York: Oxford University Press.

Jonsen, A.R. 1998. *The birth of bioethics*. New York: Oxford University Press.

Jonsen, A.R. 2007. The God squad and the origins of transplantation ethics and policy. *The Journal of Law, Medicine, & Ethics* 35(2): 238–240.

Jordi, P., and J. Smith Jr. 2022. An ethical discussion of cardiovascular disease in pregnancy: Peripartum cardiomyopathy and pulmonary hypertension. In: *Ethical issues in cardiovascular medicine*, D.M. Zientek and M.J. Cherry (eds). New York: Routledge.

Kannel, W.B., T.R. Dawber, A. Kagan, N. Revotskie, and J. Stokes. 1961. Factors of risk in the development of coronary heart disease: Six-year follow-up experience. The Framingham Study. *Annals of Internal Medicine* 55: 33–50.

Kirkpatrick, J.N., A.V. Fields, and V.A. Ferrari. 2010. Medical ethics and the art of cardiovascular medicine. *The Lancet* 376: 508–509.

Kittleson, M.M., and J.A. Kobashigawa. 2017. Cardiac transplantation: Current outcomes and contemporary controversies. *Journal of the American College of Cardiology: Heart Failure* 5(12): 857–868.

Klaidman, S. 2000. *Saving the heart*. New York: Oxford University Press.

Kohn, L.T., J.M. Corrigan, and M.S. Donaldson (eds). 1999. *To err is human: Building a safer health system*. Washington, DC: National Academy Press.

Kolata, G. 2018. Harvard calls for retraction of dozens of studies by noted cardiac researcher. *The New York Times*, October 16, 2018. Section A, Page 13.

Kolessov, V.I. 1967. Mammary artery-coronary artery anastomosis as method of treatment for angina pectoris. *Journal of Thoracic and Cardiovascular Surgery* 54: 535–544.

Mehta, N.J., and I.A. Khan. 2002. Cardiology's 10 greatest discoveries of the 20th century. *Texas Heart Institute Journal* 29(3): 164–171.

Mirowski, M., P.R. Reid, M.M. Mower, L. Watkins, V.L. Gott, J.F. Schauble, A. Langer, M.S. Heilman, S.A. Kolenik, R.E. Fischell, and M.L. Weisfeldt, et al. 1980. Termination of malignant ventricular arrhythmias with an implanted automatic defibrillator in human beings. *New England Journal of Medicine* 303: 322–324.

Moore, N.J. 2003. Regulating self-referrals and other physician conflicts of interest. *Healthcare Ethics Committee (HEC) Forum* 15(2): 134–154.

Parsi, K., and D.M. Zientek. 2022. Just distribution of cardiovascular resources: The left ventricular assist device. In: *Ethical issues in cardiovascular medicine*, D.M. Zientek and M.J. Cherry (eds). New York: Routledge.

Patel, N., R. Kalra, R. Doshi, N. Bajaj, G. Arora, and P. Arora. 2018. Trends and cost of heart transplantation and left ventricular assist devices: Impact of proposed federal cuts. *Journal of the American College of Cardiology* 6(5): 424–432.

Pavri, G. 2022. Cardiac implantable electronic device reuse: Ethical considerations and enhancing awareness. In: *Ethical issues in cardiovascular medicine*, D.M. Zientek and M.J. Cherry (eds). New York: Routledge.

Pellegrino, E.D. 2000. Decisions to withdraw life-sustaining treatment: A moral algorithm. *Journal of the American Medical Association* 283(8): 1065–1067.

Penticuff, J., and A. Clark. 2022. Ethical practice in cardiovascular nursing. In: *Ethical issues in cardiovascular medicine*, D.M. Zientek and M.J. Cherry (eds). New York: Routledge.

Persad, G., A. Wertheimer, and E.J. Emanuel. 2009. Principles for allocation of scarce medical interventions. *The Lancet* 373: 423–431.

Pinney, S.P., A.C. Anyanwu, A. Lala, J.J. Teuteberg, N. Uriel, and M.R. Mehra. 2017. Left ventricular assist devices for lifelong support. *Journal of the American College of Cardiology* 69(23): 2845–2861.

Rovelli, F., C. De Vita, G.A. Feruglio, A. Lotto, A. Selvini, G. Tognoni, and GISSI Investigators. 1987. Gissi trial: Early results and late follow-up. *Journal of the American College of Cardiology* 10(5): 33B–39B.

Shah, R.R. 2020. Genotype-guided warfarin therapy: Still of only questionable value two decades on. *Journal of Clinical Pharmacology and Therapeutics* 45: 547–560.

Sliwa, K. and P. Zilla. 2017. 50th anniversary of the first human heart transplant – How is it seen today? *European Heart Journal* 38(46): 3402–3404.

Sones, F.M. Jr., and E.K. Shirey. 1962. Cine coronary arteriography. *Modern Concepts in Cardiovascular Disease* 31: 735–738.

Spece, R.G. Jr. 2003. Conflicts of interest affecting those who participate in staff privileges matters. *Healthcare Ethics Committee (HEC) Forum* 15(2): 188–227.

Stout, S.M., and D.C. Warner. 2003. How did physician ownership become a federal case? The Stark Amendments and their prospects. *Healthcare Ethics Committee (HEC) Forum* 15(2): 171–187.

Sulmasy, D.P. 2008. Within you/without you: Biotechnology, ontology, and ethics. *Journal of General Internal Medicine* 23(Suppl 1): 69–72.

Swetz, K.M., S.E. Wordingham, D.D. Matlock, and D.M. Zientek. 2022. Deactivating cardiac implantable electronic devices at end of life. In: *Ethical issues in cardiovascular medicine*, D.M. Zientek and M.J. Cherry (eds). New York: Routledge.

Vitalsmarts. 2005. *Silence kills: The seven crucial conversations for healthcare.* https://www.aacn.org/nursing-excellence/healthy-work-environments/~/media/aacn-website/nursing-excellence/healthy-work-environment/silencekills.pdf?la=en.

Weindling, P.J. 2004. *Nazi medicine and the Nuremberg trials: From medical war crimes to informed consent.* New York: Palgrave MacMillan.

Wordingham, S.E., and K.M. Swetz. 2022. Palliative care issues in advanced cardiac disease. In: *Ethical issues in cardiovascular medicine,* D.M. Zientek and M.J. Cherry (eds). New York: Routledge.

World Health Organization. 2020. *World health statistics 2020: Monitoring health for the SDGs, sustainable development goals.* Available at: www.who.int/gho/publications/world_health_statistics/2020.

Wynia, M.K., and B. Crigger. 2011. Conflicts – and consensus – about conflicts of interest in medicine. *Narrative Inquiry in Bioethics* 1(2): 101–105.

Zientek, D.M. 2003. Physician entrepreneurs, self-referral, and conflicts of interest: An overview. *Healthcare Ethics Committee (HEC) Forum* 15(2): 111–133.

Zientek, D.M. 2022a. Conflicts of interest in daily practice. In: *Ethical issues in cardiovascular medicine,* D.M. Zientek and M.J. Cherry (eds). New York: Routledge.

Zientek, D.M. 2022b. Error, malpractice, and complication: A practical approach. In: *Ethical issues in cardiovascular medicine,* D.M. Zientek and M.J. Cherry (eds). New York: Routledge.

Zoll, P., M.H. Paul, A.J. Linenthal, L.R. Norman, and W. Gibson. 1956. The effects of external electric currents on the heart. Control of cardiac rhythm and induction and termination of cardiac arrhythmias. *Circulation* 14: 745–756.

Part I

Cardiovascular Ethical Issues at the Beginning of Life

1 Ethical Issues in Reproductive Genetic Testing for Cardiovascular Disease

Sara Cherny and Dawn Allain

I Introduction

The availability of genetic testing for inherited cardiovascular diseases has increased dramatically over the last decade, making it possible to offer diagnostic and predictive testing to affected individuals and at-risk family members. In response to the high utility of and demand for genetic testing, a genetic counselor has rapidly become an essential component of the cardiovascular team.

Conditions commonly evaluated in the Cardiovascular Genetics Clinic include inherited arrhythmia (irregular heart beat) conditions such as Long QT Syndrome and Brugada syndrome; cardiac muscle disorders such as hypertrophic cardiomyopathy, dilated cardiomyopathy, arrhythmogenic right ventricular cardiomyopathy; connective tissue disorders (connective tissue is material inside the body, such as cartilage, bone, and fat, that supports organs and other parts of the body), such as Marfan syndrome and Loeys Dietz syndrome; and familial hyperlipidemia (a condition which results in high lipids, or fats, in the blood, thus increasing the risk for heart disease and stroke). The majority of these conditions are inherited in an autosomal dominant pattern, which entails up to a 50% risk for first-degree relatives (parents, siblings, and children) to be affected. Therefore, most families have multiple affected or at-risk individuals that need genetic counseling and cardiology evaluation. The manifestation of these conditions is further complicated by reduced penetrance in which a gene carrier may be asymptomatic or subclinically affected, and by variable expressivity, which is demonstrated by the presentation of a wide range of associated symptoms, including variable age of onset, disease process, and severity within the same family.

Genetic testing for inherited cardiovascular conditions often involves large multi-gene testing panels due to the number of genes associated with each condition, as well as the possibility that a single gene might manifest in different ways within a particular family, such as by causing both hypertrophic and dilated cardiomyopathy. With any genetic testing, but even more so with large gene panels, there is a possibility of an inconclusive result referred to as a variant of unknown significance. A variant of unknown significance is a change in the DNA sequence for which there are insufficient data to determine if the variant

DOI: 10.4324/9781003240273-3

is likely to be disease-causing or benign. Thus, these variants of unknown significance cannot be used for clinical or reproductive decision-making until further data are gathered to clarify their potential pathogenicity.

Pre- and post-test genetic counseling is crucial to patient consent and ultimate adaptation to a genetic diagnosis. The genetic counselor acts as patient educator, psychosocial counselor, and advocate. Genetic counselors are trained in eliciting a targeted medical genetics family history; they are also trained in pedigree analysis. They assess risks, identify and coordinate the best diagnostic testing plan, communicate results in lay terms, and coordinate family cascade screening. Genetic counselors may see patients for cardiovascular genetic testing as part of a larger cardiovascular, maternal/fetal medicine, or genetics clinic; they often work in collaboration with a specialty cardiologist, such as an electrophysiologist. Patients may need to see a genetic counselor only once, or they may have two to three visits over the course of assessment, testing, and result disclosure. In many cases, multiple members of the same family will see the same genetic counselor either simultaneously or sequentially with regard to the familial condition.

The guiding ethical principles accepted in the practice of genetic counseling are focused on the "values of care and respect for the client's autonomy, individuality, welfare, and freedom" (NSGC Code of Ethics, 2017). Genetic counseling is rooted in the "Ethics of Care" with an emphasis on receptiveness, relatedness, attentiveness, and responsiveness (Uhlmann, Schuette, & Yashar, 2009). Autonomy, beneficence, nonmaleficence, and utility are the core bioethical principles that inform genetic counseling practice on a daily basis.

Historically, the basic tenet of genetic counseling has been to facilitate client decision-making in a nondirective manner (Weil, 2000; Uhlmann, Schuette, & Yashar, 2009). Through the use of a nondirective approach, combined with other psychosocial counseling techniques, the genetic professional elicits the values and goals of the patient to support the autonomy of their client (Weil et al., 2006). Clients are thereby aided in making complex testing choices or electing a particular management option, within the context of their personal values, experiences, and beliefs.

It is important to note that although considered a guiding principle of the genetic counseling profession, the nondirective approach has been challenged by colleagues within and outside of the profession (Kopinsky, 1992; Veach, Bartels, & LeRoy, 2002; Weil, 2003; Weil et al., 2006). According to Weil and colleagues, while nondirective counseling may be an important component of ethically based genetic counseling care, it cannot serve as the primary theoretical basis of the genetic counseling process (Weil et al., 2006). As such, while genetic counselors may endeavor to attain a nondirective approach, it may not always be done successfully nor, at times, will it be warranted (Weil, 2003; Weil et al., 2006). For example, a directive counseling approach may be necessary to promote adherence to management recommendations and increase the likelihood of better health outcomes in patients affected with genetic disorders. However, in the case of prenatal and pre-implantation counseling and testing services, the use of a nondirective approach is of particular importance as clients make reproductive decisions.

This chapter addresses ethical issues inherent in genetic counseling focused on the case of a couple considering predictive reproductive testing by preimplantation genetic diagnosis or prenatal diagnosis. The case history is presented, the methods of testing are discussed, and the ethical dilemmas introduced. We will then discuss the application of ethical principles to genetic counseling practice and considerations to take in approaching such ethically complicated situations.

II Case Description

A couple presents for preconception genetic counseling due to a previous child with idiopathic dilated cardiomyopathy. The child was found to have three genetic variants identified by a 38-gene panel for dilated cardiomyopathy.

A Pertinent History

This couple's previous child presented to the emergency department at five months of age in respiratory distress. Echocardiography showed severe left ventricular dilation and severely depressed left ventricular systolic function with an ejection fraction (EF) of 5% (normal EF >50%). His evaluation for viral illness of the heart (myocarditis) was negative. He had successful heart transplantation at six months of age. It is notable that the family history is significant for a paternal aunt who experienced a "weak heart" during her pregnancy and a paternal great uncle that drowned at fifteen years of age.

The genetic panel completed for the child identified three variants; a disease-causing variant (mutation) in the *SCN5A* (Sodium Channel, Voltage-Gated, Type V, Alpha) gene, a variant of unknown significance in the *RBM20* (RNA-Binding Motif Protein 20) gene, and a likely disease-causing variant in the *TTR* (transthyretin) gene. Parental testing showed that the *SCN5A* and *RMB20* variants were paternally inherited and that the *TTR* variant was maternally inherited.

The paternally-derived *SCN5A* disease-causing variant had been previously reported in a patient referred to the testing laboratory for Long QT Syndrome (LQTS). Mutations in *SCN5A* are associated with a number of divergent cardiac conditions, including potentially lethal inherited arrhythmias, Long QT Syndrome Type 3 and Brugada Syndrome, as well as dilated cardiomyopathy, Sudden Infant Death Syndrome, and sick sinus syndrome. The father's clinical cardiology evaluation was unremarkable. The clinical Long QT phenotype associated with this *SCN5A* variant correlates with the reported paternal family history of heart concerns during pregnancy as well as the relative that drowned at 15 years of age (drowning is suspicious for arrhythmia). Given the pathogenicity of the variant, the family history, and the crossover of phenotypes common to this gene, the family was informed that the presence of this variant increases the risk for Long QT Syndrome and that it likely is the most significant factor contributing to the child's dilated cardiomyopathy identified thus far.

The data are insufficient to determine at this time whether the paternally derived *RBM20* variant of unknown significance contributes to disease or is benign. The presence of the variant may be a disease modulator—either working in combination with a disease-causing variant to further increase risk or having a protective effect and decreasing risk.

The maternally-derived *TTR* likely disease-causing variant is associated with amyloidosis cardiomyopathy, which usually onsets in mid to late life. Amyloid cardiomyopathy results when abnormal proteins, called amyloids, replace normal cardiac muscle, leading to abnormal heart beat and heart signals. Amyloid neuropathy results when amyloids are deposited on the nerves, resulting in progressive nerve damage (neuropathy) that is manifested by various symptoms such as nerve pain, numbness, and weakness in the extremities. The mother's evaluation with medical genetics was unremarkable. There is no family history of heart disease or neuropathy to support this variant as disease-causing in this family. The *TTR* variant is interpreted as not contributing to the son's dilated cardiomyopathy. However, the presence of the variant may significantly increase the risk for adult onset amyloid conditions.

The parents wish to avoid having another child with serious childhood heart disease or an increased risk for adult onset heart disease. The parents are willing to consider pre-implantation or prenatal genetic diagnosis to ensure unaffected offspring.

B Recurrence Risk Assessment

The parents were counseled that the variants are autosomal and transmitted in a dominant manner. The risk to transmit each variant is 50% with any conception. They were informed that predictive prenatal genetic testing for the *RBM20* variant of unknown significance is not appropriate, since the clinical significance of the variant is unknown. Given this fact, prenatal testing for this *RBM20* variant of unknown significance would not be recommended. The recurrence risk for the *SCN5A* and *TTR* variants was outlined: there is a 25% chance of a conception with the normal gene complement from each parent. There is a 25% chance of a conception with both the *SCN5A* and the *TTR* variants. There is a 25% chance of a conception with only the *TTR* variant. There is a 25% chance of a conception with only the SCN5A variant. Overall, the parents have a 25% chance of an unaffected conception and a 75% chance of a conception with increased risk for childhood and/or adult heart disease.

III Methods of Reproductive Testing for Known Familial Variants

Before discussing the ethical issues inherent in this case, it is important to review some basic aspects of prenatal genetic testing and pre-implantation genetic diagnosis (PGD). Prenatal genetic testing is completed during a pregnancy and pre-implantation genetic diagnosis is completed prior to a pregnancy.

A Prenatal Genetic Testing

Amniocentesis and chorionic villus sampling (CVS) are traditional prenatal genetic testing options for couples wishing prenatally to detect a genetic condition with a previously identified genetic variant. Amniocentesis is possible at 16 or more weeks of gestation and involves obtaining a small sample of amniotic fluid to test fetal cells. Chorionic villus sampling is possible at 10 to 12 weeks' gestation and involves obtaining a small sample of placental cells. DNA is extracted from the cells obtained from either procedure and can be tested for variants in a specific gene of interest. Both procedures are invasive and pose a risk of miscarriage: ~1% risk for chorionic villus sampling and <0.5% for amniocentesis. An important factor in prenatal genetic diagnosis is that couples are then faced with a decision about whether or not to continue a pregnancy in the case of an affected fetus. With either chorionic villus sampling or amniocentesis, the stage of pregnancy may be relevant to a couple's comfort with this decision.

B Pre-implantation Genetic Diagnosis

While a discussion of the ethical considerations for pregnancy termination are beyond the scope of this chapter, it is noted that many couples wish to avoid the possibility of a pregnancy termination for religious, moral, or other personal reasons. Pre-implantation genetic diagnosis is an alternative approach to reproductive genetic testing, allowing for the diagnosis of a genetic condition before a pregnancy has been established. Pre-implantation genetic diagnosis requires couples to undergo *in vitro* fertilization (IVF), whereby multiple embryos are generated, allowed to grow and divide for about three days, and tested at the six- to ten-cell stage before transfer to the uterus. If the biopsied cell is shown to be free of the genetic variant it can be inferred that the embryo is unaffected. Only unaffected embryos are then transferred to the mother's uterus and any resulting pregnancy is unlikely to be affected with the genetic condition.

There are drawbacks to pre-implantation genetic diagnosis, however; for example, IVF has a low efficiency with a 20–30% pregnancy rate per IVF cycle. There are also technical limitations in analyzing DNA derived from a single cell that can lead to a false negative result in about 10% of cases. Invasive prenatal testing by chorionic villus sampling or amniocentesis to confirm the results of pre-implantation genetic diagnosis is encouraged because of technical limitations. Thus, despite having invested significant time, emotion, and money into pre-implantation genetic diagnosis, couples are then sometimes faced with the same disadvantages of mid-trimester prenatal diagnosis they had tried to avoid. Lastly, pre-implantation genetic diagnosis is prohibitively expensive ($10,000–$15,000 per cycle) for many couples who lack private insurance or whose insurance will not pay for testing.

In addition to the technical, psychological, and financial limitations of pre-implantation genetic diagnosis, it is important to note that some people, as well as religious and secular organizations, believe that embryos have a moral status equivalent to that of a live born child. As such, even though the use of pre-implantation genetic diagnosis allows for the avoidance of abortion, because it encompasses the "unnatural" creation of embryos, and, in some cases, the destruction of embryos, some argue that it is unethical to utilize this technology (see Engelhardt, 2000). Pre-implantation genetic diagnosis, as well as prenatal diagnosis with amniocentesis or chorionic villus sampling, also raises ethical debates regarding the eugenic implications of selecting for fetuses and embryos with certain traits. Thus, while the use of pre-implantation genetic diagnosis may help some individuals resolve ethical dilemmas around abortion, others argue that the practice remains ethically unacceptable.

C Adoption, Donor Gamete, and Nonintervention

For parents who chose not to utilize prenatal or pre-implantation diagnostic testing, there are additional options. They may choose to take the risk with each future child and hope for the best. They may also elect to use donor gametes, which, in the case of the father being the genetic variant carrier, allows for achieving pregnancy without the use of IVF and having a partially genetically related child, who is at no increased risk for the familial condition. Finally, the option of adoption also exists.

IV Discussion of Ethical Considerations

The interested parties in this case are the parents, the future child, the ordering provider, the managing pediatric cardiologist, and the testing laboratory. It is important that the primary clinical parties—the genetic counselor and the attending physician—weigh in with facts and analysis to help assure best decision-making with the interest of the parents, their first child, and future children in mind. In keeping with the ethical practices of genetic counseling, the priority is to respect parental autonomy with regard to managing decisions regarding the recurrence of heart disease, be it infantile or adult form, while the interests of other parties are considered.

A Autonomy—Testing for the SCN5A Variant

Parental interests include maintaining autonomy to make decisions in the best interests of their future children and family. Additionally, parents require informed consent delineating the benefits and limitations of testing, and an understanding of the potential outcomes of their decisions prior to proceeding with a testing plan.

In the case under consideration, the parents wish to limit recurrence of heart disease in their future children. Providers and parents agree that testing the family for the *SCN5A* variant with known pathogenicity and association with demonstrated poor outcomes is appropriate given that the variant interpretation is valid and intervention can be offered, whether it be non-transfer of embryos, termination of pregnancy, or clinical monitoring for potential future treatment. However, the *SCN5A* gene is known for reduced penetrance and variable expressivity. It is not possible to predict whether the gene-positive embryo or fetus would ever manifest a disease state. The parental decision to elect testing for the *SCN5A* variant is supported whether or not individual predictions can be made regarding prognosis or age of onset. Provision of the testing with these limitations in mind respects parental autonomy in making decisions regarding family planning.

B Presymptomatic Testing of Minors / Embryos—Testing for the TTR Variant

Testing for the *TTR* variant raises concern of revealing a presymptomatic diagnosis for an adult onset condition with uncertain penetrance. This variant predisposes to a mid-life, adult onset cardiomyopathy, rather than a debilitating childhood disease. Professional medical genetics societies and bioethicists are generally in agreement that prenatal genetic testing for an adult-onset condition is not recommended, as it is potentially damaging to the future child, increasing the chance of overmedicalization, psychological distress, and unjustly depriving the future child of their right to medical decision-making (Ross et al., 2013; NSGC Position Statement on Prenatal Testing for Adult Onset Conditions, 2018).

Respect for autonomy generally requires that a patient be respected as their own agent and that they receive adequate counseling to provide informed consent. In cases where genetic testing has a medical benefit to the child, it may be appropriate to pursue testing. In practice, genetic counselors discuss the following topics with the family as a part of the informed consent process: the medical benefit to the child (increase screening, discontinue screening, initiation of treatment, etc.), the psychosocial benefit to the family, and the professional guidelines to be considered. In most cases, through open discussion, providers and parents can manage the family's concerns and fears surrounding the recurrence risk for an adult-onset condition.

For some individuals, family trauma caused by heart disease (e.g., sudden death, loss of a parent or baby) is so distressing that prenatal testing will be beneficial whether or not termination of pregnancy is being considered as an option by the couple. Studies have shown that the ambiguity of a "possible diagnosis" of arrhythmogenic conditions can be more psychologically distressing for a longer period than the certainty of a diagnosis (Hendriks et al., 2008). Therefore, in many cases following thoughtful discussion, prenatal testing for an adult onset condition may be beneficial to family well-being. As testing in the prenatal setting includes the legal option of pregnancy termination for a gene-positive fetus, testing for conditions that will not be medically actionable in childhood is generally discouraged. In fact, there are providers who may choose not to offer testing on ethical grounds in such situations (Deans, Clarke, & Newson, 2015).

Many states have conscience clauses, which can be interpreted to cover health-care providers who refuse to provide prenatal genetic testing for adult-onset disorders.

Does parental autonomy compel proceeding with prenatal testing for conditions that may not be medically relevant in childhood? This question must be considered in the context of the interests of the other stakeholders. Parents have a legal right to proceed with testing and act on positive test results which, in some cases, may lead to termination of pregnancy. There is much discussion about the ethical dilemma of termination of pregnancy when the condition is of questionable severity or adult-onset. Some providers and laboratories (in rare cases) have decided not to participate in screening programs or targeted prenatal testing due to ethical objections to the outcome. However, in the United States, early termination of pregnancy is generally legal for any reason, including personal choice. The interest of the fetus as a future child is ultimately secondary to parental autonomy, even when the prenatal test is known to be valid and accurate, and the condition causes sufficient morbidity and/or mortality in childhood. Psychosocial considerations of the family are weighed on a case-by-case basis and may support ethical prenatal testing for adult-onset disease in a fetus or child.

C Nonmaleficence

Within the context of this case, the application of the principle of nonmaleficence with regard to the known *SCN5A* disease-causing variant is straightforward; avoiding implantation of an affected embryo will avoid the possible traumatic experience of life-threatening heart disease in the child.

With respect to the *TTR* variant, it is important to consider potential harms with regard to the psychological health of the parents. It could be psychologically distressing to the parents to know that their future child's *TTR* status is positive when there is no way to predict whether or when the child might become affected later in life. On the other hand, there may be significant psychological benefits for the parents in knowing a *TTR*-negative status. Finally, if no testing is completed, it must be considered that raising a child with uncertainty of *TTR* status may be emotionally harmful to these parents, especially since they have experienced the trauma of heart transplantation during the infancy of their first child.

Pre-implantation or prenatal testing has a significant risk of causing harm to the couple since the risk to have one or both variants is 75%. Potential outcomes must be explored prior to testing. Pretest discussion should result in a plan with which the family and provider are comfortable regarding which procedure best meets the family needs and which genetic testing gives the information the family is seeking, while balancing the rights of the future child and emotional preparation of the parents for poor outcomes, such as all embryos/fetuses testing positive. Parents may need help envisioning scenarios in which they know a future child is gene-positive for mid-life heart disease and decide whether this information is of any benefit to them or to the child. The family in the case example has a high risk for a gene-positive conception, which could provoke serious psychological distress for a couple who is already caring for a medically fragile child. Pretest counseling ought to discuss whether the potential reassurance of a negative result trumps concerns surrounding the possibility of adverse results.

D Beneficence

Pre-implantation genetic diagnosis or prenatal diagnosis for the *SCN5A* disease-causing variant and *TTR* likely disease-causing variant could result in reduced parental anxiety and emotional stress if the embryo/fetus was predicted not to have inherited these variants. Furthermore, in preventing the birth of a child predicted to have inherited the disease-causing variant, the emotional and financial toll of having to care for a child who would require continued cardiac surveillance and possibly a cardiac transplant could be avoided. There would also be an additional element of long-term psychological benefit for the parents in knowing that the child is not at increased risk for developing cardiomyopathy.

An unaffected child, potentially, could take the role of caregiver should both parents develop disease related to their genetic status. Since the father carries the same *SCN5A* gene as the child with cardiomyopathy and the mother carries the *TTR* likely disease-causing variant, both parents are potentially at risk of medical problems. Likewise, this child could potentially take the role of caregiver for a sibling, who may develop medical complications from the heart transplant in the future should the parents succumb to illness themselves. Certainly, there are a number of ethical considerations with regard to the question of whether there is an obligation to care for a family member, but the possibility of it offers potential psychological relief for the parents.

Should the parents undergo prenatal diagnosis and decide to continue a pregnancy predicted to have inherited the disease-causing variant, there is the psychological benefit of being able to prepare for the birth of a child who is at increased risk and who will require on-going surveillance. There is also the benefit of being able to prepare a surveillance plan to be followed immediately after birth and the benefit of being able financially to prepare for added medical costs. Knowing whether or not the child carries the *TTR* variant may offer peace of mind to the parents that positive or not they can be prepared for the future.

Whether there is any psychological benefit or burden that would arise for the child is less clear. It is interesting to consider how a child's perception of themselves, their self-worth or quality of life, would be affected by knowing that they are genetically predisposed to develop cardiomyopathy or Long QT Syndrome. Will this knowledge empower the child to face the risk and follow the recommended medical surveillance over their lifetime, or will it result in stigmatization and undue psychological distress as a result of the unpredictability of disease onset and medicalization for a condition that may never manifest? A recent study on predictive testing of minors found a range of benefits and absence of harms resulting from testing regardless of whether results were negative or positive. The greatest causes of stress reported occurred in the pretesting phase and were related to the uncertainty of their gene status and the counseling process required for informed consent prior to undergoing genetic testing (Mand, Gillam, Duncan, & Delatycki, 2013).

E Utility

Part of practicing nonmaleficence on the part of reproductive endocrinologists, maternal fetal medicine specialists, and genetic counselors rests in offering procedures and tests that have clinical utility; that is, a reasonable chance of successful outcome and valid test interpretation that is actionable. The odds of obtaining embryos that meet specific criteria is a relevant consideration in this regard. Testing an embryo for two mutations reduces the odds of identifying a gene-negative embryo to 25%. IVF may yield only one to eight embryos for testing. There may not be any gene-negative embryos for transfer. Natural conception and pregnancy typically yields only one conception, which in our case has the exceedingly high chance of 75% to be gene-positive. What is the utility of this testing for the parents? Should they not test for the *TTR* variant?

It is common for a genetic counselor to consider the utility of testing in the context of parental autonomy, and, in some cases, these two ethical considerations are at odds. In other words, some patients will feel strongly about obtaining information even in the case of low clinical utility. The family in our case is requesting testing for a variant (*TTR*) that is classified as "likely disease-causing" as opposed to "disease-causing". The variant has many characteristics of a disease-causing mutation; however, it has not been previously reported in other affected individuals, nor has it been shown to track with any disease in this particular family. There is the possibility that the *TTR* variant does not predispose to cardiomyopathy in this family and, therefore, has questionable relevance to the health of the future child.

As genomic testing becomes more prevalent, increasing numbers of families will be presenting with questions about testing for variants that have questionable predictive value. Is it ethical to offer prenatal testing for a variant that is unproven to be disease related in the family? This is an individual judgment call that should be based on the characteristics of the variant, the likely medical consequence, and the needs of the family.

Furthermore, in thinking through the outcomes with the parents, a genetic counselor should inform them that if an embryo is transferred with a *TTR* mutation, the resulting child will not need cardiology care until adulthood. Thus, there may be no clinical benefit of knowing the *TTR* status during childhood. In these cases, parents will likely vary widely in when they choose to disclose such genetic information to their child. This approach, however, is in conflict with medical genetic professional guidelines indicating that one should avoid presymptomatic testing of minors.

With regard to the clinical utility of such genetic testing, the cost of testing to the patient and to the medical community at large also comes in to play. Payers have an interest in covering only genetic testing that is clinically indicated. If providers classify all genetic testing as medically necessary, it will add to the already increasing cost of healthcare. This is potentially balanced by the appropriate use of genetic testing in a preventive manner.

F *Informed Consent*

Paramount in the consideration of test utility when prioritizing parental autonomy is assuring that all decisions are made in the context of informed consent. For example, the informed consent of the parents regarding the high likelihood of abnormal results, as mentioned previously, is essential. Parental informed consent about presymptomatic diagnosis and related uncertainty for the *TTR* mutation will be necessary as well as informed consent about revealing the gene-status of a future child.

It is unreasonable for any party at this time to see genetic testing as a way to avoid all heart disease or to ensure a healthy baby. The number of individuals with heart disease due to single-gene conditions is by far the minority. However, even if a child is born with no familial genetic mutations or variants, they are still at risk of developing heart disease due to numerous other factors. Moreover, the incidence of birth defects is in the range of 3–5%, which demonstrates the enduring inability to completely control reproductive outcomes.

Informed consent moves in two directions. First, the genetic counselor must make sure that the patient is aware of all facts that may be relevant for decision-making. The genetic professional must also be able to offer a comprehensive view of the potential benefits and limitations of testing or other clinical choices. In the reverse direction, the genetic counselor must be able fully to elicit the patients' concerns, as well as any misinformation or misunderstanding about the facts relating to their specific situation. This helps the genetic counselor more fully to understand the patient's perspective in order to best facilitate autonomous decision-making. In addition, to do a thorough analysis of the option of preimplantation genetic diagnosis, a genetic counselor will also discuss other reproductive alternatives, such as adoption, egg donation, or sperm donation. A discussion of all likely test result scenarios will guide decision-making, such that both the parents and clinicians reach a plan for testing or not testing that has an outcome with an appropriate management plan in place.

V Summary

Ethical issues in genetic counseling must be considered in a case-by-case fashion due to the uniqueness of each patient or set of patients, the condition(s) involved, the technical specifications, and the availability of testing. The case we have presented here demonstrates the importance of autonomous decision-making informed by facts, complete analysis of available options, and open disclosure of patient and practitioner values and clinical recommendations.

References

Deans, Z., A.J. Clarke, and A.J. Newson. 2015. For your interest? The ethical acceptability of using non-invasive prenatal testing to test 'purely for information'. *Bioethics* 29(1): 19–25.

Engelhardt, H.T., Jr. 2000. *The foundations of Christian bioethics*. Lisse: Swets & Zeitlinger.

Hendriks, K.S.W.H., M.M.W.B. Hendriks, E. Birnie, F.J.M. Grosfeld, A.A.M. Wilde, J. van den Bout, and E.M.A. Smets et al. 2008. Familial disease with a risk of sudden death: A longitudinal study of the psychological consequences of predictive testing for Long QT Syndrome. *Heart Rhythm* 25: 719–724.

Kopinsky, S.M. 1992. Value-based directiveness in genetic counseling. *Journal of Genetic Counseling* 1(4): 345–346.

Mand, C. L. Gillam, R.E. Duncan, and M.B. Delatycki. 2013. "It was the missing piece": Adolescent experiences of predictive genetic testing for adult-onset conditions. *Genetics in Medicine* 15(8): 643–649.

National Society of Genetic Counselors. 2017. *NSGC code of ethics*. https://www.nsgc.org/p/cm/ld/fid=12.

National Society of Genetic Counselors. 2018. *NSGC position statement on prenatal testing for adult-onset conditions*. https://www.nsgc.org/p/bl/et/blogaid=1042 (accessed 18 August 2018).

Ross, L.F., H.M. Saal, K.L. David, R.R. Anderson, American Academy of Pediatrics, and American College of Medical Genetics and Genomics. 2013. Technical report. Ethical and policy issues in genetic testing and screening of children. *Genetics in Medicine* 15(3): 234–245.

Uhlmann, W.R., J.L. Schuette, and B.M. Yashar. 2009. *A guide to genetic counseling*, second edition. Hoboken: John Wiley and Sons.

Veach, P.M., D.M. Bartels, and B.S. LeRoy. 2002. Commentary on GC - A profession in search of itself. *Journal of Genetic Counseling* 11(3): 187–191.

Weil, J. 2000. *Psychosocial genetic counseling*. New York: Oxford University Press.

Weil, J. 2003. Psychosocial genetic counseling in the post-nondirective era: A point of view. *Journal of Directive Counseling* 12(3): 199–211.

Weil, J., K. Ormond, J. Peters, K. Peters, B.B. Biesecker, and B. LeRoy. 2006. The relationship of nondirectiveness to genetic counseling: Report of a workshop at the 2003 NSGC annual education conference. *Journal of Genetic Counseling* 15(2): 85–93.

2 An Ethical Discussion of Cardiovascular Disease in Pregnancy

Peripartum Cardiomyopathy and Pulmonary Hypertension

Pamela Jordi and James Smith, Jr.

I Introduction

Ethical issues involving pregnancy have been a challenge for decades, even for the best politicians, lawyers, doctors, and ethicists. In many cases, courts have decided the outcome for women and their fetuses based on the rights of the fetus. This, however, calls into question the pregnant patient's autonomy and presumed rights to make medical decisions for herself and her unborn child. While it is not the physician's role to be the sole decision-maker in the patient-physician relationship, it is important to understand the culture we live in, provide necessary information, and provide appropriate medical support for the patient (Committee on Ethics 2005).

Women can and do accept the risk of complications associated with pregnancy. Certain maternal conditions increase these risks, such as autoimmune, renal, pulmonary, and cardiovascular diseases. With advancing medical technology and a focus on patient autonomy, physicians and other providers are able to care for patients with increasingly complex problems and risks during pregnancy. This attribute of contemporary obstetric practice highlights the need periodically to revisit ethical considerations involving the care of women and the neonate during and after pregnancy.

In this chapter, we will discuss two cardiovascular cases that may complicate pregnancy and raise ethical questions. We will highlight the germane medical issues, some of the social situations in which these issues exist, and the complexity of ethical issues that are brought forth. Many of the issues overlap. They represent some of the most polarizing ethical considerations in modern bioethics and may include sensitive topics such as assisted reproductive technology (ART), contraception, and pregnancy termination. Regardless of the provider's own moral position on these issues, this chapter will briefly discuss some of the more complicated ethical issues that arise in contact with a patient requiring care for complex cardiovascular conditions in pregnancy.

DOI: 10.4324/9781003240273-4

II Physiologic Cardiovascular Changes in Pregnancy

To understand the significance of cardiovascular disease processes and their impact on pregnancy, it is important to appreciate some basic physiologic changes that occur during pregnancy. Early in pregnancy, the plasma and blood volume increases and venous resistance decrease secondary to hormonal changes. Cardiac output increases 20–30% as early as five to eight weeks due to changes in heart rate, venous return, end-diastolic left ventricular volume, and stroke volume. In other words, there are changes that allow for the volume of blood that the heart is able to pump each minute to increase. Furthermore, pulmonary blood flow, that is, the blood being pumped to the lungs, increases significantly early in the pregnancy. If this increase in flow is the only change, there will be an increase in pulmonary blood pressure. However, there is a concurrent reduction in the resistance of the pulmonary vessels. The resulting physiology results in no increase in pulmonary artery pressure. By the middle of the second trimester of pregnancy, cardiac output has increased by 50% above non-pregnant state. Structural cardiac changes also occur, including heart chamber enlargement, myocardial hypertrophy, and multi-valvular regurgitation, especially during the later stages of pregnancy. During labor, significant changes in cardiovascular physiology are also noted. During uterine contractions the cardiac output is increased further to 60–80% above non-pregnant state. In the immediate postpartum period, the heart rate, systemic vascular resistance, cardiac output, and cardiac dimensions change as a result of the blood loss of childbirth and postpartum physiologic changes. These changes can be rapid and complicate patients with concomitant cardiovascular disease. Functional recovery takes place within two weeks. However, structural recovery, such as myocardial hypertrophy, can take five to six months to return to normal (Martinez and Rutherford 2013; Weiss and Hess 2000).

The two cases below illustrate the medical complexities of cardiovascular disease in pregnancy and some of the ethical issues that arise in caring for patients with these conditions.

Peripartum Cardiomyopathy: A 33-year-old healthy female delivered a healthy 7 pound 11 ounce male via uncomplicated spontaneous vaginal delivery five years previously. One week after delivery, she developed dyspnea, fatigue, and peripheral edema, and was subsequently diagnosed with cardiomyopathy by echocardiography. She had treatment with an antihypertensive and a diuretic and slowly recovered over the course of 12 months. She has been off medications for four years. Echocardiogram shows recovery of left ventricular function. She has no symptoms of cardiac dysfunction. She and her spouse have attempted pregnancy for 12 months, but have been unsuccessful. Today she and her husband are in your office with questions about infertility treatments and subsequent risks of pregnancy.

A Pathophysiology of Peripartum Cardiomyopathy

Peripartum cardiomyopathy (PPCM) is a cardiac disorder affecting women during the peripartum period. It is defined by four criteria according to the National

Heart, Lung, and Blood Institute and Office of Rare Disease of the National Institutes of Health: (1) development of cardiac failure during last month of pregnancy or within five months postpartum, (2) absence of demonstrable cause for cardiac failure, (3) absence of demonstrable heart disease before the last month of pregnancy, and (4) documented systolic dysfunction (Pearson et al. 2000, 1184–85). The diagnosis requires the absence of other pre-existing cardiac disease or dysfunction, as these may be exacerbated during pregnancy. PPCM occurs in 1/3000–1/15,000 pregnancies in the United States (Ro and Frishman 2006). Maternal mortality rates remain 9–56% despite advances in medical care. The majority of deaths occur within the first three months postpartum (Pillarisetti et al. 2014; Ro and Frishman 2006). Sudden death in these patients has been reported at 50% (Pillarisetti et al. 2014; Ro and Frishman 2006). The causes of mortality include heart failure, arrhythmias, or embolic events.

Risk factors for PPCM are multiparity, twin gestation, tocolytic therapy, pre-eclampsia, African-American race, obesity, and low socioeconomic status (Garg, Palaniswamy, and Lanier 2015; Pillarisetti et al. 2014; Ro and Frishman 2006). The etiology of PPCM is currently unknown, with several hypotheses, including connections to infectious disease, immunologic disorders, or nutritional deficiencies; it may also be drug-induced, or have a familial (genetic) component (Garg, Palaniswamy, and Lanier 2015; Ro and Frishman 2006). The diagnosis of PPCM requires a high level of suspicion as its symptoms closely mimic that of normal late pregnancy. These include dizziness, dyspnea, fatigue, or pedal edema. Diagnosis testing includes cardiac protein assays, EKG, echocardiogram, MRI, and possible endomyocardial biopsy (Garg, Palaniswamy, and Lanier 2015). Treatment includes standard therapy for heart failure with medication to reduce preload and afterload, anticoagulation, and inotropic agents. In other words, medical therapies are used to optimize cardiac function. This may involve the use of medications that improve the strength of heart muscle contraction, reduction in blood pressure to improve "forward-flow" of blood out of the heart, and anticoagulation to reduce the risk of blood clots forming from blood not flowing efficiently through the heart. Complicating therapy during pregnancy is the potential for some of these medications to cause harm to the fetus in the form of birth defects or death. Medical therapy may be insufficient in some patients. Defibrillators to correct irregular heart rates and rhythms are sometimes necessary. In the most severe cases of PPCM, in which cardiac function remains poor despite maximal medical therapy, left ventricular assist devices (LVADs) have been utilized. These devices serve as the pumping chamber for heart muscle that is not working efficiently. In some cases, heart transplant may also be considered (Garg, Palaniswamy, and Lanier 2015; Pillarisetti et al. 2014).

In cases of PPCM, multidisciplinary care ought to be coordinated among obstetricians, cardiologists, anesthesiologists, perinatologists, neonatologists, and other ancillary support personnel. These may include social workers and pastoral care providers (Ro and Frishman 2006). Postpartum prognosis is dependent on recovery of cardiac function. In women with resolution of cardiomegaly, the risk of death from congestive heart failure is low (Demakis et al. 1971). Those with persistent cardiomegaly or clinical evidence of cardiac dysfunction, however, experience a high mortality of about 85% at a median of 4.7 years (Demakis et al. 1971; Ro and Frishman 2006). Persistent symptoms beyond six months post-partum are indicative of irreversible myocardial damage and generally suggest a poor prognosis (Ro and Frishman 2006).

Recent advances offer more treatment options for PPCM. Treatment with the dopamine receptor agonist, bromocriptine, has shown improvement in recovery of left ventricular function, compared to standard heart failure treatment. The lactation inhibition action of bromocriptine limits its use in some postpartum patients. Pentoxifylline and immunoglobulins have also been studied for their effects on left ventricular function. Although these studies are promising, larger randomized controlled trials are needed to determine beneficial effects, safety, and efficacy across population subgroups (Garg, Palaniswamy, and Lanier 2015).

B Ethical Discussion

Counseling is imperative for women who have been diagnosed with PPCM in a previous pregnancy but who desire a future pregnancy (Ethics Committee of the American Society for Reproductive Medicine 2009, 2016). PPCM has a propensity to recur in subsequent pregnancies and patients are at risk for this condition if pregnancy occurs. For instance, when recovery of cardiac function following PPCM is noted, subsequent pregnancies carry a very low mortality risk despite recurrence risks. However, if cardiac dysfunction persists following a pregnancy complicated by PPCM, mortality may be almost 20% (Garg, Palaniswamy, and Lanier 2015). There is still an increased risk of recurrent PPCM during and after a subsequent pregnancy, even when complete recovery of cardiac function occurs in the antecedent interval. Current opinions regarding pregnancy following an episode of PPCM weigh in favor of avoiding pregnancy due to the increased and sometimes unpredictable risk of maternal and fetal complications (Garg, Palaniswamy, and Lanier 2015). These patients should likely be counseled against additional pregnancies and on appropriate contraception options at the time of diagnosis of PPCM and in follow up visits.

Balancing the admonitions against pregnancy in patients with a history of PPCM is the desire of many patients to have children (Committee on Ethics 2013; Committee on Ethics 2014a). Ideally, patients with a history of PPCM should present for preconception counseling, prior to a subsequent pregnancy. This allows comprehensive discussion of the medical and obstetrical risks of pregnancy, as well as the social and psychological dimensions of the patient's desire to expand her family. Alternatively, patients may present for counseling after having already conceived. In both scenarios, the risks of recurrence of PPCM are at the core of the medical discussion, but the ethical dimensions of the second scenario, in which a patient is already pregnant, involves the additional moral dimensions and tensions associated with the possible termination of pregnancy.

In the clinical situation presented, a patient with a history of PPCM has attempted pregnancy, and has been unsuccessful. Her providers are now faced with more than counseling about pregnancy and its risks, or even medical support for an ongoing pregnancy already conceived. They are now, at the request of an infertility patient with a history of PPCM, asked to assist in achieving pregnancy. While the physicians are well aware of the attendant risks of pregnancy in such a patient, they are also well aware of the desire of some patients for further children regardless of attendant risks. How then is the physician to balance concern for the overall long-term wellbeing of the patient with concern to assist her in fertility resulting in a high-risk pregnancy?

The goal of effective counseling is to allow patient decisions to be made in the absence of coercion from the counselor's biases. For instance, from a principlist perspective, respect for the patient requires promotion of autonomy in making decisions. Even with balanced and comprehensive counseling, patients can and will make decisions that are against the better judgment of the providers who have counseled them. To the extent that the providers remain involved in their care, tensions arise when the providers feel that they are proceeding on morally tenuous grounds. For providers counseling such patients, who requests assistance with conception for a pregnancy despite significant risk, it will be necessary to reflect and discern their own moral position on just how much to support the patient's request and assist her in achieving pregnancy. For some providers, this reflection may uncover previously unidentified discomfort, moral perspectives, and professional limits to participation in patient care. The development of skills to balance the perspectives of the patient, and the personal perspectives of the provider is an important professional focus in these cases.

An evolving concept in its application in reproductive medicine is that of "reproductive liberty" (Macdonald 2002). This foundational core value underpins the provision of infertility services for individuals, who determine for themselves whether and how to reproduce. Reproductive liberty does not imply that all reproductive desires or requests of individuals be met, but rather that the desire for reproductive potential should be recognized as a common human attribute that should be supported. Thus, the request of a patient for fertility treatment, despite the potential of significant morbidity risks, including an increased risk of mortality, of an ensuing pregnancy, is framed as reasonable, supportable, and compelling. In this light, discussions related to maternal and fetal/newborn risks of pregnancy in a patient with a history of PPCM are oriented toward not just the relative and absolute medical risks of recurrence, but also the personal, social, and psychological dimensions of risks, should they recur. Maternal death related to a rare but predicted cardiovascular event, leaving a newborn without a biological mother, is a scenario which is uncomfortable for patients and providers to consider; but it is a reality that ought to be discussed.

The complexities of such counseling can be challenging for providers. There are legitimate differences in providers' assessment of relative and absolute risks for patients. There are also legitimate differences in assessments of the consequences of these risks should they occur. For requests that, in the opinion of a provider, place an individual patient at unacceptable risk, referral for second opinions or follow-up care is appropriate. In such circumstances, it is reasonable for a provider to decline to participate in fertility care (Macdonald 2002).

III Pulmonary Hypertension in Pregnancy

Idiopathic Pulmonary Hypertension: Case: A 27-year-old female with idiopathic pulmonary hypertension (PH) was diagnosed by right heart catheterization at age 22. Further testing did not reveal an etiology. She has been responding well to calcium channel blockers. She presents to the clinic with a positive home pregnancy test. Vaginal ultrasound confirms viable intrauterine pregnancy at ten weeks four days. She states that she desires to continue this pregnancy.

A Pathophysiology of Pulmonary Hypertension during Pregnancy

Pulmonary hypertension (PH) is a common condition in the general population and, when defined as a systolic pulmonary blood pressure of >35 mmHg, occurs in about 20% of the population. PH is the result of a host of etiologies that result in the common finding of hypertension in the pulmonary circulation (McGlothlin 2012; Shah 2012). This hypertension may be the result of vasoconstriction, or remodeling and "thickening" of the lining of the pulmonary arteries that result in increased vascular resistance, and thus hypertension. Most cases of PH are the result of acquired chronic conditions such as chronic hypertension, chronic obstructive pulmonary disease, thromboembolism, and lung disease (Committee on Ethics 2005; Martinez and Rutherford 2013; Weiss and Hess 2000). Primary PH and PH that results from congenital cardiac disease is the least common type, but it has specific implications for pregnancy. Primary PH affects women more frequently than men, and occurs on average earlier in life than secondary forms of PH. Correction of congenital cardiac disease, such as ventricular septal defects, has reduced the etiology of PH. Primary PH remains a rare, but potentially lethal, condition with specific implications for pregnancy.

Pregnancy represents a particularly risky condition for women with PH due to normal physiologic changes in pregnancy. The most compelling are the increased blood volume that occurs in pregnancy, and the resultant increased cardiac output. In other words, the volume of blood circulating is increased during pregnancy. In women without PH, the pulmonary vessels usually accommodate this increased volume without complication. However, in patients with PH, the increased demand for space in the pulmonary circulation is met with increased vascular resistance, hypertension in the pulmonary arterial circulation, and, ultimately, right heart failure. Thus, normal physiologic changes in pregnancy can pose a direct and progressive threat to the patient with PH. Historically, this condition has led to the near-universal recommendation for termination of pregnancy. In many ways, PH has served as the "prototypic" diagnosis leading to maternal-fetal conflict.

Yet progress has been made in optimizing maternal and fetal outcomes in ongoing pregnancies. In the decade between the years 1997 and 2007, the mortality rate dropped from 30% to 17% for primary PH and from 38% to 28% for PH secondary to a congenital heart defect, when compared to the preceding two decades. The main factor noted in these improvements appears to be the use of advanced treatments, including nitric oxide, prostacyclin analogues, and calcium channel blockers, in over 70% of patients. Most maternal deaths occur in the late antepartum period or within the month following delivery (Martinez and Rutherford 2013; Weiss et al. 1998). Neonatal survival approaches 90% (Cunningham et al. 2013; Martinez and Rutherford 2013; Ward and Beachy 2003). These pregnancies represent some of the most complicated clinical situations encountered by providers, and a multidisciplinary approach with input from obstetricians, maternal fetal medicine physicians, pulmonologists, cardiologists, and neonatologists is vital. Despite improvements in outcomes, current evidence suggests that mortality rate related to pregnancy in the patient with PH remains relatively high and has not declined in the last decade or so (Meng et al. 2017; see also, Kumar and Suresh 2008; Ramani and Park 2012).

B Ethical Discussion

Ideally, the risks and complications of pregnancy in a patient with PH should be discussed prior to pregnancy. For pregnant patients with PH, 60% were diagnosed before pregnancy, while 30% were diagnosed during their pregnancy. The ethical issues related to those patients with known PH prior to a planned or unanticipated pregnancy center on the appropriateness of a continued pregnancy, when mortality is known to be increased. Many advocate termination of pregnancy due to the increased mortality (Hemmes et al. 2015). With current therapies used during pregnancy, however, successful outcomes are possible, which leads some patients to desire support for an ongoing pregnancy. Counseling related to the request for an ongoing pregnancy is complex. Fundamentally, the counseling should be based on objective evidence and best estimates of the likelihood of successful outcomes. "Successful outcomes" may mean different things to different patients. For some, a "successful outcome" includes only the term delivery of a normal newborn with no decompensation related to PH during pregnancy. For others, a successful outcome may include the delivery of a premature infant who survives despite neurologic impairment related to preterm delivery. The provider must deliver information in understandable terms, and in an evidence-based, non-discriminatory fashion, despite significant reservations. Furthermore, once the patient decides to continue the pregnancy, she will require unwavering diligence and robust management to attain the most favorable outcome.

References

Committee on Ethics. 2005. Maternal decision making, ethics, and the law. *The American College of Obstetricians and Gynecologists Committee Opinion* 321: 1–11.

Committee on Ethics. 2007. Ethical decision making in obstetrics and gynecology. *The American College of Obstetricians and Gynecologists Committee Opinion* 390: 1–9.

Committee on Ethics. 2012a. Informed consent. *The American College of Obstetricians and Gynecologists Committee Opinion* 439: 1–8.

Committee on Ethics. 2013. The limits of conscientious refusal in reproductive medicine. *American College of Obstetricians and Gynecologists Committee Opinion* 385: 1–6.

Committee on Ethics. 2014. Empathy in women's health care. *The American College of Obstetricians and Gynecologists Committee Opinion* 480: 1–6.

Demakis, J. G., S. H. Rahimtoola, G. C. Sutton, W. R. Meadows, P. B. Szanto, J. R. Tobin, and R. M. Gunnar. 1971. Natural course of peripartum cardiomyopathy. *Circulation* 44(6): 1052–1061.

Ethics Committee of the American Society for Reproductive Medicine. 2016. Provision of fertility services for women at increased risk of complications during fertility treatment or pregnancy: An ethics committee opinion. *Fertility and Sterility* 106(6): 1319–1323.

Garg, J., C. Palaniswamy, and G. Lanier. 2015. Peripartum cardiomyopathy: Definition, incidence, etiopathogenesis, diagnosis and management. *Cardiology in Review* 23(2): 69–78.

Hemmes, A. R., D. G. Kiely, B. A. Cockrill, Z. Safdar, V. J. Wilson, M. Al Hazmi, and I. R. Preston, et al. 2015. Statement on pregnancy in pulmonary hypertension from the Pulmonary Vascular Research Institute. *Pulmonary Circulation* 5(3): 435–465.

Macdonald, H. 2002. Perinatal care at the threshold of viability. *Pediatrics* 11(5): 1024–1027.

Martinez, M. V. and J. D. Rutherford. 2013. Pulmonary hypertension in pregnancy. *Cardiology in Review* 21(4): 167–173.

McGlothlin, D. 2012. Classification of pulmonary hypertension. *Heart Failure Clinics* 8(3): 301–317.

Meng, M. L., R. Landau, O. Viktorsdottir, J. Banayan, T. Grant, B. Bateman, and R. Smiley, et al. 2017. Pulmonary hypertension in pregnancy: A report of 49 cases at four tertiary North American sites. *Obstetrics and Gynecology* 129(3): 511–520.

Pearson, G. D., J. C. Veille, S. Rahimtoola, J. Hsia, C. M. Oakley, J. D. Hosenpud, A. Ansari, and K. L. Baughman. 2000. Peripartum cardiomyopathy: National Heart, Lung, and Blood Institute and Office of Rare Diseases (National Institutes of Health) workshop recommendations and review. *JAMA* 283(9): 1183–1188.

Pillarisetti, J., A. Kondur, A. Alani, M. Reddy, M. Reddy, J. Vacek, and C. P. Weiner, et al. 2014. Peripartum cardiomyopathy: Predictors of recovery and current state of implantable cardioverter-defibrillator use. *Journal of the American College of Cardiology* 63(25 Pt. A): 2831–2839.

Ro, A., and W. H. Frishman. 2006. Peripartum cardiomyopathy. *Cardiology in Review* 14(1): 35–42.

Shah, S. J. 2012. Pulmonary hypertension. *JAMA* 308(13): 1366–1374.

Ward, R. M., and J. C. Beachy. 2003. Neonatal complications following preterm birth. *BJOG* 110(Suppl. 20): 8–16.

Weiss, B. M., and O. M. Hess. 2000. Pulmonary vascular disease and pregnancy: Current controversies, management strategies, and perspectives. *European Heart Journal* 21(2): 104–115.

Weiss, B. M., L. Zemp, B. Seifert, and O. M. Hess. 1998. Outcome of pulmonary vascular disease in pregnancy: A systematic overview from 1978 through 1996. *Journal of the American College of Cardiology* 31(7): 1650–1657.

Additional Reading

Committee on Ethics. 2008. Medical futility. *The American College of Obstetricians and Gynecologists Committee Opinion* 362: 1–4.

Committee on Ethics. 2012b. Innovative practice: Ethical guidelines. *The American College of Obstetricians and Gynecologists Committee Opinion* 352: 1–7.

Committee on Ethics. 2014a. Disclosure and discussion of adverse events. *The American College of Obstetricians and Gynecologists Committee Opinion* 520: 1–4.

Committee on Ethics. 2014b. Increasing access to abortion. *The American College of Obstetricians and Gynecologists Committee Opinion* 613: 1–6.

Cunningham, F., K. J. Leveno, S. L. Bloom, C. Y. Spong, J. S. Dashe, B. L. Hoffman, B. M. Casey, J. S. Sheffield. 2013. The preterm newborn. In *Williams obstetrics, twenty-fourth edition*, F. Cunningham, K. J. Leveno, S. L. Bloom, C. Y. Spong, J. S. Dashe, B. L. Hoffman, B. M. Casey, and J. S. Sheffield (eds). New York: McGraw-Hill Education, 668–671.

Ethics Committee of the American Society for Reproductive Medicine. 2009. Fertility treatment when the prognosis is very poor or futile. *Fertility and Sterility* 92(4): 1194–1197.

Kumar, P., and G. Suresh. 2008. Complication after preterm birth: An overview for emergency physicians. *Clinical Pediatric Emergency Medicine* 9(3): 191–199.

Ramani, G. V., and M. H. Park. 2012. Pharmacotherapy for pulmonary arterial hypertension. *Heart Failure Clinic* 8(3): 385–402.

3 Severe Congenital Anomalies in the Fetus or Infant

"Best-Interests" Decisions for Ambiguous Outcomes

Dalia M. Feltman

I Introduction

Whether to provide neonatal intensive care when it is of uncertain benefit to the baby is an ethical challenge. Newborns rely on others to weigh treatment burdens and benefits in their "best-interests." These decisions are straightforward when effectiveness is predictable: efficacious (low mortality, low morbidity) treatments are indicated; inefficacious (high mortality, high morbidity) treatments are not. When life-sustaining treatments are deemed overly burdensome compared to potential benefits, they should be withdrawn or not initiated, and the goal of care is redirected toward that of comfort. Comfort care focuses on treating a baby's pain, providing warmth, and trying to optimize bonding time with parents and family until the baby dies. Unfortunately, best-interests decisions are often unclear. The American Academy of Pediatrics explains, "[if] prognosis is uncertain but likely to be very poor and survival may be associated with a diminished quality of life for the child... parental desires should determine the treatment approach" (AAP Committee on Fetus and Newborn, 2007, p. 402). Parents and physicians must collaborate to deliver medical management aligned with the child's best interests, paying careful attention to changing outcomes and management approaches.

This chapter examines treatment decisions for two high-risk newborns who, forty years ago, would have died in hospice: one born with hypoplastic left heart syndrome; the other prenatally diagnosed with trisomy 18 and ventricular septal defect. It reviews evolution of management, empirical studies of parents' and professionals' attitudes, ethical debates surrounding these changes, and necessary elements of informed consent when counseling parents. When a clear "best-interests" choice for management does not exist, physicians must assist parents in making fully-informed decisions, ensuring all ethically acceptable options and their likely outcomes are considered.

Hypoplastic left heart syndrome and trisomy 18 share several features: neither is curable, management paradigms are changing, prenatal detection has increased and, when detected prenatally, pregnancy termination is common, and whether benefits of intervention outweigh burdens are unclear. Because of marked improvement of post-surgical survival rates for hypoplastic left heart syndrome,

DOI: 10.4324/9781003240273-5

some argue that only offering comfort care is not ethical. While until recently trisomy 18 was termed a "lethal" condition for which only comfort care was offered, higher survival rates, better quality-of-life outcomes and shifting paradigms in decision-making have resulted in providing intensive care at the parents' request. After examining the medical facts (survival and neurologic outcomes) and quality of life (life-long medical management and empirical data) for each condition separately, the ethical challenges they share will be analyzed and suggestions for navigating these difficult management options will be proposed.

II Case One: Newborn with Hypoplastic Left Heart Syndrome

"Faith" is a two-day-old full-term female, born to a 21-year-old healthy mom, who required neonatal intensive care unit (NICU) transfer after becoming mottled with rapid respirations in the nursery. Prostaglandins started for a suspected ductal-dependent cardiac lesion have stabilized her condition. Echocardiogram confirms hypoplastic left heart syndrome. You are the pediatric cardiologist preparing to discuss hypoplastic left heart syndrome management with Faith's parents. The NICU social worker asks if comfort care is an option.

A What Is Known about This Condition?

Hypoplastic left heart syndrome refers to a constellation of congenital heart anomalies sharing an underdeveloped left ventricle, atretic or critically stenotic aortic or mitral valves and hypoplasia of the ascending aorta and arch; atrial-septal defect, ventricular septal defect or aortic coarctation are often present. Hypoplastic left heart syndrome accounts for 1% of congenital heart anomalies, but carries the highest neonatal mortality (Park, 2002). Co-morbid conditions (intrauterine growth retardation, genetic defects, microcephaly, and periventricular leukomalacia) exist more frequently than with other congenital heart lesions (Wernovsky, 2008). Diagnosis is made prenatally (with ultrasound suspicions confirmed by fetal echocardiography) or in the first hours or days of life. It presents as desaturations, respiratory distress, murmur, poor perfusion, or signs of heart failure after the ductus arteriosus closes, and no longer allows a way for the body to receive adequate circulation. (The ductus is a connection between the pulmonary artery and aorta that allows oxygenated blood to bypass the left heart prenatally and typically closes shortly after birth.) Immediate management includes maintaining systemic circulation by keeping the ductus open with prostaglandin E_1 infusion and supportive care of respiratory failure and metabolic acidosis. Surgical intervention is necessary for survival beyond a few weeks.

B Survival Outcomes

Hypoplastic left heart syndrome surgical interventions are "palliative" because they cannot cure malformed left-sided structures. To avoid confusion with the "palliative care" provided in conjunction with hospice, "comfort care" is used hereafter. Prior to the 1980s, surgical palliation for hypoplastic left heart syndrome did not exist. Babies died within days with comfort care. Aggressive medical management achieves a median survival time of 60 days (Pager, 2000). When staged surgical palliation was introduced, primary cardiac transplantation also became possible. Because of high mortality rates after surgery or awaiting transplant, uncertainty of long-term outcomes, and burdens of multiple surgeries, parents of babies with hypoplastic left heart syndrome were offered surgical palliation, cardiac transplantation, or comfort care. Better preoperative and intraoperative strategies now yield improved survival rates; with five-year survival rates ranging from about 50% to 70%, depending on surgical center and study years (Mercurio, Peterec, & Weeks, 2008). One-quarter of newborns awaiting heart transplantation for hypoplastic left heart syndrome die; 70% of those receiving transplants survive five years (Kon, 2008). According to the *Journal of the American College of Cardiology*'s White Paper comprehensive hypoplastic left heart syndrome review by Feinstein, et al. "current expectations are that 70% of newborns born today with HLHS (hypoplastic left heart syndrome) may reach adulthood" (Feinstein et al., 2012, p. S1).

C Neurodevelopmental Outcomes

Attention, language, and coordination problems are more common in children with hypoplastic left heart syndrome than in healthy children, as are behavioral and emotional difficulties (Paris, Moore, & Schreiber, 2012). Neuropsychological development is likely affected by decreased oxygenation of the developing fetal brain, hypothermia with circulatory arrest historically required during surgery (Feinstein et al., 2012), and ischemic injuries (seen on MRI) worsened after bypass (Paris, Moore, & Schreiber, 2012). Neurologic problems in 23 patients with hypoplastic left heart syndrome (and normal chromosomes) studied at age five included: MRI abnormalities, primarily ischemia (82%); major neurodevelopmental impairments (23%); minor neurologic dysfunction (43%); median IQ scores in normal range but significantly lower than in controls (Sarajuuri et al., 2012). Neurologic outcomes may improve as deep-hypothermia exposure is limited with improved surgical techniques and prenatal detection increases. Preventing interruption of ductal patency with prompt prostaglandin initiation may explain why prenatal detection is associated with fewer neurologic events like postoperative seizures (Feinstein et al., 2012). Wernovsky cites two more recent studies revealing improved cognition, noting that most children who have hypoplastic left heart syndrome are in mainstream education and have normal cognitive abilities (Wernovsky, 2008).

D Quality of Life

To weigh burdens and benefits of surgery for hypoplastic left heart syndrome, the ways in which lifelong management may affect quality of life ought to be examined. While some empirical quality of life studies of hypoplastic left heart syndrome patients and families exist, long-term outcomes and quality of life self-reports are limited to the first few decades of life. Patients' experiences have varied due to changing care since the advent of hypoplastic left heart syndrome surgery.

1 Lifetime Healthcare Needs

Staged surgical palliation of hypoplastic left heart syndrome requires three open-heart surgeries. A child typically undergoes the Norwood (stage I) procedure at a few weeks of life, the Glenn or hemi-Fontan (stage II) in the first year, and the Fontan (stage III) procedure between three and five years of life. (Modifications to stages exist but these aforementioned classic approaches suffice for our purposes.) While a detailed description of these surgical procedures is beyond the scope of this chapter, I will briefly describe the morbidity and mortality associated with each to facilitate an understanding of the relative benefits and burdens of surgical intervention. Stage I carries the highest mortality, although hospital survival has improved to 69–81% (Feinstein et al., 2012). The Norwood often requires deep hypothermic cardiac arrest. Stage I intraoperative complications in one study included: delayed sternal closure (75%), cardiopulmonary resuscitation (15%), and post-operative Extracorporeal Membrane Oxygenation (10%). The need for this last support, also called ECMO, is a method of pumping blood outside the body to bypass the lungs (and sometimes the heart). This system adds oxygen to the blood and removes carbon dioxide before returning it to the body and carries its own serious risks such as bleeding, clots, and infection (Feinstein et al., 2012). Post-operative complications include arrhythmia (15%), EEG-detected seizures (22%), stroke (5%), MRI ischemic changes (>20%), a serious injury to the bowel called necrotizing enterocolitis (1–18%), infection, renal dysfunction, phrenic or recurrent laryngeal nerve injury, and lymphatic injury causing chyle leakage into the lung lining called chylothorax (Feinstein et al., 2012). Mortality between stages I and II is as high as 16%. Though labor-intensive for parents, instituting home monitoring of changes in the child's weight, intake and output, and oxygenation levels has improved inter-stage survival (Feinstein et al., 2012). Before stage II, cardiac catheterization is usually required, though MRI is being studied as an alternative. Mortality after stage II and short-term post-stage III are excellent (<5%), though embolism, pleural effusion, arrhythmia, and phrenic nerve injury may occur. Five- and ten-year survival after stage III ranges from 70% to 90% (Feinstein et al., 2012). Due to high rates of wait-list deaths, primary transplantation instead of staged palliation is generally reserved for certain anatomic characteristics portending poor palliation outcomes. Primary-transplant survival rates are similar to palliation, but Kon estimates children will need repeated transplants every 10–15 years as only half of grafts survive beyond 10 years (Kon, 2008). Patients with failed palliation also require transplantation.

Morbidities are not yet known beyond a few decades of life. Adult Fontan patients require at least yearly surveillance for liver disease, protein-losing enteropathy, and plastic bronchitis. Failed palliation in adulthood may preclude cardiac transplantation or require combined heart-liver transplants. Sudden death (likely arrhythmia-related) explains nearly one-third of deaths in adult Fontan patients. While infertility and miscarriages may occur more frequently, female Fontan patients have survived the pregnancies and deliveries of healthy babies (Feinstein et al., 2012).

2 Empirical Quality of Life Data

Empirical quality of life studies reviewed by Feinstein et al. include data from non-hypoplastic left heart syndrome patients with Fontan-physiology/single-ventricle physiology. Parents of school-aged children reported lower psychosocial functioning. By contrast, adults' self-reported quality of life scores were similar to healthy respondents (Feinstein et al., 2012). Better quality of life scores by self-reporting versus parent reporting have been demonstrated in other chronic conditions (Hack et al., 2011), highlighting the importance of soliciting patient responses. Family problems, including increased divorce rates in parents of children with cardiac surgery and increased parental stress in hypoplastic left heart syndrome versus another lesion (transposition of great arteries), have been published (Mavroudis, Mavroudis, Farrell, Jacobs, Jacobs, & Kodish, 2011). Mavroudis summarizes the challenges of judging hypoplastic left heart syndrome quality of life:

> At present, discussion of possible outcomes includes not just the potential for serious adverse outcomes... but the fact that among the survivors of surgical management of hypoplastic left heart syndrome there are Eagle Scouts, college students, and two young women who 20 and 23 years after their own initial Norwood operations gave birth to infants with structurally normal hearts.
> (Mavroudis, Mavroudis, Farrell, Jacobs, Jacobs, & Kodish, 2011, p. 137)

III Case Two: Newborn with Trisomy 18 and Ventricular Septal Defect

A pregnant couple in their forties requests prenatal cardiology consultation after diagnosis of trisomy 18 with ventricular septal defect but no other major organ malformations on ultrasound. Mom tearfully recounts switching obstetricians after feeling pressured to terminate the pregnancy. Dad says they were told they would only prolong the "lethal trisomy's" suffering while burdening their three school-aged children. Their new obstetrician has agreed to provide fetus-centered obstetric care. They acknowledge "Charlotte's" low chance for live birth and her limited lifespan and developmental potential. Neonatologists have assured them their wishes for intensive care will be honored. They seek advice regarding Charlotte's large perimembranous ventricular septal defect.

What is known about this condition? Trisomy 18, or Edward's syndrome, occurs when cells have three copies of chromosome 18 instead of the usual two. In full trisomy, all cells have three complete chromosome 18s; in partial, the third copy is incomplete, and in mosaic, not all of a patient's cells have an abnormal number of chromosomes. Full trisomy accounts for most cases. After trisomy 21 (Down syndrome), trisomy 18 is the most common trisomy at birth, occurring in 0.3 in 1,000 newborn births, with greater female prevalence of about 3 to 1. Trisomy 18 often results in miscarriage or stillbirth. Prenatal detection has increased with developments in noninvasive screening. While 130 associated anomalies have been described, characteristic facial and extremity deformities, frequent cardiac defects, and profound mental and motor retardation are universal (Jones, Jones, & del Campo, 2013). Until the last few decades, trisomy 18 was considered lethal due to low survival past a few weeks of life.

A Survival

Nearly two-thirds of pregnancies with trisomy 18 end in spontaneous intra-uterine death (Burke, Field, & Morrison, 2013). A regional UK study over the years 1985–2007 revealed: increased trisomy 18 pregnancy incidence, higher proportions of cases detected prenatally, high termination rates, and fewer live births (Irving, Richmond, Wren, Longster, & Embleton, 2011). Without neonatal intensive care, trisomy 18 patients live a median 10–15 days, and most (90–100%) die by one year; with intensive care; however, Japanese and Polish studies report 25–30% of patients surviving beyond their first birthdays (McGraw & Perlman, 2008).

B Neurodevelopmental Outcomes

Trisomy 18 patients have severe mental retardation and developmental delay. Brady reports patients, on average, achieving reflective smiling by 4.7 months and sitting unassisted and walking with walkers by 39 months. While most preschool-aged children functioned at 8-month-old levels, Brady cautions that some children exhibited milestones that exceeded these averaged developmental scores: "children acquired skills such as object permanence, helping with hygiene, self-feeding, understanding cause and effect" (Carey, 2012, p. 674). Braddock reports intentional communication skills in some 10-year-olds (Carey, 2012). Parents of children with trisomy 18 or trisomy 13 (another classically-dubbed "lethal" trisomy) provided information for 23 children over age 10. Developmental milestones included: smiling (100%), laughing (96%), pointing at objects (65%), saying mama/papa (35%), and playing with toys (100%); 87% ate by mouth; 39% ate without assistance; 87% could stand assisted; 17% could stand unassisted; 74% could walk with walkers; none could walk alone (Janvier, Farlow, & Wilfond, 2012).

C *Quality of Life*

1 *Lifetime Healthcare Needs*

Studies of US trisomy 18 patients are limited by small sample sizes or by the inability to characterize individual patients' courses due to using aggregate hospitalization databases. Nelson et al. examined US hospitalizations and procedures linked to trisomy 18 or trisomy 13 diagnostic codes for five separate years between 1997 and 2009. Nearly half of birth admissions were discharged home. Children over one year represented over one-third of all admissions; over 10% of discharges were for patients over 8 years old. Children older than eight received higher rates of procedures than younger children. Changes noted over the study years included: increased admissions, longer stays, fewer inpatient deaths, and increased home-health (including hospice) referrals (Nelson, Hexem, & Feudtner, 2012). Most data on intensive care for trisomy 18 patients come from Japan where this is routinely offered. Documenting NICU courses of 24 full-trisomy 18 patients (1994–2003), Kosho demonstrated increased survival (25% beyond one year) with intensive care as compared to population-based reports. Most (88%) required mechanical ventilation and 29% were successfully extubated. Most (83%) patients lived to one month; median survival was 152.5 days (Kosho, Nakamura, Kawame, Baba, Tamura, & Fukushima, 2006).

Cardiac surgery is not performed as regularly as other surgical procedures for patients with trisomy 18, as high burdens have appeared to outweigh unclear benefits. This may be changing with improved understanding of why trisomy 18 patients die. While only 6% of major hospital procedures were cardiac, Nelson et al. observed trends suggesting more cardiac interventions with time. Atrial septal and ventricular septal defects repairs were most frequent, though complex (e.g., truncus arteriosus and Tetralogy of Fallot) repairs occurred (Nelson, Hexem, & Feudtner, 2012). Cardiac surgery was thought unlikely to improve survival because apnea was believed the leading cause of trisomy 18 deaths (Maeda et al., 2011). However, for Kosho's patients receiving intensive care (all had cardiac defects), cardiac failure was the most common (96%) cause of death, often in combination with pulmonary hypertension (78%) and respiratory failure (41%) (Kosho, Nakamura, Kawame, Baba, Tamura, & Fukushima, 2006). Kaneko examined eras of management for cardiac lesions of Japanese trisomy 18 patients; those receiving pharmacologic and surgical management survived longer than those without surgery (median survival 243 vs. 24 days) (Maeda et al., 2011). In Kaneko et al.'s analysis of 17 trisomy 18 patients undergoing surgical palliation,

> Although one patient died intraoperatively, no other patients died of heart failure after surgery. The fact that 82% of the patients were discharged home in stable condition indicates that cardiac surgery offered the majority of these patients the opportunity of enjoying their parents' cuddle and alleviation of serious cardiac symptoms.
>
> (Kaneko et al., 2009, p. 732)

While Kaneko and others prefer surgical palliation when clinically warranted over primary repair (Kaneko et al., 2009; McCaffrey, 2002), Kobayashi reports successful ventricular septal defect closure with sternotomy and cardiopulmonary bypass in five patients, with no deaths in the post-operative period. He suggests this may prolong lifespan and is technically feasible even in the setting of trisomy 18-associated physical findings such as thoracic deformity, redundant valves, and ventricular dilation/hypertrophy (Kobayashi, Kaneko, Yamamoto, Yoda, & Tsuchiya, 2010). Yamagishi's population study of 145 Japanese patients revealed improved two-year survival with surgery (45%) vs. without surgery (5%) (Yamagishi, 2010). Graham's review of a large international cardiac registry showed 35 trisomy 18 patients had undergone cardiac surgery; 91% were discharged alive, most to their homes (Graham, Bradley, Shirali, Hills, & Atz, 2004).

2 Empirical Quality of Life Data

Because profound developmental impairments preclude quality of life self-reporting by trisomy 18 patients, empirical studies rely on caregiver reporting. Researchers have surveyed parents of children with trisomy 18 or trisomy 13 who belong to Internet-based support groups. Parents' medical choices reflected varying quality of life judgments and correlated to presence of severe anomalies. For the 107 prenatally-diagnosed children, parents chose: comfort care (53%); full interventions (25%); interventions between comfort care and full (22%). Those who chose comfort care opted against life-sustaining treatments, whereas those who chose full interventions consented to treatments, as needed, including endotracheal intubation with mechanical ventilation, chest compressions and cardiac medications in case of slow heart rate, feeding tube insertion (including surgical gastrostomies), and surgical repairs of anatomic anomalies. Children with partial trisomy or absence of cardiac defects or holoprosencephaly (abnormal development of the forebrain) were more likely to receive full interventions (Guon, Wilfond, Farlow, Brazg, & Janvier, 2013). Most (75%) parents with prenatal diagnosis reported their children had positive effects on their marriage/relationship, and nearly all (91%) would hypothetically continue another pregnancy with this diagnosis. For the 97 children who had died, 91% of parents described their child's experience as positive; 77% were satisfied by the degree of interventions, though 21% wished they had been more aggressive. Well-being of children surviving beyond three months was reported: 91% described children as happy; 25% worried they suffered more pain than other children. Family stress varied: 97% agreed their child enriched their lives; 82% thought their child was a positive experience for their other children; 43% reported financial stress; one-third described child-rearing as more difficult than expected (Guon, Wilfond, Farlow, Brazg, & Janvier, 2013). In one cohort, 95% of parents whose children were alive affirmed the ability to understand their children's needs and communicate with them (Janvier, Farlow, & Wilfond, 2012).

IV Ethical Challenges

Decision-making for hypoplastic left heart syndrome and trisomy 18 requires understanding current outcomes and awareness of changing preferences. In Case One, the social worker highlights the dilemma surrounding hypoplastic left heart syndrome: Does comfort care remain an ethical option given improved survival of surgical patients? In Case Two, is the father's request for cardiac surgery overly burdensome for a patient whose overall survival and neurodevelopmental outlook are severely limited by trisomy 18? Examining how physicians *are* counseling parents and treating patients in these situations are good starting points in analyzing how we *should be* assisting families.

A Physician and Parent Preferences

Case One: Comfort Care for Hypoplastic Left Heart Syndrome?

About 20% of US fetuses diagnosed with hypoplastic left heart syndrome are terminated; this number triples for Europe (Mavroudis, Mavroudis, Farrell, Jacobs, Jacobs, & Kodish, 2011). About half of pediatric residents and nurses surveyed by Renella would terminate or choose comfort care if their child had hypoplastic left heart syndrome. Perceived favorable long-term survival and quality of life correlated to pregnancy continuation and long-term survival correlated to choosing surgery (Renella, Chang, Ferry, Bart, & Sklansky, 2007). Pediatric subspecialists posed the same hypothetical responded: if known prenatally, 48% would terminate, 30% were unsure; if diagnosed postnatally, 28% would choose comfort care, 30% were unsure. Because these physicians' preferences did not correlate with perceived outcomes, the authors concluded, "in medical scenarios with unclear prognosis and disparate viewpoints among experts concerning the 'best choice' treatment, as in the case of hypoplastic left heart syndrome, patient (or parent) values play a major role in decision making" (Kon, Ackerson, & Lo, 2003, p. 1509).

Although physicians frequently choose termination and comfort care in hypothetical hypoplastic left heart syndrome cases for their own children, comfort care is often omitted from options presented to parents of children with hypoplastic left heart syndrome. A 2004 survey of pediatric subspecialists in 14 busy cardiac centers revealed 26% of physicians do not offer comfort care. Of those that discuss it, 85% recommend surgery over comfort care, though this recommendation varies between subspecialists: 100% of surgeons and intensivists; 90% of cardiologists; 44% of neonatologists (Kon, Ackerson, & Lo, 2004). In another survey, pediatric cardiologists and surgeons discussed: surgical palliation (100%), transplantation (about two-thirds) and comfort care (about two-thirds); 76% recommended palliative surgery. Discussing nonintervention correlated with hypothetical hypoplastic left heart syndrome nonintervention for their child (Prsa, Holly, Carnevale, Justino, & Rohlicek, 2010). Some 200 physicians on PediHeart's list-serve preferred hospice for patients with co-morbidities of low birthweight, gestational age <30 weeks, chromosomal abnormalities, or end-organ dysfunction; 45% would offer comfort care for hypoplastic left heart syndrome in absence of comorbidities (Yates et al., 2011).

Case Two: Surgery for Ventricular Septal Defect in Trisomy 18?

Only 44% of neonatologists in a 2008 survey would initiate delivery room resuscitation for a baby with trisomy 18 and ventricular septal defect; maternal preference was the main reason for intervention (McGraw & Perlman, 2008). Fully 85% of obstetricians surveyed in the UK, Australia and New Zealand in 2013 identified trisomy 18 as a "lethal malformation." Moreover, inaccurate outcomes were predicted: lifespan was underestimated and 20% reported a "vegetative existence" for survivors. Ninety-five percent of these obstetricians offered termination. Eighty percent would provide fetus-centered perinatal management, and 28% would "never" discuss caesarean section to assist live birth in trisomy 18 (Wilkinson et al., 2014). No PediHeart members (sample size unknown) queried on managing ventricular septal defect in a three-month-old trisomy 18 patient would "withhold care if pushed by the family or by consideration for the child's level of distress" (McCaffrey, 2002, p. 181). Half favored the less-invasive palliative (but not curative) treatment of ventricular septal defect, pulmonary banding (noted as efficacious and less "unpleasant"); half favored ventricular septal defect closure (median sternotomy less painful than lateral thoracotomy and technique more familiar to younger practitioners) (McCaffrey, 2002). Support for cardiac surgery in trisomy 18 or trisomy 13 was highest (32%) by cardiologists and lowest (7%) by neonatologists; repairing single-ventricle physiology in these patients was rarely recommended (90%) (Boss, Holmes, Althaus, Rushton, McNee, & McNee, 2013).

B Justice and Resource Allocation

Intensive care is expensive with benefits not always clear, creating questions of proper resource allocation. Camosy includes trisomy 18 in his proposal to "make illegal the using of resources for treatment of imperiled newborns that cannot possibly benefit from the treatment" (Camosy, 2010, p. 176). Several authors reject such arguments because expenditures for adult ICU patients with similar degrees of neurologic impairment for which no such rationing exists far exceed costs of treating this rare disorder (Janvier, Okah, Farlow, & Lantos, 2011; Koogler, Wilfond, & Ross, 2003). Regarding another limited-resource issue, Kon proposes donated hearts be reserved for conditions only treatable by transplantation. He rejects primary transplantation for hypoplastic left heart syndrome if palliation yields similar success, provided a widely-endorsed policy ensured fairness among hypoplastic left heart syndrome patients (Kon, 2009).

C Elements Required for Proper Informed Consent

Proper counseling for trisomy 18 and hypoplastic left heart syndrome obviously lacks consensus. Which options should be offered? Should counseling be directive? Wernovsky's rejection of comfort care based on improved surgical outcomes rests on maximizing beneficence. While acknowledging burdens unique to hypoplastic left heart syndrome, he maintains some cardiac and non-cardiac chronic conditions not amenable to comfort care have comparable morbidities (2008). Alternately, Ross and Frader maintain comfort care is ethical for hypoplastic left heart syndrome for people calculating best-interests from the standpoint of avoiding burdens of care (non-maleficence): "The focus must be on the chance of significant morbidity that would make survival not worth having. When the risk of intolerable deficits is not miniscule, then treatment should be optional" (2009, p. 14). Others maintain comfort care is ethical based on "reasonableness." According to Kon, for example, because people would choose nonintervention for hypoplastic left heart syndrome, the option is "reasonable" (2008). Similarly, Kopelman argues that the best-interest standard "does not require what is ideal, but what is reasonable" (Ross & Frader, 2009, p. 13).

While examining whether surgery is ethical in trisomy 18 cases is, in some ways, the opposite of considering hypoplastic left heart syndrome comfort care, both cases explore the latitude given to parents' perceptions of quality of life and of benefits of medical interventions. As no longer considered "lethal," textbooks and professional associations have stopped discouraging interventions for trisomy 18 (Carey, 2012; McGraw & Perlman, 2008). McGraw and Perlman, however, criticize neonatologists who intervene for trisomy 18: "providers seem to be willing to put aside professional responsibility to direct the treatment decision and instead concede to any decision that parents may make" (2008). Janvier and Watkins maintain that the difficult quality of life estimations essential to trisomy 18 decision-making are best made by parents: health care providers "…tend to judge disability more harshly than parents and underestimate the quality of life of disabled children. They are more likely to think that being severely disabled is worse than being dead, unlike parents" (2013, p. 1113). Janvier and Watkins explain that trisomy 18 patients possess "a minimal requirement of an acceptable quality of life… the ability to interact with loved ones and to express and perceive emotion" (2013, p. 1113). Because trisomy 18 best-interests decisions are not clear, Koogler, Wilfond and Ross conclude that "parental decisions to withhold or request treatment based on benefit-burden calculations should be respected" (2003, p. 40).

For both conditions, most agree that comfort care and intensive care are ethical. Most American authors argue for shared decision-making in which parents are offered all ethical options and in concert with physicians, make decisions in their babies' best interests. Offering similar patients similar options ensures fairness; justice is threatened if parents are left to their own resources to discover unspoken alternatives (Feltman, Du, & Leuthner, 2011). Therefore, referral should be made if individual conscience precludes offering all options (Feudtner, 2008; Ross & Frader, 2009). Counseling methods also deserve attention. Those criticizing neonatologists' abdication to parental autonomy in trisomy 18 exhibit paternalism. Non-guiding approaches may place undue guilt on parents who would choose comfort care (McGraw & Perlman, 2008). Narrative accounts (Berg, Paulsen, & Carter, 2012; Thiele, 2010) and surveys of parents of children with trisomy 18 (Guon, Wilfond, Farlow, Brazg, & Janvier, 2013; Janvier, Farlow, & Wilfond, 2012) report pressure from physicians to choose nonintervention or termination. Derrington warns that language can be subtly directive: "'lethal' or 'futile' allow physicians' opinions about quality of life to interfere with the rights of parents to use their own values and choices in determining the level of care to be provided to their infant" (Derrington & Dworetz, 2011, p. 340). Koogler, Wilfond and Ross add: "a gastrostomy tube and Nissen fundoplication is 'medically indicated' in a neurologically normal child with severe reflux; it becomes 'aggressive' when the child has trisomy 18" (2003, p. 40). In hypoplastic left heart syndrome pitting quality of life against surgery may imply to parents that the two are mutually exclusive with surgery inevitably worsening the patient's quality of life (see Wernovsky, 2008). Even visual images can create bias, as seen by contrasting photographs of trisomy 18 patients from medical publications verses family albums (Guon, Wilfond, Farlow, Brazg, & Janvier, 2013).

V Conclusions and Case Recommendations

Having reviewed the survival, neurodevelopmental outcomes, and the quality of life considerations (including surgical morbidities and empirical studies), it is clear that "best-interests" decisions for babies born with hypoplastic left heart syndrome or trisomy 18 with ventricular septal defect are anything but obvious. In these situations, physicians need to engage in honest discussions with parents, both to impart information and to explore parents' goals, values, religious beliefs, family functioning, and culture. Because so much of the discussion of quality of life centers on potential medical treatments and prognoses, difficult terms must be explained and parents' comprehension assured. Optimal shared decision-making is not likely to happen with one meeting, and may require input from other members of the medical team, such as other subspecialist physicians, social workers and clinical ethicists.

Based on current survival and morbidities, for patients of hypoplastic left heart syndrome and trisomy 18, comfort and intensive care remain ethical options. As the physician, you present to Faith's mom options of comfort care and hypoplastic left heart syndrome surgery, explain promising surgical outcomes, chronic management, and indeterminate adult complications. You acknowledge the pregnant couple's desire for a meaningful life for Charlotte, explain risks and benefits of nonintervention, medical versus surgical management, and palliation versus primary repair of ventricular septal defect in trisomy 18. By eliciting these families' hopes while explaining the limits of medical knowledge you work together to find the best treatment path. Cultivating trusting relationships empowers physicians and parents to care for children born with extremely challenging conditions.

References

AAP Committee on Fetus and Newborn. 2007. Noninitiation or withdrawal of intensive care for high-risk newborns. *Pediatrics* 119(2): 401–403.

Berg, S.F., O.G. Paulsen, and B.S. Carter. 2012. Why were they in such a hurry to see her die? *American Journal of Hospice & Palliative Medicine* 30(4): 406–408.

Boss, R.D., K.W. Holmes, J. Althaus, C.H. Rushton, H. McNee, and T. McNee. 2013. Trisomy 18 and complex congenital heart disease: Seeking the threshold benefit. *Pediatrics* 132(1): 161–165.

Burke, A.L., K. Field, and J.J. Morrison. 2013. Natural history of fetal trisomy 18 after prenatal diagnosis. *Archives of Disease in Childhood Fetal and Neonatal Edition* 98: F152–F154.

Camosy, C.C. 2010. *Too expensive to treat? Finitude, tragedy, and the neonatal ICU.* Cambridge: Wm. B. Eerdmans.

Carey, J.C. 2012. Perspectives on the care and management of infants with trisomy 18 and trisomy 13: Striving for balance. *Current Opinion in Pediatrics* 24(6): 672–678.

Derrington, S.F., and A.R. Dworetz. 2011. Confronting ambiguity: Identifying options for infants with Trisomy 18. *Journal of Clinical Ethics* 22(4): 338–344.

Feinstein, J.A., D.W. Benson, A.M. Dubin, M.S. Cohen, D.M. Maxey, and W.T. Mahle et al. 2012. Hypoplastic left heart syndrome current considerations and expectations. *Journal of the American College of Cardiology* 59(1): S1–S42.

Feltman, D.M., H. Du, and S.R. Leuthner. 2011. Survey of neonatologists' attitudes toward limiting life-sustaining treatments in the neonatal intensive care unit. *Journal of Perinatology* 32(11): 886–892.

Feudtner, C. 2008. Ethics in the midst of therapeutic evolution. *Archives of Pediatrics and Adolescent Medicine* 162(9): 854–857.

Graham, E.M. 2016. Infants with trisomy 18 and complex congenital heart defects should not undergo open heart surgery. *Journal of Law, Medicine and Ethics* 44(2): 286–291.

Graham, E.M., S.M. Bradley, G.S. Shirali, C.B. Hills, and A.M. Atz. 2004. Effectiveness of cardiac surgery in Trisomies 13 and 18 (from the Pediatric Cardiac Care Consortium). *American Journal of Cardiology* 93(6): 801–803.

Guon, J., B.S. Wilfond, B. Farlow, T. Brazg, and A. Janvier. 2013. Our children are not a diagnosis: The experience of parents who continue their pregnancy after a prenatal diagnosis of Trisomy 13 or 18. *American Journal of Medical Genetics Part A* 164(2): 308–318.

Hack, M., C.B. Forrest, M. Schluchter, and H.G. Taylor et al. 2011. Health status of extremely low birth weight children at 8 years of age. *Archives of Pediatrics and Adolescent Medicine* 165(10): 922–927.

Irving, C., S. Richmond, C. Wren, C. Longster, and N. Embleton. 2011. Changes in fetal prevalence and outcome for trisomies 13 and 18: A population-based study over 23 years. *Journal of Maternal-Fetal and Neonatal Medicine* 24(1): 137–141.

Janvier, A., B. Farlow, and B.S. Wilfond. 2012. The experience of families with children with Trisomy 13 and 18 in social networks. *Pediatrics* 130(2): 293–298.

Janvier, A., F. Okah, B. Farlow, J.D. Lantos. 2011. An infant with Trisomy 18 and a ventricular septal defect. *Pediatrics* 127(4): 754–759.

Janvier, A., and A. Watkins. 2013. Medical interventions for children with trisomy 13 and trisomy 18: What is the value of a short disabled life? *Acta Paediatrica* 102(12): 1112–1117.

Jones, K.L., M.C. Jones, and M. del Campo. 2013. *Smith's recognizable patterns of human malformation*, seventh edition. Philadelphia: Elsevier Saunders.

Kaneko, Y., J. Kobayashi, I. Achiwa, H. Yoda, K. Tsuchiya, Y. Nakajima, D. Endo, H. Sato, and T. Kawakami. 2009. Cardiac surgery in patients with trisomy 18. *Pediatric Cardiology* 30(6): 729–734.

Kobayashi, J., Y. Kaneko, Y. Yamamoto, H. Yoda, and K. Tsuchiya. 2010. Radical surgery for a ventricular septal defect associated with trisomy 18. *General Thoracic and Cardiovascular Surgery* 58(5): 223–227.

Kon, A.A. 2008. Healthcare providers must offer palliative treatment to parents of neonates with hypoplastic left heart syndrome. *Archives of Pediatrics and Adolescent Medicine* 162(9): 844–848.

Kon, A.A. 2009. Ethics of cardiac transplantation in hypoplastic left heart syndrome. *Pediatric Cardiology* 30(6): 725–728.

Kon, A.A., L. Ackerson, and B. Lo. 2003. Choices physicians would make if they were the parents of a child with hypoplastic left heart syndrome. *The American Journal of Cardiology* 91(12): 1506–1509.

Kon, A.A., L. Ackerson, and B. Lo. 2004. How pediatricians counsel parents when no "best-choice" management exists: Lessons to be learned from hypoplastic left heart syndrome. *Archives of Pediatrics and Adolescent Medicine* 158(5): 436–441.

Koogler, T.K., B.S. Wilfond, and L.F. Ross. 2003. Lethal language, lethal decisions. *Hastings Center Report* March–April 33(2): 37–41.

Kosho, T., T. Nakamura, H. Kawame, A. Baba, M. Tamura, and Y. Fukushima. 2006. Neonatal Management of trisomy 18: Clinical details of 24 patients receiving intensive treatment. *American Journal of Medical Genetics. Part A* 140(9): 937–944.

Maeda, J., H. Yamagishi, Y. Furutani, M. Kamisago, T. Waragai, S. Oana, and H. Kajino et al. 2011. The impact of cardiac surgery in patients with Trisomy 18 and Trisomy 13 in Japan. *American Journal of Medical Genetics. Part A* 155(11): 2641–2646.

Mavroudis, C., C.D. Mavroudis, R.M. Farrell, M.L. Jacobs, J.P. Jacobs, and E.D. Kodish. 2011. Informed consent, bioethical equipoise, and hypoplastic left heart syndrome. *Cardiology in the Young* 21(Suppl. 2): 133–140.

McCaffrey, F. 2002. Around PediHeart: Trisomy 18, an ethical dilemma. *Pediatric Cardiology* 23(2): 181.

McGraw, M.P., and J.M. Perlman 2008. Attitudes of neonatologists toward delivery room management of confirmed trisomy 18: Potential factors influencing a changing dynamic. *Pediatrics* 121(6): 1106–1110.

Mercurio, M.R., S.M. Peterec, and B. Weeks. 2008. Hypoplastic left heart syndrome, extreme prematurity, comfort care only, and the principle of justice. *Pediatrics* 122(1): 186–189.

Nelson, K.E., K.R. Hexem, and C. Feudtner. 2012. Inpatient hospital care of children with trisomy 13 and trisomy 18 in the United States. *Pediatrics* 129(5): 869–876.

Pager, C.K. 2000. Dying of a broken heart: Ethics and law in a case of hypoplastic left heart syndrome. *Journal of Perinatology* 20(8): 535–539.

Paris, J.J., M.P. Moore, and M.D. Schreiber. 2012. Physician counseling, informed consent and parental decision making for infants with hypoplastic left-heart syndrome. *Journal of Perinatology* 32(10): 748–751.

Park, M.K. 2002. *Pediatric cardiology for practitioners*, fourth edition. St. Louis: Mosby.

Prsa, M., C.D. Holly, F.A. Carnevale, H. Justino, and C.V. Rohlicek. 2010. Attitudes and practices of cardiologists and surgeons who manage HLHS. *Pediatrics* 125(3): e625–e630.

Renella, P., R.R. Chang, D.A. Ferry, R.D. Bart, and M.S. Sklansky. 2007. Hypoplastic left heart syndrome: Attitudes among pediatric residents and nurses towards fetal and neonatal management. *Prenatal Diagnosis* 27(11): 1045–1055.

Ross, L.F., and J. Frader. 2009. Hypoplastic left heart syndrome: A paradigm case for examining conscientious objection in pediatric practice. *Journal of Pediatrics* 155(1): 12–15.

Sarajuuri, A., E. Jokinen, L. Mildh, A. Tujulin, I. Mattila, L. Valanne, and T. Lonnqvist. 2012. Neurodevelopmental burden at age 5 years in patients with univentricular heart. *Pediatrics* 130(6): e1636–1646.

Thiele, P. 2010. He was my son, not a dying baby. *Journal of Medical Ethics* 36: 646–647.

Wernovsky, G. 2008. The paradigm shift toward surgical intervention for neonates with hypoplastic left heart syndrome. *Archives of Pediatrics and Adolescent Medicine* 162(9): 849–854.

Wilkinson, D.J.C., L. de Crespigny, C. Lees, J. Savulescu, P. Thiele, T. Tran, and A. Watkins. 2014. Perinatal management of trisomy 18: A survey of obstetricians in Australia, New Zealand and the UK. *Prenatal Diagnosis* 34(1): 42–49.

Yamagishi, H. 2010. Cardiovascular surgery for congenital heart disease associated with trisomy 18. *General Thoracic and Cardiovascular Surgery* 58(5): 217–299.

Yates, A.R., T.M. Hoffman, B. Boettner, T.F. Feltes, and C.L. Cua. 2011. Initial counseling prior to palliation for hypoplastic left heart syndrome. *Congenital Heart Disease* 6(4): 347–358.

Part II

Cardiovascular Ethical Issues at the End-of-Life

4 Palliative Care Issues in Advanced Cardiac Disease

Sara E. Wordingham and Keith M. Swetz

I Overview

Patients with advanced cardiac disease have high morbidity and mortality. As the prevalence of heart failure increases, clinicians and patients must continue to navigate best practices in the management of this life-limiting condition with high symptom burden. As patients progress through the complex trajectory of advanced cardiac illness, care must be taken continually to balance the benefits and burdens of advanced illness management. For example, clinicians must help patients define the role of advanced therapies such as inotropes, transcatheter aortic valve replacement (TAVR), and mechanical circulatory support (MCS), as well as to help them choose the best supportive care, such as palliative care or hospice. Imprecise criteria for which patients can and should receive certain therapies or interventions in addition to the complex physiologic and techno-logic landscape of advanced heart failure management have provided basis for ethical deliberations about best practices. Nevertheless, symptom palliation and maximizing quality of life remains a central role of cardiologists and other clinicians. Recently, the support of patients with advanced heart disease has expanded to include increased involvement of palliative care teams.

Palliative care is a growing multidisciplinary field focusing on the supportive care needs of patients with advanced illnesses ranging from cancer to cardiac disease and other life-threatening illnesses. Palliative care physicians are board-certified subspecialists who are often members of an interdisciplinary team (including mid-level providers, nurses, social workers, chaplains, and pharmacists and more) that provides comprehensive and concurrent care of patients with life-limiting illnesses. Palliative care often focuses on symptom management, coordination of care, and advanced care planning—with the goal of improving quality of life for the patient and the family. Domains of palliative care include the physical, social, spiritual, existential, and emotional needs of a patient and family. Palliative care can be appropriate for many persons with a serious or life-limiting illness; it can be provided at any stage of an illness, along with curative or disease-directed therapies. In contrast, hospice is typically governed by an insurance benefit and a philosophy of care that focuses on comfort and quality of life for patients with an anticipated prognosis of less

DOI: 10.4324/9781003240273-7

Table 4.1 Conceptual Differences between Palliative Care and Hospice (from Swetz and Kamal, 2012)

Palliative Care vs. Hospice
Consultative palliative care
• Addresses goals of care and focuses on quality of life, family support, and symptom management
• Can begin with onset of symptoms from a serious, life-limiting disease
Hospice
• A specific type of palliative care provided when a patient is terminally ill (i.e., life expectancy < six months if the disease runs its expected course)
• Provides team-based support services to patient, family, and caregivers in the home or an institution

than six months, in the context of patients no longer receiving life-prolonging treatment (see Table 4.1).

The traditional model of palliative care was one in which patients were receiving either active, disease-directed care or comfort-oriented palliative or hospice care. The new model for palliative care promotes early involvement of the palliative care team throughout the continuum of care in advanced illness. In heart failure, some have even suggested palliative care from the time of diagnosis, which may be provided by the primary team or specialists if required. This paradigm shift supports increasing palliative care involvement as the illness progresses over the course of time, as symptoms may become more burdensome and the goals of care become more important to delineate. Disease-directed heart failure management is often critical to maximizing quality of life. Even when a patient is enrolled in hospice, it remains important to maximize supportive care of the patient, while managing heart failure symptoms with any therapy that is not burdensome to the patient (Gibbs, McCoy, Gibbs, Rogers, and Addington-Hall, 2002).

The recommendations and practice guidelines of several medical societies are increasingly supportive of palliative care in the treatment of patients with heart failure and advanced cardiac disease. The American College of Cardiology (ACC), the American Heart Association (AHA), and the International Society of Heart and Lung Transplantation (ISHLT) guidelines each support the involvement of palliative care. For example, American College of Cardiology/American Heart Association guidelines make a class I recommendation for palliative care involvement for patients with symptomatic heart failure to improve quality of life and identify palliative care as a "key component" of the plan of care for patients with advanced heart failure (Yancy, Jessup, Bozkurt et al., 2013). For patients with mechanical circulatory support, palliative care clinicians are often distinguished as a part of the multidisciplinary selection team and support patients with end stage heart failure during the mechanical circulatory support evaluation process (Feldman, Pamboukian, Teuteberg et al., 2013; see also Evangelista, Sackett and Dracup, 2009). Emerging data from implementing the American College of Cardiology/American Heart Association guidelines for early palliative care involvement found that both cardiac and palliative care providers believed that the palliative care consultation had a "significant" impact on the patient's care with increased patient satisfaction (Schwarz, Baraghoush, Morrissey et al., 2012). Care that explicitly integrates palliative care has the potential to improve the science of health care delivery, symptom management, shared decision-making, and end-of-life care for patients with advanced cardiac disease.

II Challenges in Care of Patients with Advanced Heart Disease

Recent technologic and pharmacologic advancements have changed the trajectory of many patients with advanced heart disease. Although such advanced therapies are available, complexity of patient selection and shared decision-making remain key issues. Best practices have not yet been clearly defined. Novel therapies such as continuous-flow left-ventricular assist devices (LVADs; the most common form of durable mechanical circulatory support) have improved survival for patients awaiting cardiac transplantation, with data demonstrating a one year survival rate with mechanical circulatory support doubled that of medical therapy alone (Rogers, Aaronson, Boyle et al., 2010). However, less than 1% of patients will go on to receive heart transplants—the gold standard for the management of end-stage heart failure (Go, Mozaffarian, Roger et al., 2013). With a limited supply of available donor organs it is estimated that 150,000–200,000 patients may be potential mechanical circulatory support candidates (Miller and Guglin, 2013). Careful consideration must be given to the ethics of advanced heart failure management, including respect for patient autonomy, nonmaleficence, assessment of futility of an intervention, as well as cost considerations, and distributive justice.

Greater than 50% of people diagnosed with heart failure will die within five years of their diagnosis, making the mortality rate worse than that of breast, prostate, and colorectal cancers (Askoxylakis, Thieke, and Pleger, 2010). Many patients with heart failure will progress to have a high symptom burden from their disease, including shortness of breath at rest, pain, depression, anorexia and cachexia, a complex metabolic syndrome associated with chronic illness hallmarked by weight and muscle loss (Rutledge et al., 2006; Sullivan et al., 2007). Greater than half of patients with heart disease experience pain, shortness of breath, or low mood in the last year of life, symptoms that are not uncommon in other advanced illnesses; however, approximately 30% of cardiac patients reported little to no relief of symptoms (Evans et al., 2005; Goodlin et al., 2012; Lichtman et al., 2008; Malik et al., 2013; McCarthy, Lay, and Addington-Hall, 1996). Navigating the role of advanced heart failure therapies, such as inotropes, transplantation, or best supportive care (eventually including hospice care), requires integration of an interdisciplinary team poised to assess and meet the physical, physiologic, social, psychological, and existential needs of patient and family. Existential distress is commonly noted by providers of patients with advanced and life-limiting illnesses, but remains ill-defined. Existential questions may surround life's meaning, separation versus belonging, or religious questions. Indeed, it has been demonstrated that the degree to which staff address patients' emotional and spiritual concerns strongly correlates with patient satisfaction.

III Prognostication and Dealing with Uncertainty

The disease trajectory of advance heart failure is unpredictable. With advanced heart failure, repeated exacerbations and hospitalizations often punctuate variable periods of reasonable functional status and less symptom burden, making prognostication difficult. Patients and clinicians tend to underestimate mortality in heart failure given the complex and episodic nature of the disease (Allen, Yager, Funk et al., 2008; Murray, Boyd, Kendall, Worth, Benton, and Calusen, 2002; Warraich, Mukamal, Allen, Ship, and Kociol, 2014). The incidence of sudden cardiac death in the setting of advance heart failure also adds to uncertainty (Lane, Cowie, and Chow, 2005); however, long-term survival issues are often compounded over time, as median survival decreases progressively after each subsequent hospitalization for heart failure (Miller and Guglin, 2013). Limitations of prognostic tools, coupled with high heart failure-associated mortality, amplify ethical tensions related to decision-making facing cardiac care clinicians and their patients. Evolving therapies such as LVADs can *reset* the survival curve for some patients and are increasingly available to a broader range of patients, including older patients and those with more refractory disease. As previously mentioned, survival with an LVAD in appropriately selected patients can be more than double that with medical therapy alone and can take a patient who is nearing end of life back to a more stable point in the heart failure disease trajectory. Home-based intravenous inotropes may be available for symptom palliation and are known to improve hemodynamic parameters, but are often associated with a negative effect on survival and may accelerate the progression of the underlying disease.

Despite models such as the Seattle Heart Failure Model, reliable prognostication for patients to assist with an individual's plan of care is suboptimal, leaving clinicians with the difficult task of counseling patients with significant uncertainty (Levy and Mozaffarian, 2006). Although perhaps under-recognized, many patients prefer that their clinicians initiate discussions about prognosis at the time of diagnosis and continue to do so in an ongoing fashion. In general, patients desire clinicians to be truthful about their condition and what the future may hold in terms of prognostic possibilities and outcomes, balanced and presented in a way that maintains hope (Caldwell, Arthur, and Demers, 2007).

While communication about prognosis is fundamental to discussions about advanced care planning and, ultimately, end-of-life care, there remains significant variability among providers regarding their level of comfort and their perceived responsibility in discussing prognosis and end-of-life issues. Providers have cited lack of time, fear of destroying hope, and their own discomfort as commonly encountered barriers to these discussions (Dunlay, Foxen, Cole et al., 2014), which the American Heart Association recommends be had annually (Yancy, Jessup, Bozkurt et al., 2013). Palliative care involvement has been shown to facilitate the honing of advance directives into personalized preparedness plans in the care of mechanical circulatory support patients (Swetz, Freeman, Abouezzeddine et al., 2011). Such plans allow patients and families an opportunity to have more detailed discussions with their providers about their goals for this advanced therapy. It also allows for focus on some of the ethical subtleties that exist with mechanical circulatory support at the end of life, and provides a means for patients to make their wishes known related to mechanical circulatory support-specific complications. This is important as many patients reflect on and discuss death prior to their cardiac team broaching the topic (Brush, Budge, Alharethi et al., 2010).

IV Ethical Issues Regarding Patient Candidacy for Advanced Cardiac Therapies and Goals of Care

Selecting patients who will benefit from advanced therapies including implantable cardioverter-defibrillators, home inotropes to enhance cardiac contractility, mechanical circulatory support, transcatheter aortic valve replacement (TAVR), or cardiac transplantation remains complex and should take into consideration the patient's goals and expectations for the particular therapy or intervention being considered. The American Heart Association highlights the concept of shared decision-making and acknowledges the complex trade-off of benefits and burdens (Allen, Stevenson, Grady et al., 2012; Elwyn, Edwards, Kinnersley, and Grol, 2000). Implantable cardioverter-defibrillators are considered in the setting of advanced heart failure in patients who have an anticipated prognosis of greater than one year and have a good functional status; however, this can be challenging to delineate, especially in the setting of other comorbidities (Epstein, DiMarco, Ellenbogen et al., 2013). Consider the case example discussed below.

Case 1:

A 67-year-old man with a history of ischemic cardiomyopathy (left ventricular ejection fraction 18%) with co-morbid chronic obstructive pulmonary disease is diagnosed with stage IIIa adenocarcinoma of the lung. He is New York Heart Association (NYHA) Class II functional status. The patient begins combined modality chemotherapy and radiation therapy. Eight weeks later, the patient has clinical decompensation with his heart failure and requires hospitalization. Three months later, the patient undergoes interval restaging of his lung cancer, which demonstrates a partial

response of his tumor. The patient is noted to be having difficulty tolerating his heart failure medications, specifically his renal
function is impaired and his functional status is worsening. The
patient undergoes electrophysiology consult for consideration
of resynchronization therapy with a biventricular pacemaker and
defibrillator (CRT-D device). Both cardiology and oncology independently report the patient's prognosis is greater than one year
in length if he continues to respond to treatment for both conditions. The patient undergoes attempted placement of the CRT-D
device as an outpatient; however, lead placement is suboptimal.
A few weeks later, the patient is hospitalized for epicardial lead
placement, although he is now deemed too decompensated from
a heart failure perspective to tolerate the procedure. The patient
is discharged home with hospice and dies one month later, living
a total of eight months following his cancer diagnosis and eight
weeks following his CRT-D device implantation.

Critical to understanding a patient's and family's goals and expectations is
communication between that patient and family and their clinical providers. To
assist with informed consent for LVAD, a ten-point model has been proposed to
address commonly encountered ethical considerations for patients being considered for device placement (Petrucci, Benish, Carrow et al., 2011). Although
patients hope to undergo cardiac transplantation and agree to have a total artificial heart implanted as a bridge-to-transplant, approximately 20% of such
patients do not go on to transplantation. Approaching a total artificial heart that
has essentially become a "destination therapy" (i.e., when mechanical circulatory
support is used as long-term or permanent support in patients, who are not a
candidate for heart transplantation) can be complex (Syncardia Systems Inc.,
2018). Data are limited regarding optimal care for patients with a total artificial
heart who are no longer transplant-eligible, and ethical considerations regarding
deactivation of a total artificial heart, and whether or not care can be provided
outside of the hospital setting, are just a few of such complexities.

In addition to ethical issues at the level of the individual, macro-level issues
also exist regarding therapeutic options for treatment of advanced heart failure.
Disparities exist in heart failure mortality and readmission rates based on race,
ethnicity, sex, and socioeconomic status; socioeconomic deprivation is known to
be an independent predictor of both heart failure development and adverse
outcomes in heart failure. The adjusted risk of developing heart failure in
patients with socioeconomic disparities is estimated to be between 30% and
50%. While the mechanisms of these disparities remain obscure, postulated
mechanisms include known socioeconomic disparities in hypertension and

coronary artery disease as well as limited access to healthcare in this population, and likely remain responsive to both clinical and public health interventions (Hawkins, Jhund, and McMurray, 2012). With a limited supply of human organs for transplant, practical and ethical questions arise in the allocation of this scarce resource. This limited donor pool has contributed to the rapid increase in the use of mechanical circulatory support, which increasingly is used as destination therapy, in which patients receive a mechanical circulatory support device but are not considered transplant candidates. To date, the total artificial heart is not indicated for this purpose, but, as noted above, challenges can exist where patients with total artificial heart later become ineligible for transplantation due to clinical issues. For patients who receive mechanical circulatory support as destination therapy, or for whom transplant is no longer an option, end-of life care options can be complex, and a careful understanding of the patient's goals of care and their preferences for advance care planning is essential.

V Palliative Care and Decision-Making Support

Palliative care teams seek to provide whole-person care, which can help define the role of advanced therapies for cardiac patients in the context of their preferences and values. Palliative care consultation will explore patients' symptom burden, social support, goals of care, understanding of his/her illness, spirituality, and mental health to aid in medical decision-making through comprehensive interdisciplinary evaluation. Palliative care teams can represent a connected, yet distinct part of the cardiac team to whom patients may reveal history and preferences not previously delineated that may be relevant to their care plan or a decision to pursue advanced therapies. In fact, patients have cited explaining their values to their physicians as one of the five most important items to discuss in advanced illness. Despite patient preferences and documented improvements in satisfaction with care, communication and documentation of patients' expressed preferences remains inadequate and prognostic disclosures occur infrequently among patients with serious illnesses. Patients with advanced and life-limiting illness have linked deteriorating health status to social isolation, family burden, and decreased independence. Patients perceive resources and community services as lacking. Consider the following example.

Case 2:

A 63-year-old gentleman with a history of ischemic cardiomyopathy is referred to a tertiary care setting with stage D class IV heart failure. The patient is seen in the heart failure clinic and directly admitted to the hospital for decompensated heart failure. Work up for heart transplant and a LVAD are initiated in the hospital. After seven days in the hospital, the patient is discharged to home on home inotropes and with an external defibrillator for prevention of sudden cardiac death. The patient is referred to palliative care by his cardiologist for assistance in discussing his goals of care.

The patient is seen by the palliative care team three weeks following hospital discharge. When asked, the patient reports that his most significant complaint is "all of the things he has to carry around," referring to a belt-pack containing his inotrope pump and his external defibrillator vest. He explains that he is a pastor and his defibrillator senses an abnormal rhythm every time he sings in church and he has to then push a button to prevent it from shocking him and his inotrope infusion prevents him from going in his hot tub, which is a favorite pastime. The patient goes on to say that he wants to be honest with the palliative care physician and that he does not always take his cardiac medications regularly as he feels that he is on too many pills and that his faith in God is stronger than his belief in medications. He expressed his primary goal of being able to attend his daughter's wedding that was to be held in two months and that beyond that "it was in God's hands."

During his visit with the palliative care chaplain, he revealed that he did not want to receive an LVAD, because putting "a machine" in his body is not consistent with his faith. To the social worker, his wife expressed that she is overwhelmed providing care at home, especially helping him bathe. She elaborated that she did not have loved ones that she could talk to about his condition, because they did not want to worry parishioners at his church about the patient's health. She also revealed that they did not know how to tell their children what they both knew, "that he is dying."

As a result of the palliative care consult, the patient and his wife set up a meeting to return to the palliative care clinic in two weeks with their children for help sharing news about his limited prognosis. They obtained a bath aide through home health, and the patient's wife was referred to a caregiver support group. The cardiac team was updated on the palliative care consult, specifically the patient's goals not to pursue evaluations for LVAD or transplant and the evaluations were discontinued. The patient lived for seven months on home inotropes and ultimately died peacefully at home with hospice support.

The concept of shared decision-making moves beyond informed consent to having providers and patients work together within the context of the patient's goals and values to make treatment decisions (Allen, Stevenson, Grady et al., 2012). A critical component of this process is communication and trust that evolves over time to tailor the conversation to the patient's core values. Palliative care teams may assist in this process and have advanced communication skills that may prove beneficial to the patient, family, and cardiac team. Key components of communication in shared decision-making include assessing the patient's understanding of the illness and emotional readiness to discuss the plan of care. This discussion can be aided by the "Ask-Tell-Ask" construct, in which one *asks* the patient to describe their understanding of their condition and proposed plan of care. The provider then *tells* the patient additional information that may need to be shared or clarified in the context of the perspective shared by the patient, and then *asks* the patient to reflect back what they understand and feel about the information given. Additionally, communication in shared decision-making can be aided by asking open-ended questions, offering a recommendation for a plan of care, if desired by the patient, and helping to normalize uncertainty. Extrapolating population level estimates about prognosis can be difficult to translate to an individual; providers can help acknowledge what we cannot know with certainty, by saying phrases such as "like many things in life" (see Goodlin, 2009).

VI Palliative Care and Symptom Management

It is estimated that up to two-thirds of patients with advanced heart failure have inadequate symptom relief (McCarthy, Lay, and Addington-Hall, 1996); symptoms may also occur in other advanced structural heart disease (such as aortic stenosis). Symptoms and quality of life tend to be studied most thoroughly in heart failure; however, many management principles cross etiologic domains. Dyspnea, fatigue, anxiety, depression, and anorexia/cachexia are the result of a complex physiologic interplay in which a patient with advanced heart disease may have concurrent sleep-disordered breathing, pulmonary congestion, activation of the renin-angiotensin system, increased release of pro-inflammatory cytokines, and increased catecholamines, all contributing to suboptimal quality of life (Goodlin, 2009; Smith et al., 2007; Walke et al., 2004; Weiss et al., 2001; Yu et al., 2004). It can be difficult to delineate the particular pathophysiologic etiology of a given symptom; however, approaching symptoms in a broader context of heart disease and impaired quality of life may be most helpful.

Aggressive supportive care for heart failure can occur longitudinally with disease-directed heart failure therapies. Poor symptom management in advanced heart failure has been associated with worse outcomes, and this is particularly true with depression. Depression affects up to 70% of hospitalized patients with heart failure and in one study > 90% were not receiving treatment (Koenig, 1998). Depression is associated with a higher risk of acute myocardial infarction, decreased survival, and increased readmission rates for patient with heart failure (Chamberlain, Vickers, Colligan, Weston, Rummans, and Roger, 2011). Tools to assess quality of life in heart failure include the Minnesota Living with Heart Failure Questionnaire (Rector and Cohn, 1992; Rector, Kubo, and Cohn, 1993) and the Kansas City Cardiomyopathy Questionnaire (Green, Porter, Bresnahan, and Spertus, 2000). Two common symptom inventories—the Edmonton Symptom Assessment Scale (ESAS) and the Palliative Performance Scale—are tools initially developed to assess symptom burden in patients with advanced cancer, but have been shown to correlate with heart failure-specific assessment tools (Timmons, MacIver, Alba, Tibbles, Greenwood, and Ross, 2013).

Symptom palliation has been mentioned as a key component of the management of advanced heart failure, but this becomes particularly important as a patient approaches end of life. Despite a desire aggressively to promote comfort, providers, patients, and families may be concerned regarding use of opioids to achieve these goals out of fear that opioids may hasten death. Thoughtful opioid dosing based on a patient's tolerance and hepatic and renal function has been shown to pose an extremely small risk of hastening death, as the timing of death is complex and influenced by numerous factors, many of which may not be measurable (Portenoy, Sibirceva, Smout et al., 2006). Despite this lack of evidence that opioids hasten death, clinicians may seek moral justification for providing aggressive symptom management (HPNA Position Statement, 2013) and often do so by reference to the principle of double effect.

The principle of double effect states that it is morally permissible to allow a harmful side-effect of a permissible treatment, if the harm is not intended and is not directly responsible for causing the benefit. The original formulation is credited to Thomas Aquinas in the *Summa Theologica*, and was used to justify killing in self-defense (the formal application is listed in Table 4.2). Essentially, if management of pain or other symptoms is the intent, achieving symptom amelioration is the main goal which should be achieved by the action of the medication, not by the side-effect of the medication (i.e., shortening of lifespan).

Table 4.2 Formulation of the Doctrine of Double Effect

1.	The act itself must be morally good or at least indifferent.
2.	The agent may not positively will the bad effect but may permit it. If he could attain the good effect without the bad effect he should do so. The bad effect is sometimes said to be indirectly voluntary.
3.	The good effect must flow from the action at least as immediately (in the order of causality, though not necessarily in the order of time) as the bad effect. In other words the good effect must be produced directly by the action, not by the bad effect. Otherwise the agent would be using a bad means to a good end, which is never allowed.
4.	The good effect must be sufficiently desirable to compensate for the allowing of the bad effect.

A corollary to the principle of double effect breaks the moral analysis into three key components: *intent, proportionality, markers of success.* The *intent* of the treatment, or reason for using the treatment, must be clear and unambiguous, and that intent should be relief of suffering. The dosing of the drug should be based on the patient's tolerance and metabolic factors, and thus be *proportional.* Lastly, the marker of a successful intervention should be relief of suffering, however that is achieved. However, it is ideal that *success* is achieved via relief through the good effect of the drug (i.e., symptom relief) versus the bad effect (i.e., shortening of lifespan). Consider the following example.

Case 3: DOUBLE EFFECT IN EFFECT?

Consider two patients who are approaching end of life. Mrs. A. is an 89-year-old woman with advanced aortic stenosis who is not a candidate for transcatheter aortic valve replacement (TAVR) and who has decided to enroll in hospice. Mrs. A. has symptomatic dyspnea and opioids are being considered. She has never used opioids before. Mrs. A. receives hydromorphone 1 mg orally every 4 hours with excellent relief of her symptoms. After two weeks, Mrs. A. is requiring more frequent dosing of her opioid, and the hydromorphone is being used at 2 mg orally every 2 hours as needed on the day of her death.

Another patient, Mr. B., is a 38-year-old man with a history of advanced spine arthritis chronic opioid therapy (oxycodone 40 mg extended-release three times a day at baseline). Mr. B. is found to have a patent foramen ovale in the setting of an antiphospholipid syndrome. He suffers arterial and venous emboli which result in a stroke as well as several clots in this lower extremities and abdomen, causing severe pain. Mr. B. is made "comfort care only" and "do-not-resuscitate" and is started on a morphine drip at 3 mg/hr. Over the next 4 hours, he requires frequent rescue bolus of morphine (receiving 6 mg bolus of morphine every 1 hour for each hour). The pain is not controlled, and Mr. B. is given a 12 mg bolus of morphine taking his pain from a 10 to a comfortable level at 3 out of 10. One hour later, Mr. B. dies and the nurse has concerns that Mr. B. was euthanized.

How are these cases different? In each situation, the *intent* was clear and unambiguous—to relieve suffering, not to hasten death. In both situations, the doses were *proportionate*, as Mrs. A. was opioid naïve and slowly increased on her medications, and Mr. B. had tolerance and the dosing was appropriate in that the clinician used appropriate equianalgesic conversions, doubled the bolus dose when a lower dose was ineffective, and frequently reassessed the patient. The marker of *success* for both patients was a level of comfort, not hastening of death. If Mr. B. had lived for two more days but was comfortable with pain scores around 3 out of 10, the success would have been achieved. In essence, it did not require making Mr. B. die faster to achieve success, and having either patient die sooner or later does not factor in as a marker of clinical success is comfort. As noted earlier, death is a complex process, and in Mr. B's end-of-life experience, factors such as acidosis, multiorgan system failure, and possible pulmonary embolism or intracranial infarction all played a role—likely to a substantially higher degree than a few doses of morphine.

Broad consensus exists that clinicians have a duty to provide symptom relief, including with opioid use at the end of life and that fear of hastening death does not justify the withholding of such treatment (National Consensus Project, 2013). Opioid receptors are found throughout the cardiorespiratory system and while many providers remain reluctant to utilize opioids, low-dose morphine has been shown to be safe and to improve breathlessness when compared with placebo (Currow, McDonald, Oaten et al., 2011). Opioids have been shown to relieve dyspnea, provide a sense of "calm" and improve quality of life in refractory dyspnea, but providers have reported a lack of knowledge and experience in the use of opioids for dyspnea, as well as concern for adverse effects and legal censure as barriers to their use (Rocker, Young, Donahue, Farquhar, and Simpson, 2012). Although effect may be immediate with administration, opioid-related improvement in breathlessness may not be seen until administered over a period of weeks to months in the setting of heart failure (Abernethy and Wheeler, 2008; Oxberry, Bland, Clark, Cleland, and Johnson, 2013). Interestingly, recent studies evaluating patients who receive palliative sedation at the end of life demonstrated that the use of aggressive symptom management, administered as described above, is not associated with a decrement in survival (Maltoni, Pittureri, Scarpi et al., 2009; Maltoni, Scarpi, Rosati et al., 2012).

VII Care Approaching the End of Life

Despite continued pharmacologic and technologic advancements of life-prolonging therapies, patients with advanced heart failure have significant mortality (Go, Mozaffarian, Roger et al., 2013). Hospice has a growing role in Stage D heart failure and other advanced heart disease, with cardiac disease now being the second most prevalent diagnostic group enrolled (National Hospice and Palliative Care Organization, 2018). The hospice movement developed out of caring for patients with advanced malignancy; however, it has vastly expanded to care for patients with any life-limiting disease with an anticipated prognosis of less than six months if the disease runs its normal course. Hospice care is provided by an interdisciplinary team of physicians, nurses, social workers, and chaplains, and is a philosophy of care that prioritizes comfort and quality of life for patients. The insurance benefit associated with hospice, often based on Medicare's model, prioritizes use of healthcare funds on a comfort-oriented approach, versus care that includes potentially life-prolonging interventions such as repeated hospitalizations, invasive procedures, or diagnostic tests not geared at promoting comfort. Hospice care can be provided in a number of settings, including patients' homes, skilled care facilities, or for short periods in inpatient hospice units.

Prognostic uncertainty should not be a barrier to hospice enrollment and there are no specific prognostic models that are required for hospice enrollment. Patients can remain on hospice services longer than six months as long as clinical decline is documented, and if the disease is still judged to run a survival of six months or less. Medical treatment of heart failure should *not* stop when a patient is enrolled in hospice, as continued careful management of disease-targeted medication such as beta blockers and diuretics should continue to maximally support a patient's quality of life. Rarely, patients may experience suffering near the end-of-life that is refractory to standard interventions at which time controlled sedation may be considered as the only option to alleviate suffering.

VIII Distributive Justice and Financial Considerations

The ethical challenges of caring for patients with advanced cardiac disease are not only limited to patient and clinician, but include society as a whole (Kini and Kirkpatrick, 2013). Heart failure is estimated to cost the United States more than $32 billion annually, with costs anticipated to double by 2030 (Heidenreich, Albert, Allen et al., 2013; Heidenreich, Trogdon, Khavjou et al., 2011). The costs of advanced cardiac therapies, such as transcatheter aortic valve replacement (TAVR) and LVAD have improved; however, questions remain regarding how to optimally utilize these therapies (Rogers, Bostic, Tong, Adamson, Russo, and Slaughter, 2012; Swetz, Stulak, Dunlay, and Gafford, 2012).

Recent emphasis on cost containment in healthcare has brought issues of understanding the economic burden of advanced heart disease management to the forefront. Analyses have found implantable cardioverter-defibrillators to be cost-effective (Sanders, Hlatky, and Owens, 2005); however, other factors may need to be considered, such as prognosis and quality of life. Recent analysis of cost-effectiveness of LVADs attempted to pair functionality and quality of life with survival and assessed this in terms of quality-adjusted life years (QALYs). While significantly reduced compared to older LVADs with complex care requirements, the cost of a continuous-flow LVAD approached $200,000 per QALY (Clegg, Scott, Loveman et al., 2015). Repeat analysis has shown some improvement in that figure to just under $100,000 per QALY (Clegg, Scott, Loveman, Colquitt, Royle, and Bryant, 2006; Clegg, Scott, Loveman, Colquitt, Royle, and Bryant, 2007; Hutchinson, Scott, Clegg et al., 2008), still suggesting that use of healthcare resources may be more cost-effective in different areas. While policy questions regarding optimum societal use of resources may remain, these only frame the discussion and continue to have little impact on the individual patient–clinician decision-making process.

IX Resuscitation Issues

Approaching the topic of cardiopulmonary resuscitation (CPR) in patients with advance cardiac disease is less straightforward than in other progressive advanced illnesses with more predictable outcomes. The role or anticipated outcomes of CPR may change over the course of the patient's trajectory, as patients with advanced heart failure are more likely to have experienced defibrillation in the past and some have survived CPR. However, prognostic uncertainty cannot implicitly act as a barrier to conversations between patients and providers about the role of CPR. The SUPPORT study delineated the resuscitation preferences of enrollees and found that do-not-resuscitate (DNR) orders were less common in heart failure patients than in AIDS and cancer patients—in place for only 5% of patients with heart failure, compared to 52% and 47% respectively in the other conditions (The SUPPORT Principle Investigators, 1995). Patients with heart failure also have been shown to change their minds regarding CPR preferences, in favor of resuscitation following hospital discharge (Krumholz, Phillips, Hamel et al., 1998).

More recent data have also confirmed this tendency of patients with heart failure to change their resuscitation preferences over time (Dunlay, Swetz, Redfield, Mueller, and Roger, 2014). Changes in resuscitation preference are often made in the final weeks of life in the hospital and DNR status was associated with older age, co-morbidities including COPD and history of malignancy, and reduced mobility, as opposed to heart failure-specific indicators (Dunlay, Swetz, Redfield, Mueller, and Roger, 2014). Additionally, patients may change preferences over time, but documentation of such changes via advance directives has been limited. Despite recommendations for all patients with advance cardiac disease to have an advance directive and/or engage in advance care planning, recent studies found that less than half of community dwelling patients with heart failure had an advance directive, and that most did not address important end-of-life considerations in heart failure, such as preferences regarding CPR, mechanical ventilation, or hemodialysis (Dunlay, Swetz, Mueller, and Roger, 2012).

X Conclusions

There remains significant heterogeneity in how advanced cardiac illnesses are approached, but mortality and quality of life factors remain high for patients with advanced heart failure, as well as electrophysiological and structural heart disease. Symptom management and quality of life are growing in recognition and importance, and will be increasingly highlighted in this era of patient-centered care, cost-conscious and evidence-based medicine (see, e.g., Belardinelli et al., 1999; O'Connor et al., 2009).

References

Abernethy, A.P., and J.L. Wheeler. 2008. Total dyspnoea. *Current Opinion in Supportive and Palliative Care* 2(2): 110–113.

Allen, L.A., L.W. Stevenson, K.L. Grady, N.E. Goldstein, D.D. Matlock, and R.M. Arnold et al. 2012. Decision making in advanced heart failure: A scientific statement from the American Heart Association. *Circulation* 125(15): 1928–1952.

Allen, L.A., J.E. Yager, M.J. Funk, W.C. Levy, J.A. Tulsky, and M.T. Bowers et al. 2008. Discordance between patient-predicted and model-predicted life expectancy among ambulatory patients with heart failure. *JAMA* 299(21): 2533–2542.

Askoxylakis, V., C. Thieke, S. Pleger, P. Most, J. Tanner, and K. Lindel et al. 2010. Long-term survival of cancer patients compared to heart failure and stroke: A systematic review. *BMC Cancer* 10: 105.

Belardinelli, R., D. Georgiou, G. Cianci, and A. Purcaro. 1999. Randomized, controlled trial of long-term moderate exercise training in chronic heart failure: Effects on functional capacity, quality of life, and clinical outcome. *Circulation* 99(9): 1173–1182.

Brush, S., D. Budge, R. Alharethi, A.J. McCormick, and J.E. MacPherson et al. 2010. End-of-life decision making and implementation in recipients of a destination left ventricular assist device. *Journal of Heart Lung Transplant* 29 (12): 1337–1341.

Caldwell, P.H., H.M. Arthur, and C. Demers. 2007. Preferences of patients with heart failure for prognosis communication. *Canadian Journal of Cardiology* 23(10): 791–796.

Chamberlain, A.M., K.S. Vickers, R.C. Colligan, S.A. Weston, T.A. Rummans, and V.L. Roger. 2011. Associations of preexisting depression and anxiety with hospitalization in patients with cardiovascular disease. *Mayo Clinical Proceedings* 86(11): 1056–1062.

Clegg, A.J., D.A. Scott, E. Loveman, J. Colquitt, J. Hutchinson, and P. Royle et al. 2015. The clinical and cost-effectiveness of left ventricular assist devices for end-stage heart failure: A systematic review and economic evaluation. *Health Technology Assessment* 9(45): 1–132, iii–iv.

Clegg, A.J., D.A. Scott, E. Loveman, J.L. Colquitt, P. Royle, and J. Bryant. 2006. Clinical and cost-effectiveness of left ventricular assist devices as a bridge to heart transplantation for people with end-stage heart failure: A systematic review and economic evaluation. *European Heart Journal* 27(24): 2929–2938.

Clegg, A.J., D.A. Scott, E. Loveman, J. Colquitt, P. Royle, and J. Bryant. 2007. Clinical and cost-effectiveness of left ventricular assist devices as destination therapy for people with end-stage heart failure: A systematic review and economic evaluation. *International Journal of Technology Assessment in Health Care* 23(2): 261–268.

Currow, D.C., C. McDonald, S. Oaten, B. Kenny, P. Allcroft, and P. Frith et al. 2011. Once-daily opioids for chronic dyspnea: A dose increment and pharmacovigilance study. *Journal of Pain and Symptom Management* 42(3): 388–399.

Dunlay, S., J. Foxen, T. Cole, M.A. Feely, A.R. Loth, and J.J. Strand et al. 2014. Clinician attitudes and self-reported practices regarding end of life care in heart failure. *Circulation: Cardiovascular Quality Outcomes* 7(1): A352.

Dunlay, S.M., K.M. Swetz, P.S. Mueller, and V.L. Roger. 2012. Advance directives in community patients with heart failure. *Circulation: Circulatory Cardiovascular Quality Outcomes* 5(3): 283–289.

Dunlay, S.M., K.M. Swetz, M.M. Redfield, P.S. Mueller, and V.L. Roger. 2014. Resuscitation preferences in community patients with heart failure. *Circulation* 7(3): 353–359.

Elwyn, G., A. Edwards, P. Kinnersley, and R. Grol. 2000. Shared decision making and the concept of equipoise: the competences of involving patients in healthcare choices. *British Journal of General Practice* 50(460): 892–899.

Epstein, A.E., J.P. DiMarco, K.A. Ellenbogen, M. Estes, R.A. Freedman, and L.S. Gettes et al. 2013. 2012 ACCF/AHA/HRS focused update incorporated into the ACCF/AHA/HRS 2008 guidelines for device-based therapy of cardiac rhythm abnormalities: A report of the American College of Cardiology Foundation/American Heart Association Task Force on Practice Guidelines and the Heart Rhythm Society. *Circulation* 127(3): e283–352.

Evangelista, L.S., E. Sackett, and K. Dracup. 2009. Pain and heart failure: Unrecognized and untreated. *European Journal of Cardiovascular Nursing* 8(3): 169–173.

Evans, D.L., D.S. Charney, L. Lewis, R.N. Golden, J.M. Gorman, and K.R. Krishnan et al. 2005. Mood disorders in the medically ill: Scientific review and recommendations. *Biological Psychiatry* 58(3): 175–189.

Feldman, D., S.V. Pamboukian, J.J. Teuteberg, E. Birks, K. Lietz, and S.A. Moore et al. 2013. The 2013 International Society for Heart and Lung Transplantation Guidelines for mechanical circulatory support: Executive summary. *The Journal of Heart Lung Transplant* 32(2): 157–187.

Gibbs, J.S., A.S. McCoy, L.M. Gibbs, A.E. Rogers, and J.M. Addington-Hall. 2002. Living with and dying from heart failure: The role of palliative care. *Heart* 88(Suppl 2): ii36–ii39.

Go, A.S., D. Mozaffarian, V.L. Roger, E.J. Benjamin, J.D. Berry, W.B. Borden et al. 2013. Heart disease and stroke statistics – 2013 update: A report from the American Heart Association. *Circulation* 127(1): e6–e245.

Goodlin, S.J. 2009. Palliative care in congestive heart failure. *Journal of the American College of Cardiology* 54(5): 386–396.

Goodlin, S.J., S. Wingate, N.M. Albert, S.J. Pressler, J. Houser, and J. Kwon et al. 2012. Investigating pain in heart failure patients: the pain assessment, incidence, and nature in heart failure (PAIN-HF) study. *Journal of Cardiac Failure* 18(10): 776–783.

Green, C.P., C.B. Porter, D.R. Bresnahan, and Spertus, J.A. 2000. Development and evaluation of the Kansas City cardiomyopathy questionnaire: A new health status measure for heart failure. *Journal of the American College of Cardiology* 35(5): 1245–1255.

Hawkins, N., P. Jhund, J. McMurray, and S. Capewell. 2012. Heart failure and socioeconomic status: Accumulating evidence of inequality. *European Journal of Heart Failure* 14(2): 138–146.

Heidenreich, P.A., N.M. Albert, L.A. Allen, D.A. Bluemke, J. Butler, G.C. Fonarow, and J.S. Ikonomidis et al. 2013. Forecasting the impact of heart failure in the United States: A policy statement from the American Heart Association. *Circulatory Heart Failure* 6(3): 606–619.

Heidenreich, P.A., J.G. Trogdon, O.A. Khavjou, J. Butler, K. Dracup, and M.D. Exekowitz et al. 2011. Forecasting the future of cardiovascular disease in the United States: A policy statement from the American Heart Association. *Circulation* 123(8): 933–944.

Hospice and Palliative Nurses Association. 2013. *HPNA position statement. The ethics of opioid use at end of Life* (On-line). http://clarehouse.org/wpcontent/uploads/2016/07/Challenges-in-Symptom-Managment-Addendum-2.pdf (accessed January 3, 2018).

Hutchinson, J., D.A. Scott, A.J. Clegg, E. Loveman, P. Royle, and J. Bryant et al. 2008. Cost-effectiveness of left ventricular-assist devices in end-stage heart failure. *Expert Review of Cardiovascular Therapy* 6(2): 175–185.

Johnson, M.J., and S.G. Oxberry. 2010. The management of dyspnoea in chronic heart failure. *Current Opinion in Supportive and Palliative Care* 4(2): 63–68.

Kini, V., and J.N. Kirkpatrick. 2013. Ethical challenges in advanced heart failure. *Current Opinion in Supportive and Palliative Care* 7(1): 21–28.

Koenig, H.G. 1998. Depression in hospitalized older patients with congestive heart failure. *General Hospital Psychiatry* 20(1): 29–43.

Krumholz, H., R. Phillips, M.B. Hamel, J.M. Teno, and P. Bellamy et al. 1998. Resuscitation preferences among patients with severe congestive heart failure: Results from the SUPPORT project. Study to Understand prognoses and preferences for outcomes and risks of treatments. *Circulation* 98(7): 648–655.

Lane, R., M. Cowie, and A. Chow. 2005. Prediction and prevention of sudden cardiac death in heart failure. *Heart* 91(5): 674–680.

Levy, W., D. Mozaffarian, D.T. Linker, S.C. Sutradhar, S.D. Anker, and A.B. Cropp et al. 2006. The Seattle Heart Failure Model: Prediction of survival in heart failure. *Circulation* 113(11): 1424–1433.

Lichtman, J.H., J.T. Bigger Jr., J.A. Blumenthal, N. Frasure-Smith, P.G. Kaufmann, and F. Lespèrance et al. 2008. Depression and coronary heart disease: recommendations for screening, referral, and treatment. A science advisory from the American Heart Association Prevention Committee of the Council on Cardiovascular Nursing, Council on Clinical Cardiology, Council on Epidemiology and Prevention, and Interdisciplinary Council on Quality of Care and Outcomes Research: Endorsed by the American Psychiatric Association. *Circulation* 118(17): 1768–1775.

Malik, F.A., M. Gysels, and I.J. Higginson. 2013. Living with breathlessness: A survey of caregivers of breathless patients with lung cancer or heart failure. *Palliative Medicine* 27(7): 647–656.

Maltoni, M., C. Pittureri, E. Scarpi, L. Piccinini, F. Martini, and P. Turci et al. 2009. Palliative sedation therapy does not hasten death: Results from a prospective multi-center study. *Annals of Oncology* 20(7): 1163–1169.

Maltoni, M., E. Scarpi, M. Rosati, S. Derni, L. Fabbri, and F. Martini et al. 2012. Palliative sedation in end-of-life care and survival: A systematic review. *Journal of Clinical Oncology* 30(12): 1378–1383.

McCarthy, M., M. Lay, and J. Addington-Hall. 1996. Dying from heart disease. *The Journal of the Royal College of Physicians London* 30(4): 325–328.

Miller, L.W., and M. Guglin. 2013. Patient selection for ventricular assist devices: A moving target. *Journal of the American College of Cardiology* 61(12): 1209–1221.

Murray, S., K. Boyd, M. Kendall, A. Worth, T. Benton, and H. Calusen. 2002. Dying of lung cancer or cardiac failure: Prospective qualitative interview study of patients and their carers in the community. *BMJ* 325(7370): 929–934.

National Coalition for Hospice and Palliative Care. 2013. *National consensus project clinical practice guidelines for quality palliative care.* 3rd ed. https://www.nationalcoalitionhpc.org/ncp-guidelines-2013/ (accessed January 3, 2019).

National Hospice and Palliative Care Organization. 2018. *Facts and figures hospice care in America* https://www.nhpco.org/sites/default/files/public/Statistics_Research/2017_Facts_Figures.pdf (accessed January 4, 2019).

O'Connor, C.M., D.J. Whellan, K.L. Lee, S.J. Keteyian, L.S. Cooper, and S.J. Ellis. 2009. Efficacy and safety of exercise training in patients with chronic heart failure: HF-ACTION randomized controlled trial. *JAMA* 301(14): 1439–1450.

Oxberry, S.G., J.M. Bland, A.L. Clark, J.G. Cleland, and M.J. Johnson. 2013. Repeat dose opioids may be effective for breathlessness in chronic heart failure if given for long enough. *Journal of Palliative Medicine* 16(3): 250–255.

Petrucci, R.J., L.A. Benish, B.L. Carrow, L. Prato, S.R. Hankins, and H.J. Eisen et al. 2011. Ethical considerations for ventricular assist device support: A 10-point model. *ASAIO American Society for Artificial Internal Organ Research Journal* 57(4): 268–273.

Portenoy, R.K., U. Sibirceva, R. Smout, S. Horn, S. Connor, and R.H. Blum et al. 2006. Opioid use and survival at the end of life: A survey of a hospice population. *Journal of Pain and Symptom Management* 32(6): 532–540.

Rector, T.S., and J.N. Cohn. 1992. Assessment of patient outcome with the Minnesota Living with Heart Failure questionnaire: Reliability and validity during a randomized, double-blind, placebo-controlled trial of pimobendan. *American Heart Journal* 124(4): 1017–1025.

Rector, T.S., S.H. Kubo, and J.N. Cohn. 1993. Validity of the Minnesota Living with Heart Failure questionnaire as a measure of therapeutic response to enalapril or placebo. *American Journal of Cardiology* 71(12): 1106–1107.

Rocker, G., J. Young, M. Donahue, M. Farquhar, and C. Simpson. 2012. Perspectives of patients, family caregivers and physicians about the use of opioids for refractory dyspnea in advanced chronic obstructive pulmonary disease. *Canadian Medical Association Journal* 184(9): E497–E504.

Rogers, J.G., K.D. Aaronson, A.J. Boyle, S.D. Russell, C.A. Milano, and F.D. Pagani et al. 2010. Continuous flow left ventricular assist device improves functional capacity and quality of life of advanced heart failure patients. *Journal of the American College of Cardiology* 55(17): 1826–1834.

Rogers, J.G., R.R. Bostic, K.B. Tong, R. Adamson, M. Russo, and M.S. Slaughter. 2012. Cost-effectiveness analysis of continuous-flow left ventricular assist devices as destination therapy. *Circulation* 5(1): 10–16.

Rutledge, T., V.A. Reis, S.E. Linke, B.H. Greenberg and P.J. Mills. 2006. Depression in heart failure a meta-analytic review of prevalence, intervention effects, and associations with clinical outcomes. *Journal of the American College of Cardiology* 48(8): 1527–1537.

Sanders, G.D., M.A. Hlatky, and D.K. Owens. 2005. Cost-effectiveness of implantable cardioverter-defibrillators. *The New England Journal of Medicine* 353(14): 1471–1480.

Schwarz, E.R., A. Baraghoush, R.P. Morrissey, A.B. Shah, A.M. Shinde, and A. Phan et al. 2012. Pilot study of palliative care consultation in patients with advanced heart failure referred for cardiac transplantation. *The Journal of Palliative Medicine* 15(1): 12–15.

Smith, O.R., H.J. Michielsen, A.J. Pelle, A.A. Schiffer, J.B. Winter, and J. Denollet. 2007. Symptoms of fatigue in chronic heart failure patients: Clinical and psychological predictors. *European Journal of Heart Failure* 9(9): 922–927.

Sullivan, M., W.C. Levy, J.E. Russo, and J.A. Spertus. 2007. Depression and health status in patients with advanced heart failure: A prospective study in tertiary care. *Journal of Cardio Failure* 10(5): 390–396.

SUPPORT Principal Investigators. 1995. A controlled trial to improve care for seriously ill hospitalized patients: The study to understand prognoses and preferences for outcomes and risks of treatments (SUPPORT). The SUPPORT Principal Investigators. *JAMA* 274(20): 1591–1598.

Swetz, K.M., M.R. Freeman, O.F. Abouezzeddine, K.A. Carter, B.A. Boilson, and A.L. Ottenberg et al. 2011. Palliative medicine consultation for preparedness planning in patients receiving left ventricular assist devices as destination therapy. *Mayo Clinic Proceedings* 86(6): 493–500.

Swetz, K.M., and A.H. Kamal. 2012. In the clinic: Palliative care. *Annals of Internal Medicine* 156(3): ITc2-1–TC2-15.

Swetz, K.M., J.M. Stulak, S.M. Dunlay, and E.F. Gafford. 2012. Management of advanced heart failure in the elderly: Ethics, economics, and resource allocation in the technological era. *Cardiology Research and Practice* 2012: 1–5.

Syncardia Systems Inc. 2018. *Total artificial hearts*. https://syncardia.com/patients/home/

Timmons, M.J., J. MacIver, A.C. Alba, A. Tibbles, S. Greenwood, and H.J. Ross. 2013. Using heart failure instruments to determine when to refer heart failure patients to palliative care. *Journal of Palliative Care* 29(4): 217–224.

Walke, L.M., W.T. Gallo, M.E. Tinetti, and T.R. Fried. 2004. The burden of symptoms among community-dwelling older persons with advanced chronic disease. *Archives of Internal Medicine* 164(21): 2321–2324.

Warraich, H.J., K. Mukamal, L. Allen, A. Ship, and R. Kociol. 2014. Physician estimates of prognosis in heart failure. *Journal of the American College of Cardiology* 63(12 Suppl): A951.

Weiss, S.C., L.L. Emanuel, D.L. Fairclough, and E.J. Emanuel. 2001. Understanding the experience of pain in terminally ill patients. *Lancet* 357(9265): 1311–1315.

Yancy, C.W., M. Jessup, B. Bozkurt, J. Butler, D.E. Casey, M.H. Drazner, and G.C. Fonarow et al. 2013. 2013 ACCF/AHA guideline for the management of heart failure: A report of the American College of Cardiology Foundation/American Heart Association Task Force on practice guidelines. *Circulation* 128(16): e240–327.

Yu, D.S., D.T. Lee, J. Woo, and D.R. Thompson. 2004. Correlates of psychological distress in elderly patients with congestive heart failure. *Journal of Psychosomatic Research* 57(6): 573–581.

5 Deactivating Cardiac Implantable Electronic Devices at End of Life

Keith M. Swetz, Sara E. Wordingham, Daniel D. Matlock and David M. Zientek

I Introduction

The indication for and use of cardiac implantable electronic devices (CIEDs) has steadily increased over the past quarter-century. Technology has advanced remarkably such that many CIEDs are implanted with minimal burden to patients. Implantable pacemaker use began early in the 1950s, with implantable cardioverter-defibrillators coming into use around 1980. Initial use of mechanical circulatory support (MCS) devices dates to use of the total artificial hearts during the late 1960s. In the 1990s, the United States Food and Drug Administration approved studies examining the benefits of left-ventricular assist devices (LVADs) for patients with advanced heart failure. Use of an LVAD was initially designed to be a bridge to cardiac transplantation; however, limited organ supply and observed survival benefits with LVADs led to investigation of their use as *destination therapy*—where the device would be used as a terminal treatment for patients who were ineligible for cardiac transplantation, or who did not desire it. The initial REMATCH trial, published in 2001, demonstrated that implantation of an LVAD as destination therapy (DT-LVAD) afforded patients a survival benefit over optimal medical management (Rose et al. 2001). Note, we use the term CIED to refer collectively to use of any type of implanted cardiac pacemaker, cardioverter-defibrillator, or a combination of these devices; while MCS will refer to LVAD or total artificial heart, regardless of whether implant intention was bridge to transplantation or destination therapy.

It is known that CIEDs and MCS can prolong life and increase quality of life for a majority of well-selected patients who need them. As the indications for such devices increase, the prevalence of patients with these devices will increase in the foreseeable future. At this time, nearly three million patients in the United States have CIEDs and over 350,000 devices are implanted annually (Mond and Proclemer 2011). The Interagency Network for Cardiac Devices (INTERMACS) estimates that 18,000 MCS devices have been implanted in the United States, including LVADs and total artificial hearts (Kirklin et al. 2015). With lower device costs and improving technology, an increasing number of centers are certified to implant DT-LVAD or care for patients post-operatively, and with no foreseeable change in transplantation practices, it is anticipated that more patients

DOI: 10.4324/9781003240273-8

will receive DT-LVAD. As such, more patients will be dying with CIEDs and DT-LVAD devices *in situ*, and requests for end-of-life device management including deactivation will be needed. This chapter explores the commonly articulated concerns regarding the morality and legality of deactivating CIEDs and MCSs, beginning with two case examples. The goal is to present some overall general rules and accepted practices, as well as some minority opposing viewpoints, and to discuss the clinician's role in approaching the end of life with patients who have implanted cardiac devices.

II Case Presentations

Case 1:

Mr. C is a 60-year-old male followed in the Heart Failure Clinic for the past four years. Because of refractory severe symptoms despite appropriate maximal medical therapy for non-ischemic cardiomyopathy, he was referred for consideration for cardiac transplantation. He is an excellent candidate from the standpoint of his general good health and has a strong social support system with a history of compliance with medical recommendations. However, shortly after his initial evaluation, he is diagnosed with a localized colon cancer and undergoes resection of the tumor confined to the wall of the intestine. He has a very good prognosis from his cancer, but policy requires that patients be free of cancer for five years before being placed on the heart transplantation list. Subsequently, due to worsening heart failure he undergoes placement of a left ventricular assist device (LVAD) as a "bridge to transplant" with the hope that after five years he can receive definitive treatment with transplantation.

Left ventricular assist devices require detailed care that is ongoing when returning home with one in place. Implants require anticoagulation with regular monitoring of therapeutic efficacy. If these medications are taken incorrectly, the patient is at risk of stroke or life-threatening bleeding. Meticulous care must be taken to prevent device infection. Patients must have two batteries with a backup always charged and available, in addition to contingency plans if the electricity is out for an extended period of time. Despite the complexity of care, he has done much better than expected, keeping all follow-up appointments and complying with medical advice with no device complications.

This week Mr. C presents to clinic and states that he would like to have his LVAD turned off. His cardiologist explains that he has almost reached the point where he can be placed on the heart transplantation list, and that he would likely die within hours to a few short days after turning off the device. The patient states that he is aware of this. He notes that he has thought about the LVAD and transplantation over the past several months, and he has decided that the burden of extensive medication, visits to the doctor, and the limitation of lifestyle have become excessive for him. His children are grown and established in their lives and he has discussed this decision with his wife and family. He is not willing to continue the LVAD for another year, and is well informed of the regimen of medication and follow-up needed even if he receives a transplant, and decided that he will take his chances with medication alone. His cardiologist calls the ethics committee because she is concerned that turning off the device may be equivalent to physician-assisted suicide and she is concerned about complying with a patient who has done so well.

Case 2:

Mr. K is an 84-year-old male who underwent AV node ablation and permanent pacemaker placement a year ago. At that time, he struggled with symptomatic atrial fibrillation despite attempts to control rate and symptoms with multiple medications. Approximately three months ago, he was diagnosed with metastatic adenocarcinoma of the pancreas and is admitted to the hospital now with a small bowel obstruction. The obstruction has resolved with nasogastric suction; however, he has decided to enter hospice care and not pursue further chemotherapy. The patient's pacemaker is at the end of its battery life. The patient and his family have asked that the battery not be replaced, and that it be deactivated. His cardiologist has asked for an ethics consultation because the patient is now pacemaker-dependent. Since the doctor performed the ablation procedure, he is concerned about the ethical implication of turning off the pacemaker, which will very likely hasten the patient's death in the setting of an iatrogenic (or medically created) etiology for his pacemaker dependence.

Table 5.1 Key Cases Investigating the Withholding or Withdrawing of Life-Sustaining Treatments (Swetz, Hook and Mueller 2013)

Quinlan	1975	WD ventilator
Saikewicz	1977	WH chemotherapy
Dinnerstein	1978	WH CPR
Spring	1980	WD hemodialysis
Barber	1983	WD IV fluids
Bouvia	1985	WH/WD feeding tube
Cruzan	1990	WD feeding tube
Schiavo	2005	WD feeding tube

III A Right to Be Left Alone, but Not Necessarily a Right to Die

Medical jurisprudence in the United States is replete with landmark cases that have examined the topic of what constitutes a life-sustaining treatment, and the morality and legality of withholding or withdrawing such life-sustaining treatments (see Table 5.1). The overall findings in many of these clinical cases, and subsequent court decisions, have focused on respect for patient autonomy by honoring what are often referred to as negative rights. In general, negative rights permit a patient to be left alone and refuse or request withdrawal of an unwanted intervention. The courts in the United States have consistently supported this stance, even if doing so results in a patient's death. As such, there is an obligation not to impose treatments on a patient with decision-making capacity against his or her will. The summary findings have, in essence, boiled down to the opinion that there is no ethical or legal difference between withholding and withdrawing a life-sustaining treatment, and asserted that the clinician's role is to be certain that such refusal is made by an informed decision-maker with capacity.

As corollaries to these key cases, the courts have opined further that a patient with decision-making capacity has the right to refuse or request withdrawal of life-sustaining treatments, and that a patient without such capacity maintains those rights as exercised via a surrogate decision-maker. Recent work by DeMartino and colleagues has explored the challenges that exist when patients are unable to make their own decisions, and delineated a strategy for approaching surrogate decision-making as it varies by geographic location in the United States (DeMartino et al. 2017). Interestingly, despite state-by-state variability in hierarchy of surrogate decision-makers, the Veterans Administration Health System follows a uniform standard across all sites regardless of state (Swetz, Stanton, and Lowery 2017); and other jurisdictions outside of the United States may have alternate structures for such decisions to be made.

Although some clinicians initially were concerned about liability for wrongful death if desires to withhold or withdraw treatment were honored, the courts have generally held that physicians have no liability or legal culpability for granting such requests (Swetz and Hook 2016). This protection of patients' negative rights and physicians' ability to honor such requests is distinct from a *right to die*. Collectively, the term "right to die" has been used to describe a positive right to request physician aid in dying. Although arguments have been presented that physician aid in dying should be considered morally equivalent and should be protected by Constitutional rights, the US Supreme Court has opined that this is not the case.

In the landmark 1997 decision, *Vacco* v. *Quill*, the majority opinion of the US Supreme Court concluded that there is a difference between a "right to die" and a right to be "left alone". In the brief, Chief Justice William Rehnquist noted:

> The distinction comports with fundamental legal principles of causation and intent. First, when a patient refuses life-sustaining medical treatment, he dies from an underlying fatal disease or pathology; but if a patient ingests lethal medication prescribed by a physician, he is killed by that medication…[In *Cruzan*] our assumption of a right to refuse treatment was grounded not…on the proposition that patients have a… right to hasten death, but on well established, traditional rights to bodily integrity and freedom from unwanted touching.
>
> (*Vacco* v. *Quill* 1997 at 801)

In *Vacco* v. *Quill*, the court noted that equal protection rights were not violated if a state chose to prohibit physician aid in dying, and in *Washington* v. *Glucksberg* the court further ruled that due process was not violated by a ban of physician aid in dying (*Vacco* v. *Quill* 1997; *Washington* v. *Glucksberg* 1997). However, the US Supreme Court did uphold a state's right to prohibit physician aid in dying; yet individual states could choose to legalize physician aid in dying through appropriate legislation. At this time, at least nine states have legalized forms of physician aid in dying and several more are exploring opportunities (Swetz, Barnett, Kamal, and Mansel 2017).

IV Differentiating Killing versus Allowing to Die

In evaluating end-of-life situations physician-philosopher Daniel Sulmasy (Sulmasy 1998) has cogently articulated the majority position drawing a distinction between killing and allowing to die (AMA Council on Ethical and Judicial Affairs 2016; Snyder Sulmasy, Mueller, Ethics, & Human Rights Committee of the American College of Physicians 2017). Although terms such as active euthanasia or passive euthanasia were previously used to describe the active taking of a life (or "mercy killing") versus allowing someone to die by withholding or withdrawing treatment, these terms have fallen out of favor in that the distinction appears to be between killing and allowing to die (Sulmasy 1998). Active euthanasia remains strictly prohibited in the United States and many other countries, and conflating an act of withholding or withdrawing of life-sustaining treatments as equivalent to euthanasia is confusing and has led to misunderstandings by providers and patients alike. For Sulmasy, the moral delineation between killing and allowing to die emerges in that a new pathology is introduced that is responsible for the death (Sulmasy 1998).

With the advent of multiple types of life-sustaining treatments that are both internal and external, Mueller, Hook, and others further differentiated some of the nuances between killing (i.e., euthanasia) and allowing patients to die via the withholding or withdrawing of life-sustaining treatments (Mueller, Hook, and Hayes 2003; Mueller et al. 2010; Olsen, Swetz, and Mueller 2010) (see Table 5.2). The authors note that the provision of appropriate comfort measures, including opioids or sedatives, is licit when medications are used in a proportionate fashion, with the intent of providing comfort and not with the goal of hastening death. Furthermore, a difference in the mark of success of the intervention is noted; namely, that in palliative sedation the marker of success is improved comfort and decreased pain versus the marker of success in physician aid in dying or euthanasia, which is the patient's death. Hence, the patient receives what is needed to relieve suffering and is allowed to die from the underlying cause of disease, versus a new agent being introduced to produce this effect (Mueller et al. 2003; Mueller et al. 2010; Olsen et al. 2010).

In each of these three situations, the intent or goal of the intervention is to avoid or remove a burdensome intervention or to relieve symptoms, respectively. These efforts remain legal in all of the United States. The central argument of these clinician ethicists has been that there is a fundamental moral difference with physician aid in dying and euthanasia, such that the intervention prescribed by the physician, and used by the patient or administered by the physician, has a goal or intention specifically leading to the termination of the patient's life. At the time of this publication there remains variability in states that have legalized and we anticipate this list to change in the foreseeable future (Swetz, Barnett, Kamal, & Mansel 2017).

V Fundamental Differences and Similarities with Cardiac Devices

With advances in the use and sophistication of CIEDs and MCS, questions have been raised as to whether there may be an ethical or legal difference between deactivating certain cardiac devices as compared to other life-sustaining interventions. Requests with CIEDs can range from withdrawal of currently active support to refusal of such intervention in the first place. Individual clinicians will have variable opinions about how to manage different types of CIEDs, and in a seminal 2008 paper, Sulmasy provided ethical arguments regarding these nuances (Sulmasy 2008). His initial conclusion was that there was no ethical difference between the withholding or withdrawing of life-sustaining treatments (as determined by cases in Table 5.1) and that CIEDs raised no specific new moral issues. Some have questioned duration of treatment as an issue, considering if an intervention was just initiated or if a person has utilized it for an extended period of time, but treatment with hemodialysis for a day or several

Table 5.2 Legal and Ethical Differences among Withholding and Withdrawing Life–Sustaining Treatment, Palliative Sedation, Physician–Aid in Dying, and Euthanasia (Olsen et al. 2010; Swetz and Kamal 2018)

Variable	Withhold Life-Sustaining Treatment	Withdraw Life-Sustaining Treatment	Palliative Sedation and Analgesia	Physician-Aid in Dying	Euthanasia
Cause of death	Underlying disease	Underlying disease	Underlying disease[a]	Intervention prescribed by physician and used by patient	Intervention administered by physician
Intent/goal of intervention	Avoid burdensome intervention	Remove burdensome intervention	Relieve symptoms	Termination of life	Termination of life
Legal in United States?[b]	Yes[c]	Yes[c]	Yes	Legal in some states; prohibited in some states; being considered in some states§	No

Data based on Olsen ML, Swetz KM, Mueller PS. *Ethical decision making with end-of-life care: palliative sedation and withholding or withdrawing life-sustaining treatments. Mayo Clinic Proceedings* 2010; 85: 949–54. [PHD: 208055441].

a Note "double-effect" (see text).

b Several states limit the power of surrogate decision makers regarding life-sustaining treatments.

c Refer to your state's medical guidelines for current policy.

years does not appear to be a morally decisive factor in deciding whether to withdraw this treatment at the end of life.

Another issue concerns possible differences between continuous and intermittent treatments. Treatments that are continuous are those such as being ventilator-dependent or pacemaker-dependent versus treatments that are intermittent such as demand pacing-only or hemodialysis. Yet decisions to discontinue ventilators or dialysis are traditionally made without reference to a distinction in this regard. Similarly, are there important moral differences between regulative versus constitutive treatments? A constitutive treatment takes over a function that the body can no longer provide whereas a regulative treatment is simply a guiding treatment. In constitutive therapy, such as mechanical ventilation, artificial nutrition and hydration, advanced cardiac support or hemodialysis withdrawal is not morally different from a regulative therapy such as an intermittent implantable cardiac defibrillator (ICD) or cardiac pacing device. An additional concern regards internal versus external treatments: whether something that has been fully implanted is morally different than one that has not. Others question if there is a moral difference between devices with power sources, internal versus external, which may provide an ethical quandary. Sulmasy notes that internal versus external treatment did not seem to mark the moral difference between killing and allowing to die and that definitions previously articulated make no specific reference to internal or external therapies (Sulmasy 2008).

One area in which Sulmasy notes there may be a difference between replacement and substitutive therapy where substitutive therapy is something that replaces a specific function, but replacement therapy becomes part of the patient and may be less accessible when withdrawing such support. A replacement therapy replaces a function that is pathologically lost. Features of replacement therapy include the ability to respond to changes in host and environment, ability for self-growth and repair, independence from external energy sources or expert control, immunologic compatibility and bodily integration. A commonly sighted example is the difference between the aortic valve replacement, which intrinsically becomes part of the patient versus an ICD which does not exhibit the same types of features that are noted in replacement therapies. However, as technologies evolve newer treatments such as stem cells or fully internalized MCS devices will push these boundaries.

A landmark case-series analysis by Mueller and colleagues investigated several challenges encountered with requests for CIED deactivation, prompting ethics consultation (Mueller et al. 2003). Their main findings noted that the deactivation of CIEDs is ethical if consistent with the patient's goals, preferences and values, and that these options are not akin to physician-aided dying or euthanasia because the cause of death is advanced heart disease. A call for additional research led to subsequent studies that have further examined the challenges noted with CIEDs. This is a key issue as the topic of ultimate need for deactivation is rarely discussed prior to or after implantation of such devices and that patients and surrogates often do not know that such an option is possible (Goldstein et al. 2008).

Patients can have significant concerns about experiencing defibrillation or a shock in the process of dying and other concerns often noted deal with challenges of advanced care planning. Several studies have shown that advance care planning documents often do not contain patients' goals or concerns regarding advanced therapies (Berger, Gorski, and Cohen 2006; Buchhalter et al. 2014; Swetz et al. 2011). A survey of members of the Heart Rhythm Society and industry-employed personnel from two device manufacturers in 2008 admitted that CIED deactivation requests were common and that a majority of caregivers who cared for such patients have made requests personally to deactivate such devices. Some providers did note a distinction between deactivating intermittent therapy, such as an ICD, versus a regulative therapy, such as a pacemaker (Mueller, Jenkins, Bramstedt, and Hayes 2008).

Pellegrino articulated the basic argument for the permissibility of withdrawal of burdensome treatments (Pellegrino 2000). He argued that the feasibility and efficacy of such therapy, in terms of potential benefits, falls in the purview of the clinician, but that the benefits and burdens of the therapy remain within the purview of the patient. This is a critical distinction, as what one patient is willing to endure or finds acceptable may not be the same for another patient.

VI Approaching CIED Deactivation

The shock from an ICD is perhaps a unique event in modern medicine in that it can be both beneficial and harmful depending on where a person is in their life trajectory. The decision regarding whether or not to get an ICD involves weighing a desire for longevity with the possibility for sudden death. When asked, patients often prefer both longevity and a quick death (Vig and Pearlman 2004). Recently, the American College of Cardiology/American Heart Association guidelines for heart failure added language specifically stating that this trade-off should be discussed at the time of ICD implantation:

> Counseling should be specific to each individual patient and should include documentation of a discussion about the potential for sudden death and nonsudden death from HF or noncardiac conditions. Information should be provided about the efficacy, safety, and potential complications of an ICD and the potential for defibrillation to be inactivated if desired in the future... This will facilitate shared decision making between patients, families, and the medical care team about ICDs.
>
> (Yancy et al. 2013, p. e274)

The point where an ICD shock switches from being potentially beneficial to potentially harmful depends on the patient's clinical status and their preferences. Technically, the ICD can be easily deactivated without surgery when a patient's situation approaches that point. However, research suggests that this is not always done. Despite fairly clear ethical guidance, between 20% (Kramer, Kesselheim, Salberg, Brock, and Maisel 2011) and 46% (Sherazi et al. 2010) of clinicians continue to question whether ICD deactivation is legal. While most clinicians feel it is important to deactivate the ICD near the end of life (Goldstein, Mehta, Teitelbaum, Bradley, and Morrison 2008; Hauptman, Swindle, Hussain, Biener, and Burroughs 2008; Kapa, Mueller, Hayes, and Asirvatham 2010; Marinskis, van Erven, and Committee 2010; Morrison, Calvin, Nora and Porter 2010), there is no consensus on who should do this (Hauptman et al. 2008; Kelley, Reid, Miller, Fins and Lachs 2009; Marinskis et al. 2010). Also, clinicians tend to state that they are uncomfortable having this conversation (Kelley et al. 2009; Matlock et al. 2011; Morrison et al. 2010; Mueller, Jenkins, Bramstedt, and Hayes 2008).

Consequently, patients and families are often left unprepared. Many patients do not know that the ICD can be deactivated (Lewis, Stacey, and Matlock 2014). A recent detailed series of 150 dying patients with ICDs or pacemakers had them deactivated within two days of death (Buchhalter et al. 2014). Only one of these patients had an advance directive that mentioned the ICD. As a result, surrogates were responsible for the majority of the deactivation decisions. A survey of family members of patients who had died with an ICD demonstrated that only 27% remembered ever even having a discussion about ICD deactivation (Goldstein, Lampert, Bradley, Lynn, and Krumholz 2004). Worse, half of the hospices in the United States reported having a patient receive a shock from their ICD while on hospice (Goldstein, Carlson, Livote, and Kutner 2010).

VII Return to the Cases

In light of the discussion presented, how might an ethics consultant respond to the two cases presented earlier? In the first case, the patient is requesting discontinuation of a treatment that he has decided, after careful consideration, is excessively burdensome relative to the perceived benefits. He does not appear to be requesting assistance in suicide, as he is open to continuing medical therapy, though it would be reasonable to evaluate the patient to ensure that he does not have untreated clinical depression. The consultant may recommend confirming that this decision is stable over the course of one or two further clinic follow-ups; however, the fact that the patient has done well and has the possibility of a more definitive treatment becoming available, and that the device is implanted would not preclude complying with his request.

In the second case, the fact that the patient is pacemaker-dependent as a result of a prior medical treatment would not preclude deactivating the pacemaker since the procedure was initially performed for an appropriate indication and medical circumstances have significantly changed. One might question the burden of continuing with cardiac pacing; however, in a patient entering hospice, and needing possible replacement of a depleted pacemaker battery, there would be no moral objection to deactivating the device.

References

AMA Council on Ethical and Judicial Affairs. 2016. *Code of medical ethics of the American Medical Association: Current opinions with annotations.* Chicago: American Medical Association.

Berger, J.T., M. Gorski and T. Cohen. 2006. Advance health planning and treatment preferences among recipients of implantable cardioverter defibrillators: An exploratory study, *Journal of Clinical Ethics* 17(1): 72–78.

Buchhalter, L.C., A.L. Ottenberg, T.L. Webster, K.M. Swetz, D.L. Hayes, and P.S. Mueller. 2014. Features and outcomes of patients who underwent cardiac device deactivation, *JAMA Internal Medicine* 174(1): 80–85.

DeMartino, E.S., D.M. Dudzinski, C.K. Doyle, B.P. Sperry, S.E. Gregory, M. Siegler, and D.B. Kramer. 2017. Who decides when a patient can't? Statutes on alternate decision makers, *The New England Journal of Medicine* 376(15): 1478–1482.

Goldstein, N., M. Carlson, E. Livote, and J.S. Kutner. 2010. Brief communication: Management of implantable cardioverter-defibrillators in hospice: A nationwide survey, *Annals of Internal Medicine* 152(5): 296–299.

Goldstein, N.E., R. Lampert, E. Bradley, J. Lynn, and H.M. Krumholz. 2004. Management of implantable cardioverter defibrillators in end-of-life care, *Annals of Internal Medicine* 141(11): 835–838.

Goldstein, N.E., D. Mehta, S. Siddiqui, E. Teitelbaum, J. Zeidman, M. Singson, and R.S. Morrison. 2008. "That's like an act of suicide": Patients; attitudes toward deactivation of implantable defibrillators, *Journal of General Internal Medicine* 23(Suppl 1): 7–12.

Goldstein, N.E., D. Mehta, E. Teitelbaum, E.H. Bradley, and R.S. Morrison. 2008. "It's like crossing a bridge": Complexities preventing physicians from discussing deactivation of implantable defibrillators at the end of life, *Journal of General Internal Medicine* 23(Suppl 1): 2–6.

Hauptman, P.J., J. Swindle, Z. Hussain, L. Biener, and T.E. Burroughs. 2008. Physician attitudes toward end-stage heart failure: A national survey, *American Journal of Medicine* 121(2): 127–135.

Kapa, S., P.S. Mueller, D.L. Hayes, and S.J. Asirvatham. 2010. Perspectives on withdrawing pacemaker and implantable cardioverter-defibrillator therapies at end of life: Results of a survey of medical and legal professionals and patients, *Mayo Clinic Proceedings* 85(11): 981–990.

Kelley, A.S., M.C. Reid, D.H. Miller, J.J. Fins, and M.S. Lachs. 2009. Implantable cardioverter-defibrillator deactivation at the end of life: A physician survey, *American Heart Journal* 157(4): 702–708.

Kirklin, J.K., D.C. Naftel, F.D. Pagani, R.L. Kormos, L.W. Stevenson, E.D. Blume, and J.B. Young. 2015. Seventh INTERMACS annual report: 15,000 patients and counting, *Journal of Heart Lung Transplant* 34(12): 1495–1504.

Kramer, D.B., A.S. Kesselheim, L. Salberg, D.W. Brock, and W.H. Maisel. 2011. Ethical and legal views regarding deactivation of cardiac implantable electrical devices in patients with hypertrophic cardiomyopathy, *American Journal of Cardiology* 107(7): 1071–1075.

Lewis, K.B., D. Stacey, and D.D. Matlock. 2014. Making decisions about implantable cardioverter-defibrillators from implantation to end of life: An integrative review of patients' perspectives, *The Patient* 7(3): 243–260.

Marinskis, G., L. van Erven, and EHRA Scientific Initiatives Committee. 2010. Deactivation of implanted cardioverter-defibrillators at the end of life: Results of the EHRA survey, *Europace* 12(8): 1176–1177.

Matlock, D.D., C.T. Nowels, F.A. Masoudi, W.H. Sauer, D.B. Bekelman, D.S. Main, and J.S. Kutner. 2011. Patient and cardiologist perceptions on decision making for implantable cardioverter-defibrillators: A qualitative study. *Pacing and Clinical Electrophysiology* 34(12): 1634–1644.

Mond, H.G., and A. Proclemer. 2011. The 11th world survey of cardiac pacing and implantable cardioverter-defibrillators: Calendar year 2009 — A World Society of Arrhythmia's project. *Pacing and Clinical Electrophysiology* 34(8): 1013–1027.

Morrison, L.J., A.O. Calvin, H. Nora, and S.C. Porter Jr. 2010. Managing cardiac devices near the end of life: A survey of hospice and palliative care providers, *American Journal of Hospice & Palliative Medicine* 27(8): 545–551.

Mueller, P.S., C.C. Hook, and D.L. Hayes. 2003. Ethical analysis of withdrawal of pacemaker or implantable cardioverter-defibrillator support at the end of life, *Mayo Clinic Proceedings* 78(8): 959–963.

Mueller, P.S., S.M. Jenkins, K.A. Bramstedt, and D.L. Hayes. 2008. Deactivating implanted cardiac devices in terminally ill patients: Practices and attitudes, *Pacing and Clinical Electrophysiology* 31(5): 560–568.

Mueller, P.S., K.M. Swetz, M.R. Freeman, K.A. Carter, M.E. Crowley, C.J. Severson, and D.P. Sulmasy. 2010. Ethical analysis of withdrawing ventricular assist device support, *Mayo Clinic Proceedings* 85(9): 791–797.

Olsen, M.L., K.M. Swetz, and P.S. Mueller. 2010. Ethical decision making with end-of-life care: Palliative sedation and withholding or withdrawing life-sustaining treatments, *Mayo Clinic Proceedings* 85(10): 949–954.

Pellegrino, E.D. 2000. Decisions to withdraw life-sustaining treatment: A moral algorithm, *JAMA* 283(8): 1065–1067.

Rose, E.A., A.C. Gelijns, A.J. Moskowitz, D.F. Heitjan, L.W. Stevenson, W. Dembitsky, and P. Meier. 2001. Long-term use of a left ventricular assist device for end-stage heart failure, *New England Journal of Medicine* 345(20): 1435–1443.

Sherazi, S., W. Zareba, J.P. Daubert, S. McNitt, A.H. Shah, M.K. Aktas, and R.C. Block. 2010. Physicians' knowledge and attitudes regarding implantable cardioverter-defibrillators, *Cardiology Journal* 17(3): 267–273.

Snyder Sulmasy, L., P.S. Mueller and Ethics, and Human Rights Committee of the American College of Physicians. 2017. Ethics and the legalization of physician-assisted suicide: An American College of Physicians position paper, *Annals of Internal Medicine* 167(8): 576–578.

Sulmasy, D.P. 1998. Killing and allowing to die: Another look, *Journal of Law, Medicine, and Ethics* 26(1): 55–64, 54.

Sulmasy, D.P. 2008. Within you/without you: Biotechnology, ontology, and ethics, *Journal of General Internal Medicine* 23(Suppl 1): 69–72.

Swetz, K.M., M.D. Barnett, A.H. Kamal, and J.K. Mansel. 2017. Physician aid in dying in the US south: What does the future hold? *Southern Medical Journal* 110(1): 9–10.

Swetz, K.M., and C.C. Hook. 2016. Medical ethics. In: *Mayo Clinic Internal Medicine Board Review*, 11th edition (pp. 331–336), Wittich, C.M. (ed). New York: Oxford University Press.

Swetz, K.M., C.C. Hook, and P.S. Mueller. 2013. Medical ethics. In: *Mayo Clinic Internal Medicine Board Review*, 10th edition (pp. 769–778), Ficalora, R.D. (ed). New York: Oxford University Press.

Swetz, K.M., and A.H. Kamal. 2018. Palliative care, *Annals of Internal Medicine* 168(5): 33–48.

Swetz, K.M., P.S. Mueller, A.L. Ottenberg, C. Dib, M.R. Freeman, and D.P. Sulmasy. 2011. The use of advance directives among patients with left ventricular assist devices, *Hospital Practice* 39(1): 78–84.

Swetz, K.M., A.K. Stanton, and J.S. Lowery. 2017. Surrogate decision making when patients cannot decide within the Veterans Health Administration System, *Journal of Palliative Medicine* 20(10): 1056.

Vacco v. *Quill*, No. 793, 521 (US Supreme Curt 1997).

Vig, E.K., and R.A. Pearlman. 2004. Good and bad dying from the perspective of terminally ill men, *Archives of Internal Medicine* 164(9): 977–981.

Washington v. *Glucksberg*, No. 702, 521 (US Supreme Curt 1997).

Yancy, C.W., M. Jessup, B. Bozkurt, J. Butler, D.E. Casey, M.H. Drazner, and J.L. Januzzi 2013. 2013 ACCF/AHA guideline for the management of heart failure: A report of the American College of Cardiology Foundation/American Heart Association Task Force on Practice Guidelines, *Journal of the American College of Cardiology* 62(16): e147–e239.

Part III

Allocation of Expensive/ Scarce Resources

6 Cardiac Implantable Electronic Device Reuse

Ethical Considerations and Enhancing Awareness

Behzad Pavri

I Case Scenario

Mr. JK, a 69-year-old man with sick sinus syndrome, who is easily fatigued related to chronotropic incompetence, underwent rate-responsive dual chamber (DDDR) pacemaker implantation in 2005 in Philadelphia. In 2014, nine years later, his pacemaker reached replacement voltage and he underwent generator replacement. When seen in follow-up four weeks later, it was evident that he had unfortunately developed a pocket infection; purulent material was expressed from the incision. He was admitted and administered IV antibiotics; blood cultures did not show any growth, and there was no evidence of systemic infection. He underwent pacing system extraction with removal of his pacemaker (which was one month old) and his leads (which required laser extraction). A week later, a new pacing system was implanted from the opposite shoulder without complications. *His one-month-old, rate-responsive, $6,000 explanted pacemaker was tossed in the trash.*

On the other side of the globe, in a small town in central India, SK, a 58-year-old man has experienced extreme fatigue and recurrent syncope/presyncope for the past eight months. After raising sufficient funds, he was able to travel to Mumbai to be seen at a cardiology clinic, where he was recognized as being in high-grade atrioventricular block with episodes of complete heart block and a wide-QRS escape. He was recognized as having cardiac sarcoidosis. A pacemaker was recommended, but he had no financial means to afford such an intervention. He was assessed by the social workers and nurses as being the correct patient to receive a re-sterilized pacemaker from their "Device Bank". The implanting physician donated his time, the hospital donated the operating room time, and a local pacemaker manufacturer donated a single pacing lead. He underwent implantation of a VVI pacing system (a DDD re-sterilized pacemaker with the atrial port plugged).

II Background

Advances in medical technology have translated into significant gains in reduction of human suffering with improvements in the quality and duration of

DOI: 10.4324/9781003240273-10

human life. In terms of life-prolonging technology, few inventions can parallel the cardiac pacemaker and implantable cardioverter-defibrillator, collectively referred to as Cardiac Implantable Electronic Devices (CIEDs). Pacemakers and implantable cardioverter-defibrillators are electronic devices that are surgically implanted by a small operation into patients with rhythm disturbances. The device itself, also called the pulse generator, is located under skin in the shoulder region, and is connected to the heart by transvenously placed leads. The leads are securely anchored to the pectoralis major, and then connected to the pulse generator header via set screws. At the time of replacement of the generator (whether for battery depletion or for device upgrade), the wires are typically not replaced, unless there is a lead-related problem (fracture, infection, etc.).

From an evolutionary perspective, human beings are the only species that "outlive" their projected life expectancy, based on allometric scales using resting heart rates, and it is postulated that advances in medicine (such as lifestyle changes, antibiotics, immunizations and CIEDs) have been contributory factors (Levine, 1997); however, these life-prolonging advances are not widely available in all parts of the globe. While the prevalence and mortality associated with cardiovascular disease is declining in developed nations, it is expected to increase in the developing nations of the world (Joshi, Jan, Wu, and MacMahon, 2008). As Aristotle pithily noted in 330 BC:

> Health of body and mind is so fundamental to the good life that if we believe men have any personal rights at all as human beings, they have an absolute right to such a measure of good health as society and society alone is able to give them.
>
> (Quoted in Tulchinsky and Varavikova, 2000, 56)

He sagely recognized society's role in providing this inalienable right.

III The Ethics of Inequitable Healthcare Availability Around the World

Although disparities exist in many areas of healthcare, none are as glaringly evident as in the rates of CIED utilization around the world. CIED implantation rates vary by orders of magnitude from less than 10 per million population to greater than 430 per million between developed and developing nations (Mond and Proclemer, 2011). The rates of CIED utilization are increasing rapidly in developed countries (Greenspon, Patel, Lau, Ochoa, Frisch, Ho, Pavri, and Kurtz, 2012), and this disparity of utilization rates is only likely to diverge further. These discrepancies are primarily related to the cost of such life-saving therapy, with available money being allocated to endeavors that deliver greater benefits (such as preventing and treating diarrhea in children, providing clean drinking water, and combating infectious diseases) in countries with limited resources. The most expensive CIEDs (implantable cardioverter-defibrillators) are afforded only by the richest minority in developing countries (Groh, 2012). Although arguments have been made that medical evidence rather than cost should guide CIED implantation (Delacretaz, Schlaepfer, Metzger, Fromer, and Kappenberger, 2000), these arguments may not be applicable to low- and middle-income nations, and the difficult socioeconomic conditions in these nations are unlikely to change substantially in the near future. It is estimated that more than one million patients die annually from bradycardia due to the lack of a pacemaker (Mond, Mick, and Maniscalco, 2009); some estimates put the number as high as three million.[1] By comparison, it is estimated that an average of 29,916 (range 4,310 to 63,329) persons die annually in the United States from influenza (estimates include influenza-associated deaths with both underlying pneumonia and with respiratory/circulatory causes).[2] Another comparison would be mortality from HIV/AIDS: according to the World Health Organization, an estimated 1.6 million people died of HIV/AIDS in 2012.[3] Death from bradycardia, it must be remembered, is eminently preventable. Finally, how can one reconcile the shift from the "beneficence model" to an emphasis on "patient autonomy"—a central tenet of today's medical ethics, with its emphasis on informed consent—with the complete lack of availability, let alone consenting choice, for patients in dire need of CIEDs in developing nations?

IV Medical, Practical, and Ethical Concerns Regarding Implanting Used CIEDs

There is a long history of re-sterilization and reuse of devices that are officially labeled as "Single Use Devices" (Cohoon, 2002; Dunn, 2002a, 2002b; Shuman and Chenoweth, 2012). Appropriately, much has been written about the many legitimate concerns about providing used CIEDs to poorer populations of patients.

(1) *Why should some patients, simply by virtue of socioeconomic status, get re-sterilized CIEDs?*

This has been referred to as the "taint of the second hand" by some (Farmer and Bukhman, 2012), and parallels have been drawn to the use of substandard or fake medications in underdeveloped nations, mainly antimicrobials (Fernandez, Hostetler, Powell, Kaur, Green, Mildenhall, and Newton, 2011). However, this is not an accurate analogy, since re-sterilized CIEDs are not "fake" CIEDs. Furthermore, reuse of other classes of medical devices (including surgical instruments, electrophysiology catheters, endoscopes, etc.) is sanctioned worldwide.

(2) *What are the risks of infection associated with re-sterilized, as compared to new CIEDs?*

A word on re-sterilization: There is now a substantial body of data derived from European nations (France, Sweden, Germany, Italy, Netherlands, Norway), North America (Canada, United States), Central America (Nicaragua), Africa (Nigeria) and Asia (India), and dating from 1976 to the current era, all of which confirm that explanted CIEDs can be safely re-sterilized, as evidenced by very low (<2%) rates of infectious complications after re-implantation (Havia and Schuller, 1978; Amikam, Feldman, Boal, Riss, and Neufeld, 1983; Rosengarten, Portnoy, Chiu, and Peterson, 1985; Mugica, Duconge, and Henry, 1986; Linde, Bocray, Jonsson, Rosenqvist, Radegran, and Ryden, 1998; Namboodiri, Sharma, Bali, and Grover, 2004; Baman, Romero, Kirkpatrick, Romero, and Lange, 2009; Hasan et al., 2011; Kantharia, Patel, Kulkarni, Shah, Lokhandwala, Mascarenhas, and Mascarenhas, 2012; Pavri, Lokhandwala, Kulkarni, Shah, Kantharia, and Mascarenhas, 2012; Nava, Morales, Márquez, Barrera, and Gómez, 2013). Modern sterilization techniques can destroy all microbial organisms, including viruses and spores. Concerns were raised about the inability effectively to sterilize non-metal parts such as the plastic header and the silicone grommets where the set screws reside, but all of the available data suggest that infectious issues are no different with reused CIEDs as compared to new CIEDs. Cleaning the header, especially the lead ports with pipe cleaners, is also of concern for implantable cardioverter-defibrillators, if the device is not turned off, for fear of inadvertent shock delivery during cleaning. Cleaning of the seam between the header and the body of the device may require special attention. Various re-sterilization protocols have been described, but essential steps include manual cleaning of all visible material, use of disinfectants (such as dimethlybenzyl ammonium chloride, formaldehyde, glutaraldehyde, povidone-iodone, isopropyl alcohol, phenoxypropanol/benzalconiumchloride solution, and hydrogen peroxide) and then repackaging with indicator strips for ethylene oxide gas sterilization.[4]

(3) *What are the risks of re-sterilized CIED malfunction and premature battery depletion compared to new CIEDs?*
   The majority of available data suggest that there is no significant increase in CIED malfunction (Nava, Morales, Márquez, Barrera, and Gómez, 2013). One meta-analysis (Baman et al., 2011) concluded that reused CIEDs did carry a greater risk of malfunction compared to new CIEDs (odds ratio, 5.80 [1.93 to 17.47], P = 0.002), and that this was mainly driven by abnormalities in set screws, which possibly occurred during device extraction, as well as nonspecific device "technical errors." This relatively higher odds ratio of "device malfunction" was driven by 8/793 vs. 5/2200 events accumulated from four trials from 1989, 1993, 1998 and 2003, and is not clinically worrisome enough to negate the potentially very significant benefits in terms of improved quality of life and mortality reduction in patients who undergo re-sterilized pacemaker implantation (Hughey, Baman, Eagle, and Crawford, 2013). As expected, almost all studies that have reported on longitudinal follow-up of recipients of re-sterilized CIEDs have noted shorter battery life, and this is directly proportional to the duration of device use in the first recipient. This reduction in battery life with reuse is expected, unavoidable, and acceptable, but is not to be trivialized, knowing that device replacements are associated with greater risks (Poole et al., 2010). This

information should lead to careful pairing of the appropriate reused device to the appropriate patient, after consideration of age, co-morbidities, and life expectancy. After all, clinical judgments are regularly exercised in pairing recipients to donor hearts for the purposes of orthotopic cardiac transplantation.

(4) *What is the "second shelf life" for explanted CIEDs, before they are re-implanted in the second recipient, and how well do such devices handle the rigors of transport and re-sterilization?*

There is very little data published regarding the "second shelf life" of explanted devices before they are re-implanted in the second recipient. From an engineering perspective, there is minimal battery drain when the device is not connected to any leads (an "open circuit"), except for the minimal battery drain for "housekeeping" currents and accumulation of data for counters and motion. Such drain could be further minimized by programming CIEDs to the ODO or OVO modes (pacing "OFF"). The battery drain for implantable cardioverter-defibrillators, even when programmed to the "No Therapy" mode, is still significant, because of the need for periodic capacitor reformation; each capacitor reformation reduces projected battery life by about 24 days, and 18 months of shelf time reduces overall battery life by 6.5% (personal communication, Medtronic Tachysupport). Only one study reported that the mean time from explant to re-implant was 374.0 days, with a range of 21 to 1,885 days, and this was an implantable cardioverter-defibrillator reuse study (Pavri, Lokhandwala, Kulkarni, Shah, Kantharia, and Mascarenhas, 2012). These considerations suggest that for the majority of devices, even long "second shelf life" times are not prohibitive for CIED reuse.

Regarding the mode of transportation to recipient nations, again there is virtually no detail provided in the published data, except for one study that describes how the explanted implantable cardioverter-defibrillators were transported in the personal luggage of the traveling physicians. Luggage is typically stored in the hold of a commercial aircraft, where temperatures can drop to about 45°F;[5] however, these devices continued to function normally after they were re-implanted (Pavri, Lokhandwala, Kulkarni, Shah, Kantharia, and Mascarenhas, 2012).

(5) *What are the medicolegal liabilities for the "donating" patient, the implanting physician, and the manufacturer?*

Without doubt, this is the most complicated issue that continues to cloud CIED reuse, although many clear-thinking individuals have proposed transparent guidelines to clear the way for future efforts. A major hurdle to expanded reuse of CIEDs will be to determine whether it should remain a purely charitable effort, or whether "discounted", "pro-rated", or "subsidized" pricing should be allowed. From my point of view, the answer to this question is clear: this effort should remain purely charitable, and commercialization should be robustly resisted. Financial motives would seem to negate the very purpose of this effort. This author firmly believes that grace, generosity of spirit, and political savvy—not profit— should prevail (Pavri, Lokhandwala, Kulkarni, Shah, Kantharia, and Mascarenhas, 2012).

However, the alternate view needs to be considered carefully as well. Market forces and the potential for profit, if allowed to intercede (one might argue that this is inevitable), would likely accelerate CIED reuse more quickly to a commercial scale, and formal pathways of CIED retrieval, re- sterilization, repackaging, and transport would quickly become available. One can then conceive of pro-rated pricing of CIEDs based on remaining battery longevity. This would likely result in dissemination of reused CIEDs far more rapidly than any charitable effort can achieve. Not only would this achieve more widespread distribution of life-saving medical technology, but would also achieve the ever-elusive goal of cost containment in today's healthcare environment. Of course, a commercialized process would require official sanction, something that is currently not likely. Such official sanction would likely require a large prospective trial with careful follow-up for an extended period showing the safety of re-sterilized CIEDs, and such a trial would likely be robustly resisted by the CIED manufacturers and frowned upon by the FDA, even if it were conducted outside the United States.

Informed consent, from both the first and the second recipients, would be an absolute requirement, and would address many medico-legal issues. Many have proposed (and implemented) pacemaker donation forms or a "device will" to be signed by the first recipient.[6] Such a document would clearly allow the "gifting" of a CIED (which becomes the patient's "prop- erty" once implanted) for potential reuse after the first recipient's demise, or after removal for upgrade or infection. The law should free the donors (first recipient and his or her family), the device manufacturers, and the re- sterilization facility of any liability for reused CIEDs. The recipient must have the re-sterilized nature of the donated CIED fully explained to them in their native language, and sign a consent form that describes all known and possible unknown risks in detail. It could be argued that if the effort eventually becomes commercial, the facility responsible for re-sterilization could be held liable for any breach in protocol, but this is open to debate, and might occur within a fully charitable process as well.

(6) *Who provides for the leads, since the leads cannot be reused?*
All are agreed that reuse of CIED lead(s) is not an option. However, with the exception of the latest generation of subcutaneous implantable cardioverter-defibrillators and the leadless pacemakers, the vast majority of today's CIEDs require leads. There have been multiple innovative channels used to obtain such leads for recipients of reused CIEDS. Some leads (especially those made by indigenous manufacturers) are paid for by the recipients and their families, some are donated by manufacturers, and others are provided free by the implanting hospital. The establishment of a "trust" to cover lead expenses has been proposed.

(7) *What follow-up programs and data-tracking mechanisms are available for recipients of reused CIEDs?*

Currently, no such mechanisms have been established. Follow-up data are difficult to obtain in developing nations for a multiplicity of reasons. Record keeping may not be computerized, paper charts are poorly maintained, data collection is specious or worse, and patients sometimes possess their own medical records. However, if CIED reuse is to be confirmed to be safe and effective in a systematic manner, then careful data collection and reporting will be mandatory, and would go a long way in making widespread CIED reuse a reality.

V   Potential Sources of CIEDs for Reuse

A   Battery Performance of Current Generation of CIEDs and Survival of CIED Recipients—The Potential for Post-Mortem CIED Retrieval

Today's CIEDs have outstanding battery longevity, with a cardiac pacemaker lasting greater than 10 years (up to 14 years) and an implantable cardioverter-defibrillator greater than 7 years (up to 10 years, depending on the number of leads, the percentage of pacing, and the number of high voltage therapies delivered). As life-prolonging as this technology is, significant percentages of CIED recipients die from advanced age and/or co-morbidities well before the CIED battery is consumed, and such devices often have substantial remaining serviceable battery life after the patient's demise. Older data suggested that 40% of patients die within four years after pacemaker implantation (Pyatt et al., 2002). More recent data estimate that 34.4% of pacemaker recipients die within five years of implantation (Brunner, Olschewski, Geibel, Bode, and Zehender, 2004). Another study presented in 2013 at the European Society of Cardiology meetings reported that 31% of pacemaker recipients were dead within five years of device implantation. Similar data regarding life expectancy after implantable cardioverter-defibrillator implantation are harder to find, since the mix of patients who receive implantable cardioverter-defibrillators is more diverse. One study reported that 25% of patients were dead within five years of implantable cardioverter-defibrillators implantation (Hauser, 2005). Analysis from the National Cardiovascular Data Registry showed that 42.2% of patients were dead within five years of implantable cardioverter-defibrillators generator replacement. Finally, more than 20% of all implantable cardioverter-defibrillators and CRT-D devices are implanted in patients who are older than 80 years of age (Swindle, Rich, McCann, Burroughs, and Hauptman, 2010).

After death, implanted CIEDs are routinely removed by funeral homes before cremation (to prevent explosions) (Pitcher, Soar, Hogg, the CIED Working Group, et al., 2016) and sometimes before burial; cremation rates have been steadily increasing and are projected to exceed 50% by 2025 in the United States (Cremation Association of America, 2014). These devices are collected, discarded, or returned to the decedent's family members. Available data suggest that about 20 to 33% of devices retrieved from funeral homes may have sufficient remaining battery life to allow reuse (Baman et al., 2012). Furthermore, both morticians and patients (including veterans in the United States) are open to the idea of device retrieval after demise (Kirkpatrick, Ghani, Burke, and Knight, 2007; Gakenheimer et al., 2011; Iyer and Mackall, 2013) with greater than 85% acceptance. Thus, systematic post-mortem retrieval, if legalized and sanctioned, would be the largest source for reusable CIEDs.

B Patients Undergoing Upgrade, Device Removal for Infection, Orthotopic Cardiac Transplantation or Autopsy in the Hospital

Many implantable cardioverter-defibrillators are explanted for upgrades or because of infections, although, once again, precise numbers are unavailable. Recent data suggest that rates of infection are increasing as patient comorbidities increase (Greenspon, Patel, Lau, Ochoa, Frisch, Ho, Pavri, and Kurtz, 2011). One study from a large teaching hospital reported that 8% of autopsies were on patients with CIEDs, and 30% of these devices had four years or more of remaining battery longevity (Zamani, Kirkpatrick, Litzky, and Verdino, 2012). As expected, such devices often have substantial remaining battery life (Hanzlik, Patel, Kurtz, Pavri, Greenspon, and Ochoa, 2011), but are either stored locally, discarded, or sometimes returned to the manufacturer for product analysis (Logani, Gottlieb, Verdino, Baman, Eagle, and Kirkpatrick, 2011); a small number are donated for veterinary use (Nelson, Lahmers, Schneider, and Thompson, 2006).

C Expired Product and Industry Donation

Currently, there is no public knowledge about the percentage of CIEDs that expire "on shelf", and what happens to such products. Personal inquiries with each manufacturer were met with vague responses, but on average, from less than 1% to 3% of product expires prior to utilization. Some portion of this product is either discarded, or used for training/research/veterinarian use, but the exact numbers remain unknown.

In summary, these data imply that potentially thousands of CIEDs could be harvested annually for reuse, and that there are at least three sources for CIED retrieval that could be systematically explored: (1) from funeral homes after patient demise, (2) electrophysiology laboratories that perform upgrades and device removal for infection, and (3) expired product/donations from industry (see Tables 6.1, 6.2 and 6.3).

Table 6.1 Enhancing Awareness in Donor (Developed) Nations

Patients
- "Device Living Will": A discussion to be had at the time of initial implantable cardioverter-defibrillator implantation and at generator replacement; involve families in discussion. Surveys have shown that patient acceptance of the idea of device donation is high, and this is not likely to be the major hurdle.

Physician "Mind Set"
- Develop a view that includes "global health equity"
- Enhance knowledge of immense disparities in device utilization in different nations
- Be willing to discuss device capture for reuse with their patients
- Be willing to process/transport explanted devices

Physician Education: Be Aware of the Available Data
- Risk of infectious complications is similar in new and reused CIEDs
- Modern pacemakers have battery longevity of ≈9–11 years
- Modern implantable cardioverter-defibrillators have battery longevity of ≈6–8 years
- Most CIEDs removed for upgrades/infectious reasons have substantial remaining battery life
- Explanted devices can be safely and completely re-sterilized—multiple re-sterilization "schemes" published
- Devices can withstand the rigors of re-sterilization

Funeral Home Directors/Morticians
- Data show that the majority of morticians are in favor of explanting and returning devices. Although all cremated patients must have CIEDs removed for fear of battery explosions during heating, burial does not require CIED explanation. Morticians must remove all CIEDs prior to burial, if appropriate consent exists.
- Morticians must be informed to contact physician or manufacturer before implantable cardioverter-defibrillator removal for fear of electric shocks when implantable cardioverter-defibrillator leads are cut
- Morticians need legal protection and increased awareness of "Device living will" in order to retrieve and transport explanted devices
- Standardized means of device transportation from funeral home to physicians to re-sterilization facility need to be established

---

Table 6.2 Legal Considerations in Donor Countries

- Liability concerns are the driving force that limit device reuse, and will need to be addressed first
- New laws should render donating patients, retrieving physicians, and device manufacturers free of liability
- Include specific, legally vetted statements within the device will
- Funeral homes should be freed from liability and mandated to retrieve and collect devices from deceased patients with signed device wills
- Heart Rhythm Society should NOT mandate that all explanted devices be returned to manufacturer (Carlson et al., 2006)
- Rather, HRS/AHA/ACC/ESC should endorse device reuse

Table 6.3 International/Laws

- Seek philanthropic support for costs of device reprogramming, re-sterilization, and transportation
- Transportation of devices needs to follow standardized, accepted protocols, be it courier/hand-carried/postal services
- Whether to, and how to, insure contents needs to be addressed
- Devices must be transported in accordance to customs laws, which may need to be altered, so as to avoid confiscation of devices at port of entry

---

VI A Prospective, FDA-Sanctioned Trial Is Awaited!

The "My-Heart, Your-Heart" project,[7] spearheaded by Drs. Crawford, Baman, Eagle, J. Romero, Sovitch, and A. Romero, with L. Gakenheimer, from the University of Michigan Health System has been an ongoing effort. These investigators have collected more than 10,000 CIEDs. Used CIEDs with a substantial battery will be sterilized by a commercial vendor and shipped to recipient investigators in Mexico, Philippines, Vietnam, Nicaragua, Pakistan, and Bolivia. Careful data collection and systematic follow up are planned. The study awaits final FDA approval to launch.

VII Conclusions

Ultimately, the guiding consideration should be that access to a reused CIED is better than no access to such devices, when faced with substantial mortality and morbidity from preventable causes such as heart block and ventricular fibrillation. Whereas most of the available data already strongly suggest comparable outcomes between new and re-sterilized CIEDs, there is relatively less data on equity of access, which must be the first step. Such considerations have led to calls for reappraisals of labeling CIEDs (Rosengarten, Portnoy, Chiu, and Peterson, 1985; Pantos, Efstathopoulos, and Katritsis, 2013).

Based on available data, mortality of "doing nothing" far exceeds any possible mortality associated with device reuse. This is borne out by the "appropriate use rate" of reused devices (more than 54% over 2.3 years) (Pavri, Lokhandwala, Kulkarni, Shah, Kantharia, and Mascarenhas, 2012), which far exceeds that in US populations. Individuals or groups of physicians will continue their independent efforts to send CIEDs overseas—an important, but ultimately a very small effort. Systematic CIED reuse will require collaboration with patients, funeral homes/morticians, physicians, nonprofit charitable organizations, and the FDA. Hopefully, robust data from prospective trials will become available, and free reused devices from the "taint of the secondhand."

Notes

1 https://www.heartbeatsaveslives.org/pdf/2009%20HBI%20Annual%20Report.pdf (last accessed on September 09, 2021).
2 http://www.cdc.gov/mmwr/preview/mmwrhtml/mm5933a1.htm (last accessed on September 09, 2021).

3 http://aids.gov/federal-resources/around-the-world/global-aids-overview/ (last accessed on September 09, 2021).

4 Since the initial writing of this chapter, a large, registry-based report on re-sterilized devices had been published. They concluded: "Among patients in under-served countries who received a resterilized and reused pacemaker or defibrillator, the incidence of infection or device-related death at 2 years was 2.0%, an incidence that did not differ significantly from that seen among matched control patients with new devices in Canada" (Khairy et al., 2020, p. 1823).

5 https://www.google.com/webhp?sourceid=chrome-instant&rlz=1C1FLDB_ enUS573US582&ion=1&espv=2&ie=UTF-8#q=what%20is%20the%20temperature%20 in%20the%20baggage%20hold%20of%20an%20airplane (last accessed September 09, 2021).

6 See, for example, http://media.wix.com/ugd/fd17a5_e40ad552a5f247b1a8911d-b9b732466b.pdf (last accessed on July 12, 2014) and http://www.myheartyourheart. org/ (last accessed on September 09, 2021).

7 See http://www.myheartyourheart.org/ (last accessed on September 09, 2021).

References

Amikam, S., S. Feldman, B. Boal, E. Riss, and H. Neufeld. 1983. Long-term followup of patients with re-used implanted pacemakers. In: *Cardiac pacing. Proceedings of the VIIIth World Symposium on Cardiac Pacing* (pp. 491–493). Steinbach, K., D. Glogan, A. Laszkovics, W. Scheibelhofer, and H. Weber (eds). Darmstadt: Steinkopff-Verlag-Darmstadt.

Baman, T.S., T. Crawford, P. Sovitch, P. Meier, N. Sovitch, and L. Gakenheimer et al. 2012. Feasibility of postmortem device acquisition for potential reuse in underserved nations, *Heart Rhythm* 9(2): 211–214.

Baman, T.S., P. Meier, J. Romero, L. Gakenheimer, and J.N. Kirkpatrick et al. 2011. Safety of pacemaker reuse: A meta-analysis with implications for underserved nations, *Circulation, Arrhythmia and Electrophysiology* 4(3): 318–323.

Baman, T.S., A. Romero, J.N. Kirkpatrick, J. Romero, and D.C. Lange et al. 2009. Safety and efficacy of pacemaker reuse in underdeveloped nations: A case series, *Journal of the American College of Cardiology* 54(16): 1557–1558.

Brunner, M., M. Olschewski, A. Geibel, C. Bode, and M. Zehender. 2004. Long-term survival after pacemaker implantation: Prognostic importance of gender and baseline patient characteristics, *European Heart Journal* 25(1): 88–95.

Carlson, M.D., B.L. Wilkoff, and W.H. Maisel et al. 2006. Recommendations from the Heart Rhythm Society Task Force on Device Performance Policies and Guidelines: Endorsed by the American College of Cardiology Foundation (ACCF) and the American Heart Association (AHA) and the International Coalition of Pacing and Electrophysiology Organizations (COPE), *Heart Rhythm* 3(10): 1250–1273.

Cohoon, B.D. 2002. Reprocessing single-use medical devices, *AORN Journal* 75(3): 557–567.

Cremation Association of North America. 2014 http://www.cremationassociation. org/?page=IndustryStatistics. (Accessed July 7, 2014.)

Delacretaz, E., J. Schlaepfer, J. Metzger, M. Fromer, and L. Kappenberger. 2000. Evidence rather than costs must guide use of the implantable cardioverter defibrillator, *American Journal of Cardiology* 86 (suppl. 9): 52K–57K.

Dunn, D. 2002a. Reprocessing single-use devices - Regulatory roles, *AORN Journal* 76(1): 100–127.

Dunn, D. 2002b. Reprocessing single-use devices - The ethical dilemma, *AORN Journal* 75(5): 989–999.

Farmer, P., and G. Bukhman. 2012. Reuse of medical devices and global health equity, *Annals of Internal Medicine* 157(8): 591–592.

Fernandez, F.M., D. Hostetler, K. Powell, H. Kaur, M.D. Green, D.C. Mildenhall, and P.N. Newton. 2011. Poor quality drugs: Grand challenges in high throughput detection, countrywide sampling, and forensics in developing countries, *The Analyst* 136(15): 3073–3082.

Gakenheimer, L., D.C. Lange, J. Romero, J.N. Kirkpatrick, and P. Sovitch et al. 2011. Societal views of pacemaker reutilization for those with untreated symptomatic bradycardia in underserved nations, *Journal of Interventional Cardiac Electrophysiology* 30: 261–266.

Greenspon, A.J., J.D. Patel, E. Lau, J.A. Ochoa, D.R. Frisch, R.T. Ho, B.B. Pavri, and S.M. Kurtz. 2011. 16-year trends in the infection burden for pacemakers and implantable cardioverter-defibrillators in the United States: 1993–2008, *Journal of the American College of Cardiology* 58(10): 1001–1006.

Greenspon, A.J., J.D. Patel, E. Lau, J.A. Ochoa, D.R. Frisch, R.T. Ho, B.B. Pavri, and S.M. Kurtz 2012. Trends in permanent pacemaker implantation in the United States from 1993 to 2009: Increasing complexity of patients and procedures, *Journal of the American College of Cardiology* 60(16): 1540–1545.

Groh, W.J. 2012. You shouldn't take it with you: Postmortem device reuse, *Heart Rhythm* 9(2): 215–216.

Hanzlik, J., J. Patel, S. Kurtz, B.B. Pavri, A.J. Greenspon, and J. Ochoa. 2011. *Insights into cardiac pacemaker and defibrillator revision/upgrades. Bioengineering Conference (NEBEC), IEEE 37th Annual Northeast,* April 1–3, 2011. doi:10.1109/NEBEC.2011.5778519.

Hasan, R., H. Ghanbari, D. Feldman, D. Menesses, D. Rivas, N.C. Zakhem, and C. Duarte et al. 2011. Safety, efficacy and performance of implanted recycled cardiac rhythm management (CRM) devices in underprivileged patients, *Pacing and Clinical Electrophysiology* 34(6): 653–658.

Hauser, R.G. 2005. The growing mismatch between patient longevity and the service life of implantable cardioverter-defibrillators, *Journal of the American College of Cardiology* 45(12): 2022–2025.

Havia, T., and H. Schuller. 1978. The re-use of previously implanted pacemakers, *Scandinavian Journal of Thoracic and Cardiovascular Surgery* 22(suppl. 22): 33–34.

Hughey, A.B., T.S. Baman, K.A. Eagle, and T.C. Crawford. 2013. Pacemaker reuse: An initiative to help those in underserved nations in need of life-saving device therapy, *Expert Review of Medical Devices* 10(5): 577–579.

Iyer, I.R., and J. Mackall. 2013. Patient preferences regarding device reuse and potential of devices for reuse - A study in a veteran population, *Indian Pacing and Electrophysiology Journal* 13(3): 101–108.

Joshi, R., S. Jan, Y. Wu, and S. MacMahon. 2008. Global inequalities in access to cardiovascular health care: Our greatest challenge, *Journal of the American College of Cardiology* 52(23): 1817–1825.

Kantharia, B.K., S.S. Patel, G. Kulkarni, A.N. Shah, Y. Lokhandwala, E. Mascarenhas, and D.A. Mascarenhas. 2012. Reuse of explanted permanent pacemakers donated by funeral homes, *American Journal of Cardiology* 109(2): 238–240.

Khairy, T.F., M.-A. Lupien, S. Nava et al. 2020. Infections associated with resterilized pacemakers and defibrillators. *The New England Journal of Medicine* 382(19): 1823–1831.

Kirkpatrick, J., S.N. Ghani, M.C. Burke, and B.P. Knight. 2007. Postmortem interrogation and retrieval of implantable pacemakers and defibrillators: A survey of morticians and patients, *Journal of Cardiovascular Electrophysiology* 18(5): 478–482.

Levine, H.J. 1997. Rest heart rate and life expectancy, *Journal of the American College of Cardiology* 30(4): 1104–1106.

Linde, C.L., A. Bocray, H. Jonsson, M. Rosenqvist, K. Radegran, and L. Ryden. 1998. Re-used pacemakers — As safe as new? A retrospective case-control study. *European Heart Journal* 19(1): 154–157.

Logani, S., M. Gottlieb, R.J.Verdino, T.S. Baman, K.A. Eagle, and J.N. Kirkpatrick. 2011. Recovery of pacemakers and defibrillators for analysis and device advance directives: Electrophysiologists' perspectives, *Pacing and Clinical Electrophysiology* 34(6): 659–665.

Mond, H.G.,W. Mick, and B.S. Maniscalco. 2009. Heartbeat international: Making "poor" hearts beat better, *Heart Rhythm* 6(10): 1538–1540.

Mond, H.G., and A. Proclemer. 2011. The 11th world survey of cardiac pacing and implantable cardioverter-defibrillators: Calendar year 2009—a World Society of Arrhythmia's project. *Pacing and Clinical Electrophysiology* 34(8): 1013–1027.

Mugica, J., R. Duconge, and L. Henry. 1986. Survival and mortality in 3,701 pacemaker patients: Arguments in favor of pacemaker reuse, *Pacing and Clinical Electrophysiology* 9(6 pt 2): 1282–1287.

Namboodiri, K.K.N.,Y.P. Sharma, H.K. Bali, and A. Grover. 2004. Re-use of explanted DDD pacemakers as VDD-clinical utility and cost effectiveness, *Indian Pacing Electrophysiology Journal* 4(1): 3–9.

Nava, S., J.L. Morales, M.F. Márquez, F. Barrera, and J. Gómez et al. 2013. Reuse of pacemakers: Comparison of short and long-term performance, *Circulation* 127(11): 1177–1183.

Nelson, O.L., S. Lahmers, T. Schneider, and P.Thompson. 2006. The use of an implantable cardioverter defibrillator in a Boxer Dog to control clinical signs of arrhythmogenic right ventricular cardiomyopathy, *Journal of Veterinary Internal Medicine* 20(5): 1232–1237.

Pantos, I., E.P. Efstathopoulos, and D.G. Katritsis. 2013. Reuse of devices in cardiology: Time for a reappraisal, *Hellenic Journal Cardiology* 54: 376–381.

Pavri, B.B.,Y. Lokhandwala, G.V. Kulkarni, M. Shah, B.K. Kantharia, and D.A. Mascarenhas. 2012. Reuse of explanted, resterilized implantable cardioverter-defibrillators: A cohort study, *Annals of Internal Medicine* 157(8): 542–548.

Pitcher, D., J. Soar, K. Hogg, the CIED Working Group, et al. 2016. Cardiovascular implanted electronic devices in people towards the end of life, during cardiopulmonary resuscitation and after death: Guidance from the Resuscitation Council (UK), British Cardiovascular Society and National Council for Palliative Care. *Heart* 102: A1–A17.

Poole, J.E., M.J. Gleva, T. Mela, M.K. Chung, and D.Z. Uslan et al. 2010. Complication rates associated with pacemaker or implantable cardioverter-defibrillator generator replacements and upgrade procedures: Results from the REPLACE Registry, *Circulation* 122(16): 1553–1561.

Pyatt, J.R., J.D. Somauroo, and M. Jackson et al. 2002. Long-term survival after permanent pacemaker implantation: Analysis of predictors for increased mortality, *Europace* 4(2): 113–119.

Rosengarten, M.D., D. Portnoy, R.C.J. Chiu, and A.K. Peterson. 1985. Reuse of permanent cardiac pacemakers, *Canadian Medical Association Journal* 133(4): 279–283.

Shuman, E.K., and C.E. Chenoweth. 2012. Reuse of medical devices: Implications for infection control, *Infectious Disease Clinics of North America* 26 (1): 165–172.

Swindle, J.P., M.W. Rich, P. McCann, T.E. Burroughs, and P.J. Hauptman. 2010. Implantable cardiac device procedures in older patients: Use and in-hospital outcomes, *Archives of Internal Medicine* 170(7): 631–637.

Tulchinsky, T., and E.A.Varavikova. 2000. *The new public health: An introduction for the 21st century*. New York: Academic Press.

Zamani, P., J.N. Kirkpatrick, L.A. Litzky, and R.J.Verdino. 2012. Longevity of implantable electrophysiology devices explanted from patients having autopsy in hospitals, *American Journal of Cardiology* 110(11): 1643–1645.

7 Just Distribution of Cardiovascular Resources

The Left Ventricular Assist Device

David M. Zientek and Kayhan Parsi

I Introduction

Congestive heart failure is a major cause of morbidity and mortality worldwide. In the United States, it is estimated that there are currently 5.7 million patients with heart failure with a projected increase to 8 million by 2030 (Savarese and Lund, 2017). For those patients with reduced systolic function and refractory symptoms despite optimal medical therapy, cardiac transplantation remains the "gold standard" of treatment. Candidates for transplantation typically must meet age requirements and be sufficiently healthy; only around 2,200 patients a year receive transplantation in the United States due to these requirements and the limited availability of donor hearts (Miller and Guglin, 2013). In the early 1960s, the National Heart Lung and Blood Institute (NHLBI) initiated a program to develop an artificial heart for such patients (Institute of Medicine, 1991). While a device completely able to replace the failing heart has not yet become practical, the program has led to the development of a more limited but useful technology, the left ventricular assist device (LVAD), which has revolutionized the care of patients with advanced systolic failure.

The LVAD is a pump surgically implanted in the patient's chest to assist the failing heart in providing adequate blood flow to the patient's other organs. The device is attached through the chest wall to an external battery. The cost of initial implantation of these devices in one recent study was greater than $175,000 (Shreibati et al., 2017). While there have been significant improvements since they were first introduced for clinical use, potentially devastating and costly complications remain. These include stroke, bleeding and thrombosis or infection of the device (Estep et al., 2015; Pinney et al., 2017). The devices were initially indicated for temporary placement in patients expected to recover from an acute reversible illness, or as a "bridge" to transplantation in patients awaiting a suitable donor heart. In 2003, however, Medicare approved the use of LVADs as a "destination," or permanent, therapy for patients who were not candidates for transplantation by virtue of their age or co-morbidities (Hernandez et al., 2008). Between 2009 and 2014 the annual number of hospitalizations with implantation of an LVAD increased from 2,205 to 3,645, with the annual associated cost increasing from about $400 million to

DOI: 10.4324/9781003240273-11

approximately $800 million. Medicare and Medicaid covered over half of these costs (Patel et al., 2018).

Given this background, several questions about the just distribution of this expensive technology arise. At the "macro" societal level, given the high cost of these devices, is taxpayer funding of such a large program a wise use of resources? If so, is it reasonable to provide these devices to Medicare recipients by virtue of their insurance coverage while denying the technology to younger patients who may be uninsured or underinsured, but are more likely to survive longer with destination therapy, or at least long enough to undergo transplantation? At the "micro" level, how can local healthcare systems and hospitals justly apportion such expensive technologies, especially to patients who may not have insurance coverage? This chapter will present two brief case reports demonstrating the ethical issues that may arise surrounding just distribution of expensive technology, and will then discuss the ethical issues first at a "macro" or societal level and subsequently at a "micro" or hospital level.

II Cases

Case 1:

Mr. Ramirez was a 36-year-old male, who was admitted with a malfunction of his left ventricular assist device (LVAD). The patient was healthy until 2009 when he began to experience increasing shortness of breath and ankle edema. He was evaluated and found to have a non-ischemic, dilated cardiomyopathy and moderate congestive heart failure (NYHA Class III). He was treated with ACE inhibitors, low-dose beta blockers and aldosterone antagonists, but was poorly compliant with his medications. Because of morbid obesity, Type 2 diabetes, and alcohol and cocaine abuse, Mr. Ramirez was considered a poor candidate for heart transplantation. His heart failure symptoms worsened, and he was admitted for an elective LVAD and automatic internal cardioverter-defibrillator (AICD) implantation as a potential "bridge-to-transplant," if he became compliant with his medications and abstained from cocaine and alcohol. Despite this advice the patient continued to gain weight, and was admitted for a "pump exchange" due to a driveline fracture. He was ultimately discharged from the hospital to home after a complicated post-operative course, but was re-admitted for LVAD malfunction due to thrombus formation. Following the patient's wishes and after consultation with psychiatry, the LVAD was disconnected and the AICD turned off. While in the coronary care unit, symptoms were managed with diuretics and dobutamine until he became increasingly short of breath and lethargic. Due to end-stage heart failure, Mr. Ramirez passed away overnight, surrounded by his family.

Case 2:

Mr. Johnson is a 45-year-old carpenter, who presented 18 months ago with new onset non-ischemic cardiomyopathy, likely due to a viral illness. Despite maximal doses of beta blockers, ACE inhibitors and diuretics, his ejection fraction remains at 25% and he has an AICD placed prophylactically for ventricular arrhythmias. He has been followed in the hospital's heart failure/transplantation clinic and has been compliant with all medications, dietary restrictions and follow-up visits. Over the past three months he has had four admissions for decompensated heart failure. His cardiac team recommends consideration for an LVAD as a potential "bridge-to-transplant." Unfortunately, due to his disability over the preceding year, Mr. Johnson has been unable to work and has lost insurance coverage. The hospital often provides charitable procedures for patients and feels an obligation to Mr. Johnson as a longstanding patient; however, there are concerns about the ability of the hospital to absorb the costs of the LVAD implant and the ongoing management of the device as an outpatient.

III Societal Distribution of Scarce or Expensive Medical Therapy

In a morally pluralistic society, such as the United States, there is no single agreed-upon approach for assessing just means for allocating scarce or expensive technology. In the cases presented, one patient, by virtue of his insured status, received complex and expensive medical interventions despite the fact that his social situation and co-morbidities make him a less than optimal candidate for these measures. Ultimately, the outcome was much as it would have been with continued medical therapy. In the second case, a patient who is an excellent candidate for implantable devices based on his medical condition and proven ability to comply with complex medical regimens is potentially denied a device because of a lack of sufficient funding. We will consider three prominent ethical approaches to respond to these types of distributive justice questions at the societal level: a libertarian approach, a utilitarian approach, and a fair equality of opportunity approach.

A libertarian approach to justice emphasizes preserving the individual's freedom and rights to property as long as these do not unduly infringe upon another's similar rights. Given the multiplicity of views about what constitutes beneficial and just healthcare in Western society, it is impossible for a government to impose a universally acceptable plan for providing healthcare. While one may choose to aid others out of personal charity, there is no obligation or justification for governmental entities to correct inequalities resulting from one's station in life. Rather, the focus should be on fair procedures and laws allowing the market to determine the distribution of goods. For the libertarian, justice consists in the appropriate operation of just procedures, not in the production of particular outcomes assumed to be just (see, e.g., Engelhardt, 1996; Beauchamp and Childress, 2013).

This perspective leads one to object not only to Medicare coverage of LVADs but also to federal funding of research leading to the development of LVADs in the first place. The development of new technologies is morally best left to market forces. Given the prevalence of heart disease and the profits to be made from developing innovative treatment for such patients, there is no libertarian justification to force citizens to subsidize research. Indeed, the market may be more likely to direct resources to the development of technology that could be less costly and, hence, available to a broader patient population. Once available, no matter how expensive, there would be no objection to such technology being made available, as long as it is the individual's obligation to bear the cost through either individual savings or privately purchased insurance. This view would have the benefit of minimizing taxation and government spending, allowing individuals greater discretion in how they choose to utilize their resources in procuring healthcare. In this way, the overall cost and availability of healthcare would reflect individual choices rather than governmental decisions.

A critique of such a perspective might claim that government funding is more likely than private funding to be directed to large projects with a very long timeline such as the artificial heart. Such projects, like the space program of the 1960s, are more likely to develop "spin off" technologies that may have unexpected benefits and applications providing benefits ultimately greater than the research cost. But this is a set of empirical questions. Market forces have led to significant technological developments, such as microchips, pharmaceuticals, and implantable devices. Other objections include alternate visions of justice: some judge the fact that the first patient received an expensive device, because he had access to financial resources, as unjust.

A utilitarian approach to justice would require maximizing some measure of overall social welfare. Important to this approach is the choice of the pertinent benefit to be measured, including both direct and indirect benefits of any technology. This perspective is popular in setting broad health policy because it lends itself to quantitative measures of the cost versus the chosen social benefit or utility for various therapeutic options. A widely used tool in medicine is the Quality Adjusted Life Year (QALY), which attempts to determine the value of a given treatment by determining the number of years of life the treatment can add while discounting value for the amount of disability a patient will suffer during those additional years (Persad et al., 2009).

For example, when considering federal funding of the artificial heart program, one would have to evaluate the cost of research compared to the actual long-term benefits. One of the challenges to such an analysis is the difficulty in predicting the direct and indirect benefits at the outset of a research project, as noted with spinoff technology from the space program. In addition, from a policy perspective the analysis is complicated by trying to compare the benefits of research on artificial hearts to, for example, research on vaccines that may be significantly less costly but applicable to an even broader population.

While the number of patients who might benefit from an LVAD is very large, the number of years of life the typical patient will gain given current technology is limited and the likelihood of substantial disability from associated complications remains significant (Pinney et al., 2017). A recent study suggested that LVAD implantation would increase QALYs for low-risk patients with advanced heart failure from 2.67 to 4.41, but because of more frequent and costly readmissions for complications of LVADs the incremental cost compared to medical therapy would be $209,400 per QALY gained (Shreibati et al., 2017). This is well in excess of what most economists would consider cost-effective per life of year gained. Based on such an economic analysis, there would seem to be little justification for federal funding of end-of-life interventions such as the LVAD.

An important critique of the utilitarian perspective from those who argue that justice requires correcting inequalities in healthcare is that focusing on benefits to the population as a whole, including the use of QALYs, to guide funding decisions may harm vulnerable groups. Funding may be directed to diseases that affect large proportions of the population, while those with far less common conditions, or significant pre-existing disabilities, would be less likely to receive research funding, or payment for technology once available (Powers and Faden, 2006). Such a criticism might also apply to a libertarian approach of allowing the market to allocate resources. Insofar as the market ignores less common conditions or significant pre-existing disabilities, such care will not be available.

A third approach to justice frequently cited in the United States is a fair equality of opportunity approach. Norman Daniels perhaps best develops this perspective for the healthcare context. Proponents argue that a just society gives all members an equal opportunity for the goods available in that society. Daniels sees health as a special good without which citizens cannot achieve other goals, and for which all should have an equal opportunity: "by keeping people close to normal functioning, health care preserves for people the ability to participate in the political, social, and economic life of their society" (Daniels, 2001, p. 3). While this approach does not require equality of outcome, providing equal opportunity to achieve one's best level of functioning may require giving preference to worse-off members of society. He recognizes that there will be limits to the amount of healthcare provided to all citizens. In determining what interventions will be available, a fair process will be required that includes: (1) publicly announcing coverage decisions and the rationale for those decisions, (2) an appeals process to challenge the decision, and (3) a means of enforcing the fairness of the process (Daniels, 2001).

In our judgment, such a perspective would have no specific objection to public funding of research for ventricular assist devices as long as they are made equally available to all. In this light, Daniels' approach would find the different abilities of the patients in the two cases we have presented to access a potentially lifesaving technology unjust. The ideal would be universal coverage of healthcare with decisions to provide LVADs to all eligible patients or none using a process outlined above. It would be explicitly recognized that rationing would be a part of universal coverage. In the absence of universal coverage, legitimate criteria would need to be developed to favor governmental support of those most likely to benefit and who cannot afford the cost of the technology on their own, much as the decision to provide dialysis to all patients requiring therapy regardless of age. Such an approach has the benefit of avoiding the situation presented where a patient is denied coverage because of lack of insurance. The drawback of such an approach is that it will be difficult to constrain costs, if governmental entities decide to compensate for technology such as LVADs, and it has even been argued that providing universal coverage encourages individuals to seek healthcare independently, weakening the traditional financial and social support provided to the ill by their families (Engelhardt, 2012).

Our discussion demonstrates the difficulty of developing coherent policies that provide a significant proportion of the population with potentially lifesaving therapy, while moderating the cost of healthcare. This analysis would suggest that all three conceptions of justice would find objections to the current Medicare funding of LVADs, albeit for very different reasons. In the absence of a consensus at a societal level about how justly to make decisions about funding and availability of costly medical care, regional and local healthcare providers are placed in the position of deciding how best to allocate these resources within their institutions. We will now turn to a consideration of principles to guide decisions at this "micro" level.

IV Institutional Distribution of Scarce or Expensive Medical Therapy

The two cases presented in this chapter demonstrate the conundrum often faced by local healthcare providers. While the patient in case 1 has insurance covering the LVAD, there are significant costs for the hospital and society in providing this technology to a patient unlikely to derive long-term benefit. These include operating room and intensive care utilization, in addition to the burden on caregivers with extensive clinical obligations to other patients. On the other hand, while most institutions simply will not consider charitable care for LVADs, the caregivers of case 2 may feel obliged to make this technology available to the patient, who has been cared for in their system for a significant period of time. What ethically appropriate principles should guide decisions regarding who may be a candidate for expensive technology, and who might be a candidate for charitable care given the institution's resources?

Early in the era of renal dialysis and cardiac transplantation, Rescher put forward a two-step approach that has been adopted in modified form by Beauchamp and Childress (Rescher, 1969; Beauchamp and Childress, 2013). First, a pool of candidates is chosen from all patients with the particular disease process based on three criteria: constituency, progress of science and prospect of success. The constituency factor is based on the group of patients typically cared for by the institution, such as those within a certain geographic area, or veterans for a Veterans Administration medical center. The second factor, pertinent for research, is choosing patients based on medical or demographic criteria important for answering a scientific question about the role of a scarce resource. Finally, considering the prospect of success, or prognosis of the patient if they receive the scarce intervention, prioritizes those most likely to benefit and avoids wasting resources on those who derive only marginal benefit.

Once a general pool of patients is identified, more patient-specific criteria are used for determining those patients to whom the intervention will be offered. Here Rescher included: the relative likelihood of success, life expectancy, family role, potential future contributions, and past service (Rescher, 1969). These criteria, particularly the final three, may be controversial. The first criterion is a more in-depth consideration of prognosis in light of a patient's characteristics than in the initial screening. For example, Human Leukocyte Antigen (HLA) and blood-type matching for transplant patients may give one patient preference over another for a particular organ. Life expectancy with the intervention, the second criterion, may be controversial if a strict age cutoff is used for offering an expensive or scarce resource, though most transplant programs have an upper age limit beyond which they are reluctant to proceed with cardiac transplantation.

The next three criteria are far more susceptible to value judgments and moral controversy. Rescher suggested that it would be legitimate to favor the parent of minor children over a patient with no children, or to favor those most likely to provide significant beneficial services to society in the future or who have provided significant service in the past. A 1962 *Life* magazine article describing the committee in Seattle in the early days of dialysis that would choose patients for the then very scarce intervention using similar criteria engendered significant debate about the moral legitimacy of these criteria (Jonsen, 2007). Public review of this rationing method influenced the decision years later to cover dialysis under Medicare (Blagg, 2007). While these criteria of "social utility" are rarely explicitly invoked in the current climate, Beauchamp and Childress argue that they may be appropriate in some instances (Beauchamp and Childress, 2013). An often-cited example is giving preferential treatment or vaccination to healthcare workers during an influenza pandemic, enhancing their ability to care for other patients. While the value of one's role in the family is not typically considered in transplantation decisions, evidence of a quality social support system is often considered. In addition, some groups, such as veterans, are given benefits by virtue of their prior sacrifice for the nation.

After this second step in patient selection, there may remain more patients who are relatively equally good clinical candidates for the therapy than there are available organs or resources. At this stage, Rescher argues that a random process is appropriate for selecting the final candidates for therapy (Rescher, 1969). From a perspective of justice, random allocation has the advantage of giving "equals" (medically) an equal chance of receiving the therapy, avoiding the controversy of allowing those with greater wealth or social standing to take precedence over other patients. Two means of random allocation are typically considered. First is a lottery in which patients from the pool are randomly chosen for the intervention. The second approach is a first-come, first-served approach.

Lotteries are the most truly blind method and may be useful to allocate limited supplies of drugs or vaccines when there is a large pool of potential candidates. Some have argued that the second method, a first-come, first-served scheme, is a flawed form of random allocation because it is more susceptible to manipulation. For example, the wealthy or powerful may have earlier access in their disease process to the healthcare system, than a patient with poor or no insurance coverage. In the case of transplantation, a wealthy patient may have the resources to travel and be listed for transplantation at several different locations, enhancing the opportunity to receive an organ (Persad et al., 2009). Yet, the reality is that for most illnesses, such as congestive heart failure, there is often not a pool waiting for treatment. Rather, patients present randomly over time and progress at various rates to a stage requiring mechanical support or transplantation. Hence a first-come, first-served allocation method is often the only reasonable option, at least initially, in settings such as the intensive care unit.

Another limitation of this second method of random allocation is that if the first patient to receive a scarce resource does not improve quickly, or his or her prognosis worsens despite treatment, there may be a reluctance to remove the intervention in favor of a subsequent patient who is more likely to benefit. Truog uses extracorporeal membrane oxygenation (ECMO), a form of heart-lung bypass that may be used to support patients with severe respiratory failure, as an example. Many patients may be supported by ECMO for months, but the chance of being successfully weaned from the device may significantly decline after the first few weeks. Since most institutions have a limited number of devices and trained personnel for round-the-clock care of these patients, subsequent patients who might benefit from the treatment may be denied access if physicians are reluctant to withdraw therapy from patients already on ECMO who are unlikely to improve. Truog suggests that it is reasonable for institutions to have a policy whereby patients are informed before instituting therapy, such as ECMO, that if certain criteria are met demonstrating a very poor prognosis with continued treatment, and if another patient presents who would likely benefit from the treatment, the first patient may be removed from continuing support (Truog, 1992).

While many have criticized the United Network for Organ Sharing (UNOS) system for allocating organs for cardiac transplantation, it incorporates many of the features discussed above for allocation. Given that the patient population overlaps with candidates for LVADs, it may provide a useful template for allocation of LVADs. As described above, patients typically go through a multistep screening process. Most institutions give preference to patients within their usual service area, though, as noted, it is possible for some patients to gain an advantage by being listed at several institutions. Prognosis or probability of success with transplantation plays a significant role in screening patients. Recent advances in medical therapy and devices such as implantable defibrillators have significantly impacted mortality and morbidity. Hence, patients often undergo stress testing with peak oxygen consumption to help determine those who will have a significantly better chance of survival with transplantation versus those who continue medical therapy. Patients are also evaluated for severe irreversible pulmonary hypertension, which might cause the new heart to fail acutely. In addition, other factors impacting prognosis are considered; for example, patients with a significant history of cancer may not be considered for transplantation until they have been free of recurrence for 5 years.

Once patients have demonstrated that they might benefit from transplantation, a more detailed screening of medical prognosis and social factors is undertaken. Co-morbid conditions are carefully analyzed. Patients with severe obesity, diabetes with evidence of end-organ damage, and those with renal dysfunction will be carefully assessed to determine the impact of these medical issues on the likelihood that transplantation will provide long-term benefit. Factors such as ongoing tobacco use, alcohol use, or illicit drug use may be considered as potential contraindications for transplantation. Finally, patients often undergo extensive psychosocial evaluation to determine if they will be able to comply with the complex medical regimen and have the social support system necessary to do so (Mehra et al., 2006).

Once patients are accepted as candidates for transplantation they are placed on a list awaiting available organs. This is a modified form of first-come, first-served allocation. For cardiac transplantation, the UNOS network gives preference to a sickest-first criterion, whereby the most acutely ill patients are moved to the front of the waiting list. This system may be subject to abuse, however, as transplant centers may modify reporting to make their patients appear more acutely ill (Persad et al., 2009). Less weight is given to patients who have been on the list for a longer period of time, though this is still a consideration.

Having considered these models, how might an institution structure an LVAD program to avoid wasting resources on candidates unlikely to benefit from the technology and possibly provide some charitable support for those needing the device? It seems reasonable to consider a modified screening process akin to that for transplantation, given that many candidates for LVADs will have been screened for transplantation and may still be candidates should a heart become available.

First, it seems reasonable for an institution to limit offering complex and costly technology, especially for charitable care, to those living in its service area. This would be particularly important because if an institution was one of the few to provide charitable LVADs, there would be a high likelihood that unfunded patients would travel to the institution in hopes of receiving a device, straining the ability to provide care for local patients. In addition, patients with advanced heart failure should be screened medically, as suggested above, with stress testing and based on symptoms to determine those who may do as well with continued medical therapy rather than LVADs or transplantation.

Once a decision has been made that a patient could benefit from mechanical assistance or transplantation, institutions could undertake an evaluation similar to that for transplantation. A more in-depth consideration of prognosis would identify those acceptable for transplant listing, including those who would be candidates for LVADs as a bridge to transplantation. A significant number of patients turned down for transplant listing may still be candidates for destination LVAD therapy. Those with co-morbidities such as diabetes with end-organ injury or greater degrees of renal insufficiency, and those with advanced age or the presence of an untreated cancer, are still candidates for permanent device placement. It would still be appropriate for the institution to place limits on LVAD placement for patients who have extremely poor prognosis, such as those with terminal comorbidities, who are not expected to survive beyond six months even with device placement.

Psychosocial assessment should also be a part of the evaluation for LVAD placement. As with transplantation, the LVAD requires a strong social support system and the ability to follow a rigorous medical regimen. Without these, patients may conceivably be worse off with a device, as they may be more likely to develop infection, strokes, or significant bleeding. Such patients may be better managed with medical therapy, including periodic infusion of inotropes for symptom relief and possible hospice or palliative care support. Such an evaluation may have avoided the brief and ultimately unsuccessful attempt to stabilize the first case with implantable devices. Some centers have recommended that candidates for LVADs have a palliative care or ethics consultation prior to placement to inform patients of the possible complications and begin a discussion of how the patient would want to be managed should they suffer a catastrophic stroke or unmanageable bleeding (Swetz et al., 2011).

Finally, if a patient is viewed as a good LVAD candidate based on this evaluation, those with adequate funding will be able to proceed with the procedure. However, how is the institution to deal with the second patient presented? First the institution must decide what patient populations and treatments will take precedence. This will require a value judgment of whether allocating resources to advanced heart failure benefits the community more or if resources should be directed to other diseases or treatment options. It may well be reasonable to decide that charitable devices will not be provided. If, on the other hand, the institution has adequate funds and has an obligation to patient two, it should have a clear policy on charitable care. For example it may be most appropriate to use a first-come, first-served policy, taking only as many charitable patients as possible up to the limit of available funds. It would also be reasonable to expect patients to pursue any available sources of funding for ongoing care. Finally, if a first-come, first-served method is used to allocate charitable funds, it may be reasonable to follow Truog's views on ECMO. Patients would be informed prior to charitable LVAD placement that if prognosis significantly worsens, or if the patient is noncompliant, and other patients need charitable device placement, the device may be deactivated, or the patient will be required to come up with outside funding to continue treatment. If an institution decides to provide charitable allocation, it would be appropriate to have a transparent process outlined to avoid ad hoc decisions that may appear unjust to the hospital's patient population.

V Conclusion

In summary, there is no consensus in the United States currently about the best principles to guide just distribution of medical resources. As a consequence, there is no agreed-upon framework for making decisions such as the funding of LVADs by Medicare for destination therapy. As we have seen, three common, but very different approaches to justice could all find grounds to object to the decision to fund LVADs at the end of life. Subsequently, local healthcare systems are left to determine how to best allocate expensive or scarce medical interventions in a system with multiple different levels of insurance coverage for such therapy, and a significant number of patients who may have no coverage at all. We propose, based on existing methods for evaluating candidates for transplantation, a means for institutions to determine who may be appropriate for LVAD placement and how to determine if charitable care can be provided for some patients.

References

Beauchamp, T.L., and J.F. Childress. 2013. *Principles of biomedical ethics*, seventh edition. New York: Oxford University Press.

Blagg, C.R. 2007. The early history of dialysis for chronic renal failure in the United States: A view from Seattle. *American Journal of Kidney Diseases* 49(3): 482–496.

Daniels, N. 2001. Justice, health, and health care. *American Journal of Bioethics* 1(2): 1–16.

Engelhardt, H.T., Jr. 1996. *The foundations of bioethics*, second edition. New York: Oxford University Press.

Engelhardt, H.T., Jr. 2012. Fair equality of opportunity critically reexamined: The family and sustainability of health care systems. *The Journal of Medicine and Philosophy* 37(6): 583–602.

Estep, J.D., R.C. Starling, D.A. Horstmanshof, C.A. Milano, C.H. Selzman, K.B. Shah, M. Loebe, N. Moazami, J.W. Long, J. Stehlik, K. Vigneshwar, D. Haas, J.B. O'Connell, A.J. Boyle, D.J. Farrar, and J.G. Rogers. 2015. Risk assessment and comparative effectiveness of left ventricular assist device and medical management in ambulatory heart failure patients: Results from the ROADMAP study. *Journal of the American College of Cardiology* 66(16): 1747–1761.

Hernandez, A.F., A.M. Shea, C.A. Milano, J.G. Rogers, B.G. Hammill, C.M. O'Connor, K.A. Schulman, E.D. Peterson, and L.H. Curtis. 2008. Long-term outcomes and costs of ventricular assist devices among Medicare beneficiaries. *Journal of the American Medical Association* 300(20): 2398–2406.

Institute of Medicine. 1991. A chronology of the national heart, lung, and blood institute artificial heart program and related events. In: *The artificial heart: Prototypes, policies, and patients*, Hogness, J.R. and M.VanAntwerp (eds). Washington, DC: National Academies Press. Available from: https://www.ncbi.nlm.nih.gov/books/NBK234439/

Jonsen, A.R. 2007. The god squad and the origins of transplantation ethics and policy. *The Journal of Law, Medicine, & Ethics* 35(2): 238–240.

Mehra, M.R., J. Kobashigawa, R. Starling, S. Russell, P.A. Uber, J. Parameshwar, P. Mohacsi, A. Augustine, K. Aaronson, and M. Barr. 2006. Listing criteria for heart transplantation: International society for heart and lung transplantation guidelines for the care of cardiac transplant candidates—2006. *Journal of Heart Lung Transplantation* 25(9): 1024–1042.

Miller, L.W., and M. Guglin. 2013. Patient selection for ventricular assist devices: A moving target. *Journal of the American College of Cardiology* 61(12): 1209–1221.

Patel, N., R. Kalra, R. Doshi, N. Bajaj, G. Arora, and P. Arora. 2018. Trends and cost of heart transplantation and left ventricular assist devices: Impact of proposed federal cuts. *Journal of the American College of Cardiology* 6(5): 424–432.

Persad, G., A. Wertheimer, and E.J. Emanuel. 2009. Principles for allocation of scarce medical interventions. *The Lancet* 373: 423–431.

Pinney, S.P., A.C. Anyanwu, A. Lala, J.J. Teuteberg, N. Uriel, and M.R. Mehra. 2017. Left ventricular assist devices for lifelong support. *Journal of the American College of Cardiology* 69(23): 2845–2861.

Powers, M., and R. Faden. 2006. *Social justice*. New York: Oxford University Press.

Rescher, N. 1969. The allocation of exotic medical lifesaving therapy. *Ethics* 79(3): 173–186.

Savarese, G., and L.H. Lund. 2017. Global public health burden of heart failure. *Cardiac Failure Review* 3(1): 7–11. Available at: http://doi.org/10.15420/cfr.2016:25:2.

Shreibati, J.B., J.D. Goldhaber-Fiebert, D. Banerjee, D.K. Owens, and M.A. Hlatky. 2017. Cost effectiveness of left ventricular assist devices in ambulatory patients with advanced heart failure. *Journal of the American College of Cardiology* 5(2): 110–119.

Swetz, K.M., M.R. Freeman, O.F. AbouEzzeddine, K.A. Carter, B.A. Boilson, A.L. Ottenberg, S.J. Park, and P.S. Mueller. 2011. Palliative medicine consultation for preparedness planning in patients receiving left ventricular assist devices as destination therapy. *Mayo Clinic Proceedings* 86(6): 493–500.

Truog, R.D. 1992. Triage in the ICU. *The Hastings Center Report* 22(3): 13–17.

8 The Cardio-Ethics of Endocarditis

Alexandra Charrow and James N. Kirkpatrick

I The Case

A 42-year-old male presents to the emergency room with worrisome symptoms a year after his first mitral valve replacement. He complains of low-grade fevers and shortness of breath, and an exam demonstrates purpuric lesions at his fingertips and nail beds. A transesophageal echocardiogram reveals endocarditis with features consistent with need for urgent mitral valve replacement. The patient's initial valve replacement one year prior had been performed after a heroin-use relapse. Subsequent infections left his mitral valve perforated and showering vegetative material, which caused a transient ischemic attack. Now that the patient has returned with new infection of his porcine valve and cutaneous signs of recent intravenous drug use, the question to you as the consulting cardiologist is how to proceed. The patient is seeking treatment and is willing to undergo any intervention which will prolong his life. The patient, let's call him Mr. Wallace, is an out-of-work construction worker with two estranged children. Now in the midst of his third drug relapse in as many years, his current drug-use calls into question whether he will adequately care for his next mitral valve.

As a physician, you have a moral and legal obligation to provide care for your patients. However, parallel to your patient obligations is a duty to all of your other patients as well as to society as a whole to ensure that scarce resources, such as valves, surgeons, and funding, are available should they be needed. This case's details may seem specific, but the moral questions at play are applicable to all patient–physician interactions, namely: (1) What is the extent of a cardiologist's obligation to his patients? (2) What is the extent of a cardiologist's obligation to society? (3) How do the cardiologist's dual obligations to patient and society intersect with resource limitation? (4) How does the cardiologist determine when treatment is futile, and is she obligated to provide futile treatment? (5) How can physicians be mindful of their own biases when confronting patients who use intravenous drugs?

The case of the intravenous drug user stricken with repeated episodes of endocarditis is also an excellent case study in utilizing the principles of bioethics and ethical reasoning to answer the above questions. The discussion below will

DOI: 10.4324/9781003240273-12

highlight how to balance those bioethical principles and explore their limits. While traditional ethical norms have articulated that the obligation of the physician is to his patient primarily and societal stewardship secondarily, there are ways to advocate for one while respecting both.

II Fiduciary Responsibilities

Mr. Wallace needs an expensive intervention, one he has already received once before. A mitral valve surgery requires specialized expertise (cardiac surgeon, anesthesiologist, cardiac surgery operating room staff), a highly specialized environment (cardiac surgery operating room) and the prosthetic valve, all of which carry considerable expense. If every patient with valve surgery were to engage in behaviors which contribute directly to a recurrence of the disease or loss of valve function (whether refusing to take anticoagulation for a mechanical valve or using IV drugs), surgical valve replacement would become an even more onerous financial burden to society (either because of increased costs passed on by insurance companies to consumers, direct costs to government-funded insurers, or increased costs absorbed by hospitals and passed on to payers). Because medical resources and funds are ultimately finite, the use of medical resources to "rescue" patients who have made choices which lead to adverse consequences inevitably means there are, or will be, fewer resources available to other priorities. What emerges from this line of logic are two conflicting principles of bioethics that must be balanced – obligations to the individual patient and obligations to all of society.

In their landmark book on bioethics, Tom Beauchamp and James Childress outline four principles that they believe underlies and guides moral decisions (1994). The four principles are: autonomy (respect for persons and their desires), beneficence (doing good for others), nonmaleficence (doing no harm), and justice (equity). This form of bioethical principlism proposes moral rules, ideas, and intuitions underlying ethical conflict, and then, by balancing relevance, applicability, and import, distills these principles into a final decision (1994). It should be noted that there are many other ways of engaging in moral reasoning to make decisions in the clinical context, but we address the four principles as they are particularly salient to the case of Mr. Wallace. Most apropos is the principle of beneficence that dictates treating Mr. Wallace with the most effective therapy to prevent morbidity and mortality. Autonomy plays a critical role as well, since Mr. Wallace has exercised his right to make poor decisions but has also indicated his willingness to undergo any procedure that will prolong his life. Mr. Wallace is unable to pay for a valve replacement, so, ultimately, society would end up paying. While few cost analyses exist for mitral valve replacement surgery, costs for an aortic valve replacement range from $25,000 to $50,000 dollars, depending on complication rates (Osnabrugge, Speir, Head, Fonner, Fonner, Ailawadi, Kappetein and Rich 2013; Starr and Grunkemeier 2007). Does this financial responsibility also give society the right to refuse to provide valve replacement or to dictate Mr. Wallace's actions – perhaps by requiring him to participate in a drug rehab program – as a condition for receiving life-prolonging interventions? Justice, in terms of the fair distribution of resources, plays a role in this scenario as well. Resources expended on Mr. Wallace will not be available to treat patients whom society might deem more deserving. Principlism isolates much of the tension in fiduciary duty to the physician's duty to her individual patient versus her duty as a steward of expensive resources. The American Medical Association, in their Code of Medical Ethics, outlines in opinion 1.1.1 that the physician has "ethical responsibility to place patients' welfare above the physician's own self-interest or obligations to others, to use sound medical judgment on patients' behalf, and to advocate for their patients' welfare" (2019a). However, the American Medical Association also describes the role of physician as steward of health care resources, explaining in code 11.1.2 that "Managing health care resources responsibly for the benefit of all patients is compatible with physicians' primary obligations to serve the interests of individual patients" (2019b). There are times when the good of all patients is incompatible with the good of an individual patient, particularly in regards to the use of scarce resources, but the American Medical Association assigns primary importance to the interest of individual patients. The American College of Physician recognizes these tensions, but is also explicit about physician obligations:

> The physician's primary commitment must always be to the patient's welfare and best interests, whether in preventing or treating illness or helping patients to cope with illness, disability, and death. The physician must respect the dignity of all persons and respect their uniqueness. The interests of the patient should always be promoted regardless of financial arrangements; the health care setting; or patient characteristics, such as decision-making capacity, behavior, or social status.
>
> (Sulmasy and Bledsoe 2019)

The 2020 American Heart Association/American College of Cardiology Consensus Conference of Professionalism and Ethics similarly opined, "Clinicians must balance the interests of patients and the stewardship of valuable resources through transparency, focus on quality, SDM, and patient-centeredness in the development and implementation of new models of care delivery" (Benjamin et al., 2021, p. 3117).

Similarly, the American College of Cardiology has weighed in on stewardship and patient advocacy. Their 29th Bethesda Conference Report concluded that while cardiologists have dual obligations, stewardship can only be demanded once an agreed-upon code of ethics has been established within a system by cardiologists. As the report explains, "only with the establishment of a code of managed care ethics can physicians in such systems be stewards of society's resources and patient advocates" (Parmley, Passamani and Lo, 1998, p. 931). The alternative, that such codes be developed by legislature or management, is untenable given that such institutions lack understanding of individual patients and their diseases (Parmley, Passamani and Lo, 1998).

III Rationing and Financial Stewardship

In cases of limited resources, there is a need to ration care: to determine either who will get a limited resource or in what order a limited resource should be allocated. Transplanted organs, for example, are rationed based on a set of criteria, and given their cost, perhaps other scarce and expensive resources like heart valves could be similarly disseminated on the basis of expected patient follow-up, adherence, support, and reliability. From a bioethics perspective, however, organ transplantation is perhaps the clearest, though not necessarily most the straightforward, version of rationing. It demands such standards because organs are doubly scarce in ways that valves are not; organs are both costly and rare. This specific scarcity, along with an organ's connection to the life and death of another human, make the imperatives surrounding its use paramount. To waste a donated organ is to violate an implicit agreement with the donor, or the donor's family, and society as a whole. The donor and the donor's family have a right to expect that their gift will be used well. Because donated hearts are scarce resources, when a heart goes to one person, it cannot (by its very limited nature) be used by another. From a utilitarian perspective, the graft should be used in such a way as to provide the greatest benefit. When a recipient does not take his medications and the graft fails, the recipient harms himself but also decreases the overall utility of the graft, which likely would have survived longer in a compliant patient. The utility of valves can also be diminished by nonadherence, but valves otherwise do not carry the same implications. To waste a valve is to waste financial resources, but valves are not otherwise innately scarce. More valves can be made, and since valve manufactures do not provide them as a gift, they have no expectation that values should be well-cared for. (Indeed, in light of increased sales, they may prefer the opposite.)

An alternative to the scarcity model that is perhaps more apropos is rationing based on costs relative to medical benefit or medical necessity. The American College of Cardiology 29th Bethesda Conference Report takes the position that physicians serve as the only appropriate gatekeepers for medical care (Parmley, Passamani and Lo, 1998). Ubel and Arnold (1995) are among the scholars who agree with this position and have suggested that there are circumstances under which a physician might compare costs and ration care accordingly. Ubel and Arnold compare bedside rationing conducted by physicians to other methods of cost-containment before determining it to be more nuanced and patient-centered than the alternative top-down or system-wide approaches. Financial stewardship is part of every physician's dual duties to patient and society: when benefits are minimal and costs are large, physicians must consider their duty to the general population as well as to the patient in front of them (Ubel and Arnold 1995; Ubel and Jagsi 2014). Although the fact that physicians may be too close to patients to consider properly the interests of society (or may have their judgment about medical benefit similarly clouded), Ubel and Arnold argue they are better positioned as stewards than bureaucrats. If rationing is inevitable as costs rise, it is better for the physicians to steer the course than those forces less favorable to (or completely inconsiderate of) the patient, especially since physicians are better suited to determine the relative benefits of the rationed care in the individual patient's situation. In doing so, the physician need not approach the decision from the perspective of choosing which patients will receive and which will go without.

Even if bedside rationing became common practice among clinicians, Ubel and Arnold would likely agree that a cardiologist must be careful in considering bedside rationing under the circumstances of the vignette above. They (as well as others in favor of bedside rationing) argue that it can only be conducted on or between opportunities that are *marginally beneficial*. *Marginally beneficial* interventions are defined in terms of their benefits and costs to the patient and society, as well as their costs and benefits in comparison to other interventions. By way of example, Ubel and Arnold cite organ transplantation as an intervention that, while costly to the individual and society, has great benefit to the patient (especially as compared to the alternative –death). On the other hand, yearly pap smears are only marginally beneficial as compared to pap smears conducted every three years, providing only one year of life gained for every million dollars spent (Eddy 1990). Patient preference is given consideration here as well, specifically as it relates to outcomes and values. If a patient needing valve replacement values the benefits afforded by a porcine valve over a mechanical valve, while accepting the limited longevity of a biological valve, such values should be taken into consideration. However, rational patient preferences are placed in contrast to patient preferences without medical justification, such as a euvolemic patient's demand for more furosemide. A rational value is worth consideration, while an irrational demand is not.

Under such a system, mitral valve replacement is more akin to transplantation in terms of its benefits and costs: it is a costly intervention with significant benefits to the patient. In choosing between a mitral valve replacement and attempting medically to control symptoms related to valvular dysfunction, there is a clear benefit to surgery from a longevity perspective. The "second-best" option is not only marginally but substantially less beneficial than the standard of care. If, however, Mr. Wallace were so sick that he would likely not survive surgery, referral to hospice may provide superior quality and quantity of life. Alternatively, if there were less costly, non-surgical options, that gave Mr. Wallace a marginally reduced life expectancy, mitral valve replacement would be open to bedside rationing in this case. If there were an antibiotic, for instance, that could penetrate an abscess, and if a percutaneous option was available to reduce mitral regurgitation resulting from valvular dysfunction to moderate rather than severe, Ubel and Arnold might argue that surgery could be appropriately denied in favor of this "second-best" but cheaper option. (The cost saving in this case, of course, would depend on the cost of the percutaneous option and the antibiotic.) An analogous situation is the performance of balloon aortic valvuloplasty in patients for whom transcatheter or standard aortic valve replacement is expected to be of marginal benefit (patients with symptomatic aortic stenosis but <1 year prognosis from comorbidities, or patients with significant frailty).

Others argue that such decisions about rationing should be made at the level of the system and not the physician. Sulmasy argues, for example, that inequalities will naturally evolve as clinicians ration, to the detriment of patients (1992). The 2020 AHA/ACC Consensus Conference on Professionalism and Ethics states that clinicians should not be placed in a position to balance the benefits of a treatment with the societal opportunity costs of providing care. Ultimately, it is a societal responsibility to determine this balance when scarcity may prohibit the delivery of the care determined to be in the best interests of the individual patient.

(2021, p. 3116)

The "God Committees" that rationed the few hemodialysis machines in existence in the late 1960s and early 1970s demonstrated that physicians, whether in committee or as individuals, are likely to make rationing decisions based on subjective notions of social worth (Jonsen 2007). Even though the explicit, institutionalized rationing of the "God Committees" is a thing of the past, physicians are still subject to unconscious biases, likely in favor of those patients who are better socially and economically well off, exacerbating the current disparities in access to quality care. Physicians who attempt to be fair in rationing would be counterbalanced by those who advocate for their patients. In such a situation, rationing would be based more on physician than patient factors, or may devolve into a popularity contest.

Weinstein adds to the critique of bedside rationing by pointing to the patient–physician relationship as a paramount reason to promote rationing at a higher level than that of the clinician (1990). Maintaining a trusting relationship between patient and physician is paramount in clinical care. For instance, studies have demonstrated that patients are more likely to adhere to medications and treatments if they trust their physician (Safran, Kosinski, Tarlov, Rogers, Taira, Lieberman and Ware 1998). For a patient like Mr. Wallace, maintaining adherence is critical to his success and part of that adherence is dependent on his trust in his clinicians. Administrative rationing keeps patients and their physicians on the "same side." The current insurance system, which usually requires justification for referral to specialty care, precertification for certain diagnostic tests or medications, and appeal of prospective denials of payment for procedures and tests, can be seen as a form of administrative rationing based on cost and medical indication that firmly establishes the physician as the patient's advocate.

Lauridsen (2009) decouples this dichotomy between patient and society, offering a compromise known as administrative gatekeeping. Combining the physician role of Ubel and Arnold with that of Sulmasy, Lauridsen argues that physicians should follow whatever guidelines are set at the system level to ration care while never considering cost at the bedside (2009). Hull and Jadbabaie (2014) provide a more expanded view of administrative gatekeeping. They argue that physicians are obliged to serve as system-level rationers at times and patient advocates at others. Hull and Jadbabaie argue that physicians should both develop the guidelines for when to opt for a procedure or surgery versus medical management and provide the best care for individual patients (2014).

Administrative gatekeeping and related concepts provide a useful role for the cardiologist and other subspecialists. Subspecialists are uniquely positioned to provide high-level understanding of the issues involved in rationing care. They can serve on the committees that decide how to ration care at the system level, while advocating maximally for their individual clinic and ward patients. In many cases, serving on committees may be a way to redress rationing-induced inequalities they witness in clinical practice. They are thus able to serve their dual obligations as stewards and advocates, while maintaining the integrity of their relationships to both society and the individual.

However as Sprung, Eidelman and Steinberg (1995) specify, while physicians can play a role in developing system-level rationing schemes, because of the risk of patient–physician trust degradation, they cannot do so while they are serving patients' whose care will imminently be rationed. Dual duties could, therefore, cause physicians to advocate for one practice at the committee level while pushing for another in clinic; but, because the physician's dual obligations conflict in expressly this way, such conflict of interest may be inescapable.

In any form of administrative rationing, criteria need to be clearly articulated to patients, whether at the local (hospital) level or at the level of a subspecialty society or insurance company. Justification in terms of rationing based on marginal benefit should be spelled out, along with the "second-best" alternatives, emphasizing that patients will still receive palliative interventions to treat symptoms and improve quality of life. Ideally, rationing criteria and rationales would be publically vetted, with opportunities for input from all stakeholders, including patients, family members, clinicians and other providers and insurers, not just panels of experts, whether employed by insurance companies or assembled by subspecialty societies. However, the specific nature of each element to be rationed may make this level of input untenable. There should be an opportunity for appeal for extenuating circumstances.

IV Bias

Administrative gatekeeping allows not only for a balance of obligation and work against physician level bias in rationing, but may also prevent a slide into cycles of bias and blame in the physician–patient relationship. Trusting patients with treatments they do not follow can leave physicians not only disappointed but feeling betrayed and prepared to guard against future feelings of betrayal by profiling patients based on drug use and associated demographics. Under such circumstances, physicians are likely to view the intravenous drug user not as a treatment partner but as an adversary.

Even healthcare professionals who routinely work with intravenous drug users can develop bias against them causing significant burnout and inhibiting equitable care (Von Hippel, Brener and Von Hippel 2008; Brener, Von Hippel and Kippax 2007). Patients from ethnic minority populations and poorer patients, who already receive worse care because of cost and access differentials (Braverman, Cubbin, Egerter, Williams and Pamuk 2010; Adler and Rehkopf 2008), may find their situation exacerbated by a system that puts them even more at the mercy of physicians' unconscious biases.

Self-harming behavior exists in many forms in cardiology. Patients with coronary artery disease who do not adhere to a diet low in saturated fats, who do not take their medications as prescribed, and who do not exercise though physically able are, in fact, harming themselves. Granted, the impact that dietary and medication adherence and physical activity behaviors have on progression of disease is difficult to quantify and may be less direct than the line drawn between intravenous drug user and infective endocarditis. However, the relative degree of bias against patients with different types of self-harming behavior may not reflect the relative degree of self-harm produced by these behaviors, especially as it may be difficult to predict. Not all IV drug use relapses lead to infective endocarditis. Conversely, a patient who has been sober for years but relapses once can develop endocarditis. Furthermore, viewed as a disease with a potential (though small) for treatment instead of exclusively as a moral failing, both intravenous drug user and dietary/medication/exercise indiscretion may be placed in the larger treatment context. Blame for moral failings aside, a pragmatic solution necessitates aggressively addressing and treating risk factors concurrent to treating the ailment itself, be they dietary indiscretion or intravenous drug user.

V Futility

Mr. Wallace's medical situation highlights not only a physician's dual obligations in the face of bias and bedside rationing but forces the question of how far those obligations extend. There is a line at which point any and all cardiologists should refuse to pursue treatments demanded by patients, and that line is one of medical futility (Schneiderman, Jecker and Jonsen 1990).

Futility is defined most notably by Schneiderman et al. as "any effort to achieve a result that is possible but that reasoning or experience suggests is highly improbable and that cannot be systematically produced" (1990, p. 951). If, out of 100 similar patients, zero have been successfully treated with a particular intervention, then that treatment is futile according to Schneiderman. It would meet such criteria of futility for a patient with irreversible and end stage liver and kidney failure to receive ECMO for cardiopulmonary failure, for instance, because in similar patients, it is almost always unsuccessful and restricts a patient to the ICU indefinitely (Schneiderman, Jecker and Jonsen 1996).

Pope elaborates further on Schneiderman et al.'s concept of futility by contrasting physiologic futility with quantitative futility, and qualitative futility. Physiologically futile interventions are those that are incapable of affecting change, given the disease, like shocking a patient with clear asystole. Pope notes that while physiologically futile cases are an agreed-upon reason for refusing treatment, such cases are few and far between. Quantitative futility is defined in a similar manner to Schneiderman's characterization—the probability of success is low. In contrast, an intervention is qualitatively futile if it fails or is highly unlikely to achieve a meaningful outcome, often defined as an acceptable quality of life. This definition highlights the fact that both "low probability" and "success" are subjective. The difference between a 1 in 100 chance and a 5 in 100 chance depends on one's perspective in declaring quantitative futility. If a treatment serves only to preserve a patient's unconscious status or dependence on Intensive Care Unit level care, many but not all would deem it qualitatively futile. In general, however, qualitative futility is more difficult to define than physical impossibility or improbability and is attended by significant controversy (Pope 2007).

Reflecting then on Mr. Wallace's case, valve replacement will have a physiological effect. Though the chances of long-term freedom from re-infection in an actively using intravenous drug user are low, they are not negligible and are hard to define. Depending on the definition of "success", Mr. Wallace's endocarditis can be successfully treated with a redo valve replacement more than 1% of the time. Additionally, the vast majority of such patients will not require indefinite or even prolonged ICU-level care, and it is often difficult to identify those who will (Leontyev, Borger, Davierwala, Walther, Lehmann, Kempfert and Mohr 2011). Therefore, valve replacement does not meet the Schneiderman et al. definition of futility, or of Pope's physiological or quantitative futility, though an argument could be made for qualitative futility from the perspective of society, but not on the basis of a low probability of achieving an acceptable quality of life for the patient.

There is another component to the futility argument in Mr. Wallace's case. Some estimates suggest that intravenous drug users lose 18 years of life due to their addiction. In many studies, relapse rates following intensive drug treatment are as high as 70% (Gossop, Green, Phillips and Bradley 1989; Frater 1990; Smyth, Hoffman, Fan and Hser 2007). Those who oppose giving Mr. Wallace a valve are likely to admit that surgery is not futile in the strictest of physiologic or quantitative or qualitative terms. His clinical course, however, may be one of multiple and inevitable failures, hardships, illnesses, and recidivism. These outcomes suggest qualitative futility. Mr. Wallace, the argument goes, has already demonstrated that he is not responsible enough to care for a prosthetic valve, has brought valvular dysfunction on himself, and will do so again, due to his underlying addiction. As DiMaio, Salerno, Bernstein et al. (2009) suggest, without an expanded definition of futility recognizing not only the procedural issues but also the addiction, cardiologists run the risk of continuing to pump resources into patients who will repeatedly fail. Perhaps Mr. Wallace deserves a first shot at surgery, but futility is reached if continuous intravenous drug using ensures that he will be back for another valve replacement, potentially returning at death's door in need of an intensive care unit-level of care, eventually with no tissue to which a new prosthetic valve could be sewn.

But at what point should futility be declared? Certainly the lack of viable tissue would constitute physiological futility, but should futility be declared at the point of the second presentation, or the third presentation? What if Mr. Wallace agrees to an inpatient drug rehab program after valve replacement? What if the duration between relapses is six months? One year?

Some have demanded that physicians develop guidelines to limit overuse and futile treatment (Hull and Jadbabaie 2014). Efforts legally to define and codify the procedures surrounding application of futility have been in place in Texas since the late 1990s and early 2000s. Texas law outlines a process by which a hospital can unilaterally withdraw life-sustaining care when such care is deemed medically inappropriate (Fine and Mayo 2003). The process involves ethics consultation as well as opportunities for appeal and transfer to another hospital or physician willing to provide the treatments or interventions deemed futile, including cardiopulmonary resuscitation. If quantitative or qualitative futility is considered in Mr. Wallace's case, there may be a role for ethics consultation and/ or hospital-level discussion (La Puma, Cassel and Humphrey 1988), aided by input from addiction medicine specialists to help with treatment plans and prognostication.

VI Conclusion

Bedside rationing of valves in intravenous drug users raises serious ethical difficulties related to unequal care and trust in the doctor–patient relationship. However, cardiologists may be called to play an increasingly important role as administrative gatekeepers, helping to develop fair policies for rationing care at the population level, while providing equitable care at the individual level. While cardiologists need not provide treatments they believe to be futile, futility justifications should not be invoked without a clear understanding of what is meant. The impact of unconscious bias and blame must be acknowledged. Ethics and addiction medicine consultants may play an important role.

References

Adler, N.E., and D.H. Rehkopf. 2008. US disparities in health: Descriptions, causes, and mechanisms, and mechanisms, *Annual Review of Public Health* 29: 235–252.

American Medical Association. 2019a. Code of medical ethics opinion 1.1.1: Patient-physician relationships. https://www.ama-assn.org/delivering-care/ethics/patient-physician-relationships.

American Medical Association. 2019b. Code of medical ethics opinion 11.1.2: Physician stewardship of health care resources. https://www.ama-assn.org/delivering-care/ethics/physician-stewardship-health-care-resources.

Beauchamp, T., and J. Childress. 1994. *Principles of biomedical ethics*, fourth edition. New York: Oxford University Press.

Benjamin, I.J. et al. 2021. 2020 American Heart Association and American College of Cardiology Consensus Conference on Professionalism and Ethics: A consensus conference report. *Journal of the American College of Cardiology* 2021(77): 3079–3133.

Braverman, P.A., C. Cubbin, S. Egerter, D.R. Williams, and E. Pamuk. 2010. Socioeconomic disparities in health in the United States: What the patterns tell us, *American Journal of Public Health* 100 (suppl 1): S186–S196.

Brener, L., W. Von Hippel, and S. Kippax. 2007. Prejudice among health care worker towards injection drug users with hepatitis C: Does greater contact lead to less prejudice? *International Journal of Drug Policy* 18(5): 381–387.

DiMaio, M.J., T.A. Salerno, R. Bernstein, K. Araujo, M. Ricci, and R.M. Sade. 2009. Ethical obligations of surgeons to noncompliant patients: Can a surgeon refuse to operate on an intravenous drug-abusing patient with recurrent aortic valve prosthesis infection? *Annals of Thoracic Surgery* 88(1): 1–8.

Eddy, D.M. 1990. Screening cervical cancer, *Annals of Internal Medicine* 113(3): 214–226.

Fine, R.L. and T.W. Mayo. 2003. Resolution of futility by due process: Early experience with the Texas Advance Directives Act. *Annals of Internal Medicine* 138(9): 743–746.

Frater, R.W. 1990. Surgical management of endocarditis in drug addicts and long-term results, *Journal of Cardiac Surgery* 5(1): 63–67.

Gossop, M., L. Green, G. Phillips, B. Bradley. 1989. Lapse relapse and survival among opiate addicts after treatment. A prospective follow-up study, *British Journal of Psychiatry* 154(3): 348–353.

Hull, S.C., and F. Jadbabaie. 2014. When is enough enough? The dilemma of valve replacement in a recidivist intravenous drug user, *Annals of Thoracic Surgery* 97(5): 1486–1487.

Jonsen, A.R. 2007. The God squad and the origins of transplantation ethics and policy, *Journal of Law, Medicine, and Ethics* 35(2): 238–240.

La Puma, J., C.K. Cassel, and H. Humphrey. 1988. Ethics, economics, and endocarditis: The physician's role in resource allocation. *Archives of Internal Medicine* 148(8): 1809–1811.

Lauridsen, S. 2009. Administrative gatekeeping – A third way between unrestricted patient advocacy and beside rationing, *Bioethics* (23)5: 311–320.

Leontyev, S., M.A. Borger, P. Davierwala, T. Walther, S. Lehmann, J. Kempfert, and F.W. Mohr. 2011. Redo aortic valve surgery: Early and late outcomes, *Annals of Thoracic Surgery* 91(4): 1120–1126.

Osnabrugge, R.L., A.M. Speir, S.J. Head, C.E. Fonner, E. Fonner Jr, F. Ailawadi, A.P. Kappetein, and J.B. Rich. 2013. Cost for surgical arotic valve replacement according to preoperative risk categories, *Annals of Thoracic Surgery* 96(2): 500–506.

Parmley, W.W., E.R. Passamani, and B. Lo. 1998. 29th Bethesda conference: Ethics in cardiovascular medicine (1997), *Journal of the American College of Cardiology* 31(5): 917–925.

Pope, T.M. 2007. Philosopher's corner: Medical futility, *Mid Atlantic Ethics Committee Newsletter* 15(1): 6–7.

Safran, D.G., M. Kosinski, A.R. Tarlov, W.H. Rogers, D.A. Taira, N. Lieberman, and J.E. Ware. 1998. The primary care assessment survey: Tests of data quality and measurement performance. *Medical Care* 36(5): 728–739.

Schneiderman, L.J., N.S. Jecker, and A.R. Jonsen. 1990. Medical futility: Its meaning and ethical implications, *Annals of Internal Medicine* 112(12): 949–954.

Schneiderman, L.J., N.S. Jecker and A.R. Jonsen. 1996. Medical futility: Response to critiques, *Annals of Internal Medicine* 125(8): 669–674.

Smyth, B., V. Hoffman, J. Fan, and Y.I. Hser. 2007. Years of potential life lost among heroin addicts 33 years after treatment, *Preventive Medicine* 44(4): 369–374.

Sprung, C.L., L.A. Eidelman, and A. Steinberg. 1995. Is the physician's duty to the individual patient or to society? *Critical Care Medicine* 23(4): 618–620.

Starr, A., and G.L. Grunkemeier. 2007. The cost and value of cardiothoracic procedures, *The Journal of Thoracic and Cardiovascular Surgery* 133(3): 601–602.

Sulmasy, D.P. 1992. Physicians, cost control, and ethics, *Annals of Internal Medicine* 116(11): 920–926.

Sulmasy, L.S., and T.A. Bledsoe. American College of Physicians Ethics, Professionalism, and Human Rights Committee. 2012. American College of Physicians ethics manual: Seventh edition, *Annals of Internal Medicine* 170 (Supplement): S1-S32.

Ubel, P.A., and R. Arnold. 1995. The unbearable rightness of bedside rationing: physician duties in a climate of cost containment, *Archives of Internal Medicine* 155(17): 1837–1842.

Ubel, P.A., and R. Jagsi. 2014. Promoting population health through financial steward-ship, *New England Journal of Medicine* 370(14): 1280–1281.

Von Hippel, W., L. Brener, and C. Von Hippel. 2008. Implicit prejudice toward injecting drug users predicts intentions to change jobs among drug and alcohol nurses, *Psychological Science* 19(1): 7–11.

Weinstein, M.C. 1990. Principles of cost-effective resource allocation in health care orga-nizations, *International Journal of Technological Assessment of Health Care* 6(1): 93–103.

Part IV

Professionalism in Cardiovascular Practice

9 Conflicts of Interest in Daily Practice

David M. Zientek

I Introduction

From its inception, the practice of medicine has involved conflicts of interest. It has been argued that "Conflict of interest is the central ethical problem of a profession, and indeed the problem that gives a profession its defining characteristic" (Hazard 1996, p. 85). When a patient experiences illness, he or she is unable to resolve a problem striking at one's very existence or conception of the self. The physician or health professional who has specialized knowledge and skills unavailable to the patient and who professes to put those abilities at the service of the patient is in a unique position of power relative to the patient's vulnerability and subsequently has special moral obligations to the patient (Pellegrino 1979). One of these obligations is the fiduciary responsibility to put the patient's interests above those of the physician and above those of the institutions the physician may represent.

Many definitions have been suggested for conflicts of interest, yet their variety and complexity may defy a simple all-encompassing definition (see, e.g., Rodwin 1993; Thompson 1993; Erde 1996; Khushf and Gifford 1998; Zientek 2003). Erde, for example, has suggested that one may best describe a variety of situations providing a "family resemblance of cases and criteria," though ultimately he recognizes that a short formula may be helpful (Erde 1996, p. 33). For the purposes of this chapter, I will adopt the understanding that a conflict of interest is present when a physician places himself or herself, or is placed, in a situation in which he or she may be likely to act against the primary interest of a patient to benefit a personal interest, or the interest of an institution. This definition does not necessarily imply that the physician has actually acted against the patient's interest, but rather that there is a significant potential motivation to do so. In addition, it does not imply that the secondary interest is illegitimate. The physician may have legitimate interests in achieving a good income to support a family or in helping a hospital or other institution remain financially viable, yet in almost all instances the professional should see these interests as secondary to the patient's. It is also important to recognize that the interest need not be financial. The goal of increasing professional prestige, advancing academic rank, loyalty to one's group or institution, or supporting a cherished clinical or intellectual belief may compromise one's ability to act fully in the patient's best interest.

DOI: 10.4324/9781003240273-14

The past century has witnessed significant changes in the type and complexity of medical diagnostics and therapeutics, the structure of medical practice and the financing of healthcare that have intensified the potential for conflicts of interest and the importance of their management (Rodwin 1993). A great deal of attention has focused on the dangers of conflicts faced by researchers (Bodenheimer 2000; Klaidman 2000), physician owners of healthcare facilities (Zientek 2003), and physician entanglements with the pharmaceutical and device industry (Shimm and Spece 1996; Klaidman 2000). Yet, the very structure of medical practice, including the way physicians are compensated, their relationships with hospitals and other institutions, and the ways in which they seek to increase their share of the healthcare market, create tensions among patients, physicians, and institutions. This chapter will focus on these more mundane, but no less important, conflicts of interest and their management.

II Case Report

Dr. G joined a practice of seven cardiologists approximately two years ago just after completing a fellowship. He has gradually been building a practice in general and interventional cardiology. His group experienced a significant decline in revenue due to changes in reimbursement reducing payments for diagnostic procedures, such as echocardiograms and nuclear stress tests performed in their office, while reimbursement for those performed in a hospital setting remained stable. In addition, the group worried about the cost of adopting electronic medical records as mandated by federal regulations. As a result, the group decided to sell their practice to a hospital system. The physicians are compensated based on productivity, though consideration is underway for establishment of an integrated Accountable Care Organization under which a significant proportion of patients may be covered by bundled payment for their disease processes with some physician compensation based on meeting certain quality measures. On a quarterly basis, the hospital system provides the cardiologists with a report of each physician's volume of office visits and hospital visits with the percent of these visits that generate procedures, such as nuclear stress tests or cardiac catheterizations, so that members of the group can determine if they are ordering an appropriate volume of studies. In addition, the hospital system advertises a screening CT scan to determine the presence of coronary artery calcifications indicative of coronary artery disease to the general public for which many potential patients often pay out of pocket. If patients have calcium detected, they are notified and encouraged to visit one of the hospital's cardiologists. Dr. G has had several patients who are post coronary artery bypass surgery who have purchased this study and come to him with the positive results.

III Management of Conflicts of Interest

There are four traditional methods for managing conflicts of interest. First is prohibition of the practice that creates the conflict, if it is of such magnitude that the likelihood of compromising an important obligation to the patient is high. For example, if physicians were directly selling products to patients when there is no sound scientific backing for the products, professional associations or regulatory agencies may legitimately ban such a practice. Similarly, if a physician works within an organization that consistently puts profitability ahead of quality patient care, and the physician is unable to convince the leadership of the organization to change the practice, he or she may be faced with a decision to leave the organization. Second is disclosure of the conflict of interest to patients. This has been a mainstay of contemporary management of conflicts of interest; however, one may question how likely it is that a physician will routinely inform patients of the means for compensating members of a practice, or the specifics of how the practice is organized. In addition, patients often may not have enough information to judge the significance of a conflict or their insurance provider may limit their ability to choose alternative caregivers even if they perceive a significant conflict. Third, another technique is promulgation of professional standards which guide decision-making, such as appropriate use criteria published by professional organizations for ordering echocardiograms or other diagnostic and therapeutic procedures to minimize overutilization at the patient or insurer's expense. Fourth, consultation with other professionals to obtain a "second opinion" about appropriate management of the conflict can be useful. For example, a clinician may seek out a trusted colleague or mentor to review a situation in which that clinician feels there may be significant potential to act against his or her patient's best interests (Hazard 1996, p. 88).

To determine the management technique most appropriate to a given conflict, it is necessary to consider the gravity of the potential harm and its likelihood. Five factors have been suggested as relevant for determining the likelihood of a transgression when there is potential for significant harm to the patient's interest (Khushf and Gifford 1998, pp. 359–60). First, determine how immediate the self-interest may be. For example, if a physician is compensated based on the volume of patients referred to an imaging center, the risk of unnecessary procedures is significant. Here, the clinician is aware of a direct and immediate relation between the number of referrals and personal income. This is one of the arguments for the Stark regulations controlling physician ownership of and compensation by healthcare facilities to which they refer patients (Stout and Warner 2003). Second, the degree to which a physician's self-interest is aligned with obligations to a patient will impact the odds of acting against a patient's good. The push for compensating physicians based on quality metrics rather than volume of procedures is an attempt to align physician interests with patient well-being. Third, another factor is the character of the physician. Professional codes of ethics and attempts to educate and raise clinician awareness of potential conflicts and their management may help reduce the danger of harm to patients. Fourth, the greater the uncertainty about appropriate indications for a procedure, the more likely a physician may be to order a given diagnostic or therapeutic intervention if he or she stands to benefit financially. The increased application of appropriate use criteria and professional society guidelines are attempts to reduce this likelihood; however, as will be discussed below, the inherent uncertainty in many areas of medicine may limit the impact of guidelines. Fifth, the likelihood of sanctions should the clinician violate obligations to a patient will impact the odds that a physician will act against the trust the patient has placed in him or her. Peer review of appropriate ordering patterns, while rarely done may be a future direction to address this factor and reduce the likelihood of patient harm. For more invasive procedures with a significant risk of complication, the possibility of malpractice liability may serve as a potential sanction to prevent unnecessary utilization of such techniques.

IV The Nature of Conflicts in Clinical Practice

The case of Dr. G illustrates a variety of potential conflicts of interest that most physicians will face at some point in their career. The ubiquity of the conflicts may in fact desensitize the clinician to their presence, allowing them to continue unaddressed until some outside observer brings them to light. There are three broad arrangements under which physicians practice that may be a source of conflict with a patient's interests: practice structure, insurance reimbursement and compensation methods, and the means used to increase patient volume and market share.

A Practice Structure

The past decade has seen significant shifts in the structure under which physicians organize their practices. As of 2007, approximately "90% of cardiologists were in an independent private practice," however, likely as a result of changes in compensation, by 2010 fully 61% of physicians had dissolved their private practices and integrated themselves into hospital systems (Jaskie and Rodgers 2014, p. 350). Physician-owned private practices and hospital ownership of physician groups each raise their own potential conflicts of interest.

In private practice, cardiologists have traditionally derived a significant portion of income from doing procedures. Several of these, such as echocardiography, stress testing and nuclear cardiology studies, can easily be incorporated in a private practice office. This may benefit the patient because of the convenience of receiving these diagnostic procedures along with recommended therapy in the same location and at the same time as their physician visits. Yet, concerns have been raised that physician ownership of this diagnostic equipment leads to overutilization as clinicians directly benefit from their use (Mitchell 1996; Schneider, Ohsfeldt, Scheibling and Jeffers 2012). In addition, in a small practice with limited administrative resources, it may be difficult to ensure the maintenance of equipment and quality control needed to provide accurate results for some of the studies, potentially putting patients at risk for incorrect diagnoses.

To lower the risk of overutilization, Medicare reduced compensation for many diagnostic studies performed in physician offices relative to those performed in hospitals. This has been cited as a major factor in the realignment of physicians with hospitals (Jaskie and Rodgers 2014, p. 351). In theory, the move to hospital employment by physicians may benefit patients by reducing the administrative burden on physicians allowing them to focus more on patient care. In addition, the large volume of procedures and the resources to provide the most up-to-date equipment and maintenance may improve the quality of studies provided. However, this change may conflict with patients' interests in other ways. The inconvenience of traveling to the hospital or another site remote from the physician's office for procedures may be a significant burden for patients with limited mobility or transportation issues. Moreover, it is not clear that moving the venue for testing will significantly reduce cost or utilization. A recent study of commercial Health Maintenance Organizations (HMO) enrollees in California found that when corrected for patient illness severity and other factors, hospital-owned physician organizations had higher expenditures per patient than physician-owned organizations (Robinson and Miller 2014). Similarly, early experience with Accountable Care Organizations (ACOs) suggests greater cost savings for independent physician groups compared with hospital-integrated ones (McWilliams, Hatfield, Chernew, Landon and Schwartz 2016). Medicare has begun to shift to a "site neutral" reimbursement policy so that physician-hospital alliances will not be able to charge a greater technical component for outpatient procedures relative to independent physician practices, and the Supreme Court has refused to hear a challenge to this policy by the American Hospital Association (American College of Cardiology Foundation, 2021).

Another concern is that financial incentives and loyalty to the hospital employer may induce physicians to admit patients to the hospital with which they are affiliated or refer only to specialists within the system, rather than a competing hospital or specialist which may be better equipped to handle certain complex issues (DeCamp and Lehmann 2015; Graber, Bhandary and Rizzo 2016). Physicians may not inform patients of the alternate institution and thus impair the process of informed consent. Indeed, one of the private practice physician's strongest tools to protect patients and insist on high quality care in hospitals has traditionally been the ability to direct patients elsewhere.

B Insurance Reimbursement and Compensation Methods

The second way in which practice arrangements may put physician and patient interests into conflict on a daily basis are the various forms of reimbursement for clinician services and the ways in which physicians compensate themselves or are compensated by a hospital from the revenue generated by those services. The primary structures under which physicians have been paid over the past half-century include fee for service, capitated payments, and, most recently, accountable care type arrangements.

Fee for service is the longest-standing method for paying physicians and remains a major force in medical financial arrangements. Under this system physicians or institutions are compensated based on the number of patients seen and procedures performed (both diagnostic and therapeutic). Here, the primary concern is that this system encourages overutilization of testing and procedures since physician income is directly proportional to the number of patients treated or procedures performed (Rodwin 1993). Traditionally, procedures have been compensated more generously than patient visits, leading to a potential overemphasis on using costly technology rather than simpler treatment and diagnostic techniques, and at the cost of clearly communicating the risk and benefit to patients of these procedures. Physicians stand to benefit financially from the provision of services even if the procedure is unnecessary, only marginally beneficial, or harms the patient.

In an attempt to reign in the perceived abuses of fee for service, various forms of capitated payment have been proposed. The majority has taken the form of HMOs, which flourished in the late twentieth century. Under these types of compensation plans, physicians are typically paid by capitation, a set price per patient to care for all healthcare needs. In this way, the physician shares financial risk with the insurer. The patient's primary physician is supposed to serve as a gatekeeper, referring patients for specialized consultation and testing only when clearly indicated, because with the fixed payment the physician did not stand to gain by doing additional unnecessary or only marginally beneficial testing. This practice, however, raised concerns that the physician now had an incentive to deny services, even if clearly indicated, as they stood to benefit from the unused portion of the patient's premiums (Rodwin 1993, pp. 135–175). In addition to capitation, managed care has utilized other techniques to rein in costs. These include removing physicians from provider panels who are felt to be economically inefficient while patients are typically required to see physicians within the managed care panel, and employing utilization review in which costly procedures may be denied for payment based on some preset criteria for choosing a particular test. Concerns have been raised that such techniques limit physician autonomy to act in a patient's best interest, and by focusing on limiting expensive procedures, fail to look at instances in which appropriate testing or therapeutic procedures are in fact underutilized (Rodwin 1993, pp. 135–175).

To compensate for the potential for denying needed care under various managed care structures, many have proposed that various quality measures be incorporated into payment schemes, which will provide incentives to physicians who provide care meeting certain quality metrics, thus insuring that appropriate interventions are not neglected (Rodwin 1993, pp. 135–175; Porter and Lee 2013). The most prominent means currently for achieving this goal is the Accountable Care Organization (ACO). In these organizations, groups of providers, often a sponsoring hospital and multiple physician specialty groups, come together to provide coordinated care and take on many of the functions of a traditional insurance company. Three characteristics of ACOs differentiate them from other financing arrangements (Berenson and Burton 2011). First, they depend on shared savings in which providers receive bonuses for designing efficient means of providing care if the cost of healthcare they provide falls below a certain amount based on their historic level of spending, whether high or low in the past. It is hoped that having institutions and multiple physician specialties within the organization will streamline care and avoid duplication of testing or therapeutic measures. Second, the amount of the shared savings the providers receive is dependent on meeting a variety of quality measures such as reducing the frequency with which patients with heart failure are readmitted to the hospital, presumably measuring the quality of care provided. Finally, patients in an ACO are free to see providers outside the ACO if they are covered by their insurance, hopefully reducing the impact of economic profiling of physicians on a patient's ability to choose their provider.

While ACOs may have some benefits over previous means of financing healthcare, there are foreseeable conflicts of interest with these organizations as well. First, while the focus on quality measures is designed to avoid the most egregious abuses, the largest financial benefit for caregivers at this point still comes from reducing the cost of care. There will still be a temptation to minimize costly interventions that may benefit a patient. To benefit the most costly patients (those with multiple chronic illnesses or complex social situations) without harming their interest in receiving indicated care will require complex analysis and targeting of the needs of particular patient populations that will vary by location, type of insurance, and patient demographics (Powers and Chaguturu 2016). The focus on an ACO's costs being below a historical threshold may punish those who have already been providing appropriate levels of care. Given that quality metrics to date have primarily been those that are easily measured, these groups may be forced to avoid providing more complex and costly procedures deemed appropriate, but not included in quality measures, to improve their financial standing (Graber, Bhandary and Rizzo 2016). Even for those groups who need significantly to reduce excessive utilization, at some point, they will presumably reach an appropriate level of spending, and at that point will also be tempted to further avoid appropriate procedures to improve profitability. Even though ACOs allow patients to see physicians out of the network, the close integration of hospitals and multiple caregivers in an ACO, while streamlining care, may place patients at risk of only being referred to the involved hospital, or affiliated consultants even if alternate caregivers might be more appropriate or of higher quality (DeCamp and Lehmann 2015; Graber, Bhandary and Rizzo, 2016).

Tying compensation to quality measures may also introduce potential conflicts of interest between caregivers and patients. Up to this point, "most quality metrics do not gauge quality; rather, they are process measures that capture compliance with practice guidelines" (Porter and Lee 2013). Many of these quality measures have been items such as the percentage of patients with heart failure or coronary artery disease who receive certain guideline-recommended medications. While these may be important to track, they do not invariably lead to improvement in what patients may value, such as return to work, functional ability, and cost of care (Porter and Lee 2013). There are dangers that such simplified measures may induce physicians to place patients on treatments that may not be optimal for their situation, such as continuing statin medications in a patient with significant muscular pain impacting lifestyle. Alternatively, the physician may "game the system" by recognizing that this patient has stopped taking the statin, but continue to list it in electronic records as a prescribed medication for reporting purposes, rather than exploring alternate options for lipid lowering such as lifestyle modification or other medications. The use of patient satisfaction surveys as a quality metric may be particularly prone to conflicts. If a patient, informed by the Internet, presents to the clinic demanding a treatment the physician deems inappropriate for their condition, the clinician may be inclined to provide the treatment rather than incite the patient's displeasure (Graber, Bhandary and Rizzo, 2016).

Using adherence to guidelines as quality measures may induce another conflict due to uncertainty in many recommendations. Typically guideline recommendations are rated by a classification system with class I being treatments or procedures based on evidence or general agreement that are "useful and effective." Class III includes treatments and procedures that are not effective and may even be harmful. Class II treatments and procedures are those for which there is conflicting evidence or divergence of opinion about effectiveness, with class IIa being those where the weight of evidence or opinion favors the procedure, and class IIb being those where efficacy is less well-established by the evidence or expert opinion (American College of Cardiology Foundation, American Heart Association, 2010). Given that a significant percentage of common procedures fall into class II, there is significant potential for conflicts of interest in appealing to guidelines. Class IIb procedures are typically ones that the majority of cardiologists would utilize infrequently. A physician concerned about liability might be induced frequently to order a IIb-rated diagnostic procedure as part of practicing "defensive medicine" and would have the added incentive of being reimbursed for the procedure, while the patient would be exposed to any risks and costs of the procedure.

The limitations of current quality measures may have other impacts on patients. It has been argued that it is unethical to refer a patient to a cardiac surgeon with less than the best mortality reported to a state database (Brown and Clarke 2012). However, others have argued that such gross measures of quality may not adequately reflect the case mix of providers, would potentially limit access to care as the top rated physicians may become overwhelmed with volume, and that these measures ignore other factors such as caregiver personality and location which patients may value highly (Shahian and Normand 2012). Finally, there is some evidence that in states where mortality figures are publicly reported, physicians may refuse to take on the sickest patients, or may modify medical records to make patients appear more acutely ill than they actually are to improve their quality statistics (Kolker 2005).

The ways in which physicians are compensated as members of a group tend to parallel the different types of insurance reimbursement with similar potential conflicts of interest. Many groups, as with Dr. G's organization, are compensated based on productivity, often directly proportional to the income they generate for the group or some measure of patients seen and procedures performed. This type of compensation would be subject to similar conflicts of interest to those outlined under fee for service insurance. A second means of compensating physicians within a group is by fixed salary. While this method separates compensation from the volume of procedures and has the advantage of removing an incentive to over utilize testing, there are potential conflicts with the patient's interests. As with capitation, the physician may not have the incentive to procure testing or therapy that requires significant expenditure of time or effort. For example, the salaried physician may be less likely to take the time to argue for and provide documentation for beneficial procedures that are denied by a utilization review organization. There will also be less incentive to work in an urgent patient when the clinic is already fully booked (Kirsch 2010). As a result, many groups are now going to a hybrid type of compensation in which a base salary is guaranteed with potential bonuses for productivity above a certain level and/or meeting certain quality metrics determined by the practice. As with ACOs, this is likely an improvement, but still risks having incentives that go against the patient's interest. In these compensation models, it will be important to achieve a balance between bonuses for productivity and quality so that one does not significantly outweigh the other in physician perception. As with ACOs, the quality measures at this point are likely to be simplistic and subject to gaming of the system. Hence a great deal of attention should focus on developing truly meaningful quality metric standards that reflect beneficial outcomes for patients.

C Advertising and Marketing of Medical Procedures

In the increasingly competitive healthcare environment, marketing of medical groups has become increasingly common. Prior to 1975, advertising by physicians was prohibited by the American Medical Association (AMA); however, in that year, the Federal Trade Commission sued the AMA, arguing that such a prohibition was an antitrust violation (Tomycz, 2006; Fuster 2015). Since that time advertising by physicians, hospitals and other institutions, and direct marketing to patients by pharmaceutical companies has become standard fare in the media. For physicians and hospitals, advertising may be direct, in the form of advertising newly recruited physicians, services provided, or location. Indirect advertising, in which physicians and institutions seek out local media reporting on new techniques, treatments, or research being utilized by their group, is increasingly common.

   Whether or not one believes advertising has been beneficial to patients or the profession, its widespread utilization raises a new set of conflicts of interest in the daily practice of healthcare. Unlike a careful informed discussion between physician and patient of the indications, alternatives, and risks of a given diagnostic or therapeutic intervention, advertising lends itself to presenting a limited and typically positive perspective on the intervention. This "may increase the cost of health care and create unrealistic expectations that will further weaken the relations between doctor and patient" (Tomycz 2006, p. 27). A study of advertising encouraging self-referral for computed tomographic and magnetic resonance imaging found that a significant number of advertisements contained claims lacking documented scientific evidence and that appeals to emotion as an inducement to seek out the advertised tests were common (Illes et al. 2004). Not only does such advertising represent a potential financial conflict of interest in terms of inducing a patient to undergo a costly procedure which may be unnecessary, but given concern about the increasing exposure to radiation from medical imaging, patients may well be exposed to potential medical harm (Fazel et al. 2009).

V Review of Case Report

Dr. G is faced with many structural conflicts of interest in his practice. There are several considerations relating to his group practice sale to a local hospital system. Before entering into such an arrangement, the group must carefully consider the impact on its patients. While it seems obvious that the group would want to join the hospital when compensation for procedures in an individual practice decline relative to those done within a hospital system, is this sufficient reason to make the change? First, the group must determine how much a change in location of testing may impact a large proportion of their patients, in terms of inconvenience and out-of-pocket cost. If the decline in revenue truly imperils the survival of the group, it may be necessary to join the hospital system; however, if the impact on finances is not large, the group may have to weigh impact on patients more heavily. Groups must consider that compensation formulas are continually changing, and as the Centers for Medicare and Medicaid Services and other insurers change reimbursement for procedures to contain costs, it may be important to avoid changing practice patterns in pursuit of short-term economic benefit. For example, physicians should choose imaging techniques for diagnosing coronary artery disease based on characteristics of the patient and local expertise, rather than on the reimbursement rate for the procedure relative to others. For example, groups might be induced to order more nuclear stress tests versus stress echocardiograms based on the relative reimbursement in a given year, and change patterns if reimbursement changes. Alignment with a hospital may have sufficient benefit to patients in aspects other than cost and convenience, but Dr. G and his partners will have to weigh carefully the potential for conflicts between physicians and their patients' interests in all areas.

If the group decides after careful review that an alignment is appropriate, it will be important carefully to negotiate the arrangement with the healthcare system to preserve physician independence allowing physicians to disclose their relationship with the hospital system and any alternate caregivers or hospitals outside the network which may potentially offer better care or convenience to the patient for particular conditions. It is important for physicians to maintain some degree of control of compensation measures. In a productivity-based model, the publication of procedure ordering patterns could present a dangerous conflict of interest between physicians and their patients. Unless such data is accompanied by accurate analysis to support which partners are ordering studies according to guidelines, there will be pressure to match the ordering patterns of the highest earning members, even if these individuals are over-utilizing resources. Dr. G may help minimize the risk of his acting against his patient's interests by following professional guidelines and consulting with respected outside physicians if there are questions about the appropriateness of a procedure he is considering. However, if the potential impact of such reporting appears sufficiently strong, he should argue for ending the practice of publishing ordering profiles to the group, and if the pressure for productivity is so great that he feels he cannot exercise appropriate judgment in the interests of his patients, he may even need to consider leaving the group. As discussed in the review of methods for dealing with conflict of interest, the character or virtue of the physician plays a role in the likelihood of harm from conflicts of interest, and Dr. G. ought to play a role in influencing his partners by raising awareness of the issues faced by his group.

If the group does move to an ACO model, it will be important for members of the group to be actively involved in determining the quality measures to be used. It will be important to ensure that those measures truly reflect aspects of care that impact patients' mortality and quality of life. In the compensation plan, it will be essential that the weight of quality measures be sufficient to balance the emphasis on reducing cost of care. Physicians will need to restructure care delivery within the ACO to be sure that changes are truly beneficial to patients rather than only the institution.

Finally, the hospital system's advertising of coronary calcium scoring without a prior evaluation raises significant issues of conflicts of interest. Such advertising certainly benefits the hospital and the cardiology group by inducing a significant number of patients to have testing, with a proportion of those patients then being referred to the group for further testing. However, the role of coronary calcium testing remains controversial and has primarily been studied for risk stratification of asymptomatic patients at risk for coronary disease, and is not recommended for patients with known disease (Sanz 2015). The fact that Dr. G has had several patients who have already had coronary artery bypass undergo the expense and radiation exposure of the test should spur a response by his group. Members of the group should approach the institution to end marketing of the procedure to the general public, or at the very least make clear in the advertising those patients for whom such testing is appropriate.

VI Conclusion

As illustrated by our case, conflicts of interest are inherent in the very structures used to provide medical care. Physicians are faced with conflicts between their interests and those of their institutions on the one hand, and their patients in an ongoing basis. As the healthcare system changes, the nature of the conflicts will evolve, but will not go away. It will be crucial to patient trust in the healthcare system that their interests are protected even as physicians and institutions look after their own interests. Where conflicts are of sufficient weight and immediacy, it may be appropriate to ban particular practices or perhaps conscientious physicians may need to leave a particular group practice or institution. The ongoing promulgation of guidelines where possible and an increasing emphasis on quality, while still in its infancy, will help regulate those conflicts which may not be of sufficient weight to require an outright ban. Given that conflicts of interest will always be present, physician character and awareness of these conflicts must serve as a crucial protection for patients. As a profession, healthcare must be willing to discuss openly the conflicts of interest we face and consult both within the profession and with outside experts on the most appropriate measures to mitigate their impact.

References

American College of Cardiology Foundation, American Heart Association. 2010. Methodology manual and policies from the ACCF/AHA task force on practice guidelines. https://professional.heart.org/professional/GuidelinesStatements.

American College of Cardiology Foundation 2021. Supreme Court declines to review site-neutral payment policy. https://www.acc.org/latest-in-cardiology/articles/2021/07/07/19/24/supreme-court-declines-to-review-site-neutral-payment-policy.

Berenson, R.A., and R.A. Burton. 2011. *Accountable care organizations in Medicare and the private sector: A status update.* Washington DC: Urban Institute.

Bodenheimer, T. 2000. Uneasy alliance—Clinical investigators and the pharmaceutical industry, *New England Journal of Medicine* 342 (20): 1539–1544.

Brown, D.L., and S. Clarke. 2012. Cardiac surgeon report cards, referral for cardiac surgery, and the ethical responsibilities of cardiologists, *Journal of the American College of Cardiology* 59(25): 2378–2382.

DeCamp, M., and L.S. Lehmann. 2015. Guiding choice — Ethically influencing referrals in ACOs, *New England Journal of Medicine* 372(3): 205–207.

Erde, E.L. 1996. Conflicts of interests in medicine: A philosophical and ethical morphology. In: *Conflicts of interest in clinical practice and research* (pp. 12–41), Spece, R.G., D.S. Shimm, and A.E. Buchanan (eds). New York: Oxford University Press.

Fazel, R., H.M. Krumholz, Y. Wang, J.S. Ross, J. Chen, H.H. Ting, N.D. Shah, N. Khurram, A.J. Einstein, and B.K. Nallamothu. 2009. Exposure to low-dose ionizing radiation from medical imaging procedures in the United States, *New England Journal of Medicine* 361(9): 849–857.

Fuster, V. 2015. The hazards of physician advertising, *Journal of the American College of Cardiology* 66(22): 2561–2562.

Graber, A.D., A. Bhandary, and M. Rizzo. 2016. Ethical practice under accountable care, *HEC Forum* 28(2): 115–128.

Hazard, G.C. 1996. Conflict of interest in the classic professions. In: *Conflicts of interest in clinical practice and research* (pp. 85–104), Spece, R.G., D.S. Shimm, and A.E. Buchanan (eds). New York: Oxford University Press.

Illes, J., D. Kann, K. Karetsky, P. Letourneau, T.A. Raffin, P. Schraedley-Desmond, B.A. Koenig, and S.W. Atlas. 2004. Advertising, patient decision making, and self-referral for computed tomographic and magnetic resonance imaging, *Archives of Internal Medicine* 164(22): 2415–2419.

Jaskie, S., and G. Rodgers. 2014. Current trends in U.S. cardiology practice, *Trends in Cardiovascular Medicine* 24(8): 350–359.

Khushf, G., and R. Gifford. 1998. Understanding, assessing, and managing conflicts of interest. In: *Surgical Ethics* (pp. 342–366), McCullough, L.B., J.W. Jones, and B.A. Brody (eds). New York: Oxford University Press.

Kirsch, M. 2010. Conflicts of interest and conflicting views on physician compensation: Fee-for-service versus salaried medicine, *Clinical Gastroenterology and Hepatology* 8(8): 666–668.

Klaidman, S. 2000. *Saving the heart: The battle to conquer coronary disease.* New York: Oxford University Press.

Kolker, R. 2005. Heartless, *New York Magazine*, October 24.

McWilliams, J.M., L.A. Hatfield, M.E. Chernew, B.E. Landon, and A.L. Schwartz. 2016. Early performance of accountable care organizations in Medicare, *New England Journal of Medicine* 274(24): 2357–2366.

Mitchell, J.M. 1996. Physician joint ventures and self-referral: An empirical perspective. In: *Conflicts of interest in clinical practice and research* (pp. 300–317), Spece, R.G., D.S. Shimm, and A.E. Buchanan (eds). New York: Oxford University Press.

Pellegrino, E.D. 1979. Toward a reconstruction of medical morality: The primacy of the act of profession and the fact of illness, *The Journal of Medicine and Philosophy* 4(1): 32–56.

Porter, M.E., and T.H. Lee. 2013. The strategy that will fix health care, *Harvard Business Review* 91(12): 24–41.

Powers, B.W., and S.K. Chaguturu. 2016. ACOs and high-cost patients. *New England Journal of Medicine* 374(3): 203–205.

Robinson, J.C., and K. Miller. 2014. Total expenditures per patient in hospital-owned and physician-owned physician organizations in California, *JAMA* 312(16): 1663–1669.

Rodwin, M.A. 1993. *Medicine, money, & morals: Physicians' conflicts of interest.* New York: Oxford University Press.

Sanz, J. 2015. Coronary calcium score and the new guidelines: Back to square one? *Journal of the American College of Cardiology* 66(15): 1669–1671.

Schneider, J.E., R.L. Ohsfeldt, C.M. Scheibling, and S.A. Jeffers. 2012. Organizational boundaries of medical practice: The case of physician ownership of ancillary services, *Health Economics Review* 2(1): 7.

Shahian, D.M., and S.T. Normand. 2012. Autonomy, beneficence, justice, and the limits of provider profiling, *Journal of the American College of Cardiology* 59(25): 2383–2386.

Shimm, D.S., and R.G. Spece. 1996. Conflicts of interest in relationships between physicians and the pharmaceutical industry. In: *Conflicts of interest in clinical practice and research* (pp. 321–357), Spece, R.G., D.S. Shimm, and A.E. Buchanan (eds). New York: Oxford University Press.

Stout, S.M., and D.C. Warner. 2003. How did physician ownership become a federal case? The stark amendments and their prospects, *HEC Forum* 15(2): 171–187.

Thompson, D.F. 1993. Understanding financial conflicts of interest, *New England Journal of Medicine* 329 (8): 573–576.

Tomycz, N.D. 2006. A profession selling out: Lamenting the paradigm shift in physician advertising, *Journal of Medical Ethics* 32(1): 26–28.

Zientek, D.M. 2003. Physician entrepreneurs, self-referral, and conflicts of interest: An overview, *HEC Forum* 15(2): 111–133.

10 Ethical Challenges for Cardiology Societies

Conflicts of Interest and Clinical Practice Guidelines

Mark A. Hoffman and James N. Kirkpatrick

I Introduction

Conflicts of interest are inherent in complex avenues of human endeavor. They find universal expression in those activities in which an individual, or group of individuals, undertakes to act for the benefit of others under circumstances where self-dealing is a risk. On its face, such conflict suggests a disconnection between the interests of the individual or group, and the interests of others, to whom there is owed an obligation of loyalty or fidelity. Self-dealing and self-interest are the operative challenges in the ultimate analysis of conflict of interest.

The analytic framework for assessing potential or actual conflicts of interest examines: (1) the presence or absence of special duties or obligations; (2) the context in which these special duties and obligations arise; (3) the values rehearsed or invested in these duties or obligations; and (4) the status of the individual or group to whom these duties and obligations are ultimately owed. Resolutions of conflict of interest focus on mechanisms to eliminate or effectively neutralize the intrusive influence of competing interests in favor of selflessness.

This chapter examines the relationship of professional medical societies which promulgate clinical practice guidelines to corporate entities within the pharmaceutical, biological, and medical device industries. The topic is not unique to the field of cardiology; it finds expression across all medical disciplines. There is, however, a spectrum of responses among medical societies which range from no position or laissez-faire approaches to highly restrictive and proscriptive codes of conduct. This topic has garnered recent attention along several lines of inquiry, and has generated a robust body of scholarly analysis (Norris et al. 2011, 2012).

II Medicine and Industry: An Ethical Framework of Analysis

The medical profession's relationship with the pharmaceutical, biological, and medical device industries exist across a broad interface of clinical and academic activities. The common boundaries include medical research, grant support and funding for continuing medical education programs, and more personal

DOI: 10.4324/9781003240273-15

relationships between physicians and industry by way of speaker bureaus, stock and patent ownership, physician participation on scientific advisory boards, and physician recruitment by companies to serve as key opinion leaders and key thought leaders. These relationships, in many respects, are a byproduct of the complexities of patient management and the increasing dependence of patient care on pharmaceutical, medical devices and other products. In the modern era of medical practice, these relationships form an uneasy symbiosis of necessity, and become particularly challenging in areas of product research and development. Patient enrollment and participation in clinical research studies and the clinical phases of product development, for example, are essential components of bringing pharmaceuticals and medical products to market. Industry funding of physicians and institutions conducting clinical trials is indispensable, and ensures a sustained and evolving inventory of safe and effective drugs, biologics, and devices.

Support for physician educational activities in areas of pharmaceutical products and medical technology inure to both the physician and manufacturer, and presumptively, to the patient. These programs should result in the effective and appropriate use of newer products, while generating an expanded profile for, and broader acceptance of, the product within the medical community.

Residual discomfort, however, persists with respect to the relationship between industry and the medical profession, and is colored by skepticism and possible overtones of greed or self-interest. A disquieting loss of independence surfaces when physician–industry relationships trend toward product endorsements, promotional or marketing activities, or under circumstances of an apparent or suspected *quid pro quo*. Intimations of bias, self-dealing, self-interest, undue influence, or compromised academic or intellectual integrity can compete or conflict with the core values of professionalism expected from physicians and their representative professional societies.

The practice of medicine is fundamentally a "moral enterprise" informed primarily by the doctor–patient relationship (Pelligrino and Relman 1999). More than a millennium of tradition and historical precedent underscores the heightened and self-effacing duties owed by the physician to the patient. Such duties are defined by the medical profession's role as practitioners of the "healing arts," and the inherent and palpable manifest asymmetry of the doctor–patient relationship.

The notion of physician as fiduciary pervades the moral and legal doctrinal underpinnings of professional obligations (Furrow and Molinoff 2009). This fiduciary obligation

is rooted in the vulnerability of patients when they are sick, the discrepancy in expertise between physicians and patients, and the difficulties patients may have in judging physicians' recommendations. This fiduciary duty to act in the patient's interests distinguishes the profession of medicine from a mere business.

(Parmley, Passamani and Lo 1998, p. 923)

An alignment of fundamental interests in the doctor–patient relationship is a central guidepost of medicine. Indeed, it is a touchstone of patient care readily distinguishable from the more pedestrian arms-length relationships found in other activities.

> Most believe that becoming and practicing as a physician is a somewhat different matter, morally, from simply setting oneself up in business. Business people are expected to be ethical—for instance, not to shortchange their customers or to deliver an inferior product when the customer has paid for top quality. But an ethical businessperson is supposed to put aside her own self-interest, with the goal of serving the customer, only to a limited extent. The customer is assumed to know what is in his own interest and to act accordingly. Physicians, by contrast, are expected to put aside many of their own personal interests, and to devote themselves instead to promoting the interests of their patients.
>
> (Brody 2007, p. 23)

Three general principles of bioethics animate medicine as a "moral enterprise," and provide a general framework that expresses the values underlying rules in common morality and the guidelines of professional ethics (Beauchamp, Walters, Kahn and Mastroianni 2014). They include: respect for autonomy, beneficence, and justice, which find common ground in the physician's axiomatic commitment to "primum non nocere" ("above all, do no harm") (Beauchamp, Walters, Kahn and Mastroianni 2014).

The Hippocratic Oath proscribes self-dealing and self-interest: "In every house where I come I will enter only for the good of my patients, keeping myself far from all intentional ill-doing" (http://en.wikipedia.org/wiki/Hippocratic_Oath). While the nature of this commitment has dramatically evolved since the time of Hippocrates, the lens of conflict of interest analysis remains unchanged: a conflict of interest arises when there is a misalignment of priorities. Specifically, the misalignment is characterized by the subjugation of the primary interest—the well-being of the patient—to the draw of prohibited collateral considerations which detract from this primary interest (Molinoff 2009). The Institute of Medicine succinctly defines such a conflict of interest as "a set of circumstances that creates a risk that professional judgment or actions regarding a primary interest will be unduly influenced by a secondary interest" (2009, p. 46).

The guideposts and vitality of a fiduciary relationship reside in the moral principles of loyalty and fidelity. The philosopher Josiah Royce explained:

> In loyalty, when loyalty is properly defined, is the fulfilment of the whole moral law. You can truthfully centre your entire moral world about a rational conception of loyalty. Justice, charity, industry, wisdom, spirituality, are all definable in terms of enlightened loyalty... Loyalty shall mean...

The willing and practical and thoroughgoing devotion of a person to a cause... In any case, when the loyal man serves his cause, he is not seeking his own private advantage.

(1908, p. 15; see also DeMott 2006)

Loyalty is the defining paradigm of the doctor–patient relationship. The loyal physician "must not deal secretly with others who are contrary in interest to the patient and must at any time reasonably account to the patient for his or her activity on their behalf" (Carlisle 2004, p. 166). In its purist form of practice, "[m]edicine purports to uphold certain interests such as the good of the patient, objectivity, scientific integrity and accuracy" (Kirkpatrick, Kadakia, and Vargas 2012, p. 259). Compromise of these primary interests violates the "social contract" by which physicians are accorded "trust, prestige and a handsome income in exchange for maintaining a disinterested professionalism" (Kirkpatrick, Kadakia, and Vargas 2012, p. 259).

Conflicts of interest, whether actual or perceived, place the legitimacy of the medical profession on trial, and raise a myriad of concerns on the part of healthcare practitioners and patients alike. When motives enter into the calculus for physician activities, there is a distinct and potentially profound diminution of authenticity bordering on betrayal. Indeed, betrayal is a core phenomenon when a fiduciary duty is breached.

III Industry and Cardiology

Cardiology as a medical specialty is intensely dependent upon both technology and pharmaceuticals across various subspecialties within the field. Examples of this dependency are abundant and obvious, and include both diagnostic and therapeutic aspects of clinical cardiology (e.g., implantable electronic devices (pacemakers, defibrillators, ventricular assist devices, bridging devices to transplantation, heart valves); pharmaceutical management of cardiac risk factors (statins); antiarrhythmics; and cardiac imaging and catheter-based interventions (angiography, percutaneous coronary artery procedures and stenting; structural heart procedures such as transcatheter valve interventions, electrophysiologic mapping and ablation)). The technological and pharmacologic advancements in patient care commands the *de facto* alliance at very basic levels of physicians industry (Cadet 2011).

Additionally, more sophisticated tiers of specialization within cardiology provide a key driver for narrower and more concentrated touch-points between industry and specialists (Cassel and Reuben 2011). As practitioners tailor their area of expertise in more specific and higher-order technological areas, their dependence upon the pharmaceutical and device manufactures intensifies, thereby increasing the intimacy of the relationships.

Misgivings over these relationships have a vibrant history. In 1961, Charles May, a pediatrician at Columbia University, cautioned that "the traditional independence of physicians and the welfare of the public are being threatened by the new vogue among drug manufacturers to promote their products by assuming an aggressive role in the 'education' of doctors" (quoted in Fye 1996, p. 190).

> [May] questioned the wisdom of the profession's becoming "greatly dependent upon pharmaceutical manufactures for support in scientific journals and medical societies. Claiming that they spent $750 million on promotion (including $125 million on journal ads and direct mail in 1959, May urged "ethical drug firms" to "reconsider the appropriateness of attempting to influence physicians by subtle infiltration into the educational process."
>
> (Fye 1996, p. 190)

"The traditional independence of physicians" and "the welfare of the public" are common threads that course through conflict of interest debates. Notions of physicians selling out to corporate interests are clarion cries.

An expanding relationship between industry and medicine led Arnold Relman, longtime editor of the *New England Journal of Medicine*, to observe in 1980:

> As the visibility and importance of the private health-care industry grow, public confidence in the medical profession will depend on the public's perception of the doctor as an honest, disinterested trustee. That confidence is bound to be shaken by any financial association between practicing physicians and the new medical-industrial complex.
>
> (Relman 1980, p. 967)

Relman warned that

> pecuniary associations with pharmaceutical and medical supply and equipment firms will also be suspect and should therefore be curtailed ... the medical profession would be in a stronger position, and its voice would carry more moral authority with the public and the government, if it adopted the principle that practicing physicians should derive no financial benefit from the health-care market except from their own professional services.
>
> (Relman 1980, p. 967)

A comprehensive congressional response to this problem was a public mechanism for exposing industry relationships with medical practitioners. The Physician Payments Sunshine Act (Grassley 2013a) (also called "Open Payments") mandates public reporting of payments by pharmaceutical companies to doctors for consulting fees, travel, speeches, meals and other activities (Grassley 2013b). The Act went into effect on April 9, 2013, and requires "applicable manufactures of drugs, devices, biologicals, or medical supplies... to report annually to the Secretary [of Health and Human Services] certain payments or transfers of value to physicians and teaching hospitals."[1] Such payments or other transfers of value will be posted annually on a publically available website.[2] This federally mandated disclosure mechanism allows specific information on these payments and other transfers of value to physicians (and advance practice providers) to be available for review by patients, other clinicians, health insurers, employers healthcare service companies, regulators and law enforcement officials.

A salient question, however, arises: how does mandatory industry reporting cure conflicts of interest within medical organizations and societies, or safeguard or protect the presumptive beneficiary of clinical practice guidelines—the patient?

IV Professional Organizations and Societies

Professional medical societies represent groups of physicians whose interests and agendas are advanced through a structured and enduring organizational framework. Societies provide a unified voice to the membership and address a variety of shared needs across a range of activities: publications and journals; educational meetings and continuing medical education events; political action committees and lobbying; public health and patient care initiatives; and networking. Normatively, such societies and organizations should give expression to the core values inherent in medical practice and patient care responsibilities. Such associations are *medical* associations, and should therefore be grounded in the same ethical firmament as the *medical* profession. This extrapolation of purpose, *a fortiori*, is expressed in the various mission statements, visions, and core values espoused by these societies, which universally and uniformly endorse professionalism, research, education, public health, and dedication to patient care. (See Table 10.1.)

Medical organizations are, in many aspects, composites of moral actors. Their grounding in patient welfare should theoretically place them above the wrangling of self-interest and self-dealing.

> Effacement of self-interest is the distinguishing feature of a true profession that sets it apart from other occupations. It is the heart of the *professing* of medicine, i.e., the public declaration and promise that physicians can be trusted to use their skills for something other than their own benefit. Individual physicians privately make this promise whenever they invite trust by offering their skills to help someone who is ill. When physicians form professional associations, they should make this promise collectively. They become members of a moral community dedicated to the primacy of those who need their help.
>
> (Pelligrino and Relman 1999, p. 984)

Medical societies and organizations, however, operate within the larger context of industry interests, and are often the benefactors of industry largesse and operational support. While some organizations receive *di minimis* industry financing, others traditionally receive upwards of 40% or more of their financial support

Table 10.1 Mission, Vision and Values of the American College of Cardiology
(https://www.acc.org/About-ACC)

Mission
To transform cardiovascular care and improve heart health.

Vision
A world where innovation and knowledge optimize cardiovascular care and outcomes.

Core Values
- Patient Centered.
  - Advocate on behalf of the cardiovascular patient population in promotion of the public good
  - Practice organizational altruism — the safety and needs of cardiovascular patients are central to everything we do
  - Support and educate patients and clinicians in the practice of shared decision-making
  - Encourage the patient as part of the care team
- Teamwork and Collaboration.
  - Embrace diversity by encouraging and supporting different perspectives, backgrounds, and thought
  - Build strategic partnerships
  - Practice clear communication and transparent decision-making
  - Encourage a culture of trust, respect, and safety with all colleagues, regardless of position or title
  - Develop leaders and individuals to enhance team performance
- Professionalism and Excellence.
  - Promote a culture of continuous improvement and lifelong learning
  - Be the trusted voice for the cardiovascular community
  - Hold ourselves and our profession to the highest standards of evidence and knowledge
  - Constructively challenge the status quo through innovation
  - Strive to achieve and support balance and well-being in our roles

---

from industry (Weber and Ornstein 2011). Such support, even when deemed "unrestricted" in nature, raises fundamental concerns about the influence wielded by industry over professional societies. Recognizing the financial entanglement between medical societies and industry, Relman noted that professional associations "are confident that their own independence is wholly unaffected by all of this—although surveys reveal that they are less sanguine about other doctors' ability to resist industry's blandishments" (Relman 2003). Such skepticism invites a conversation about the propriety of industry relationships with medical societies, especially those societies which formulate clinical practice guidelines which apply to and influence the use of devices and pharmaceuticals.

V Clinical Practice Guidelines

The American College of Cardiology, the National Institutes of Health Consensus Development Program, the US Preventive Services Task Force, the

Blue Cross and Blue Shield Association, and the ECRI Institute and the Rand Corporation were front-line leaders "in devising systematic methods for assessing the evidence and developing clinical recommendations for practitioners, patients, payers, and others" in the 1980s (Lo and Field 2009, p. 191). The Institute of Medicine defines clinical practice guidelines as "statements that include recommendations intended to optimize patient care that are informed by a systematic review of evidence and an assessment of the benefits and harms of alternative care options" (Institute of Medicine 2011, p. 18). A broader view also includes "medical technology assessments, clinical opinions, and other evidence-based clinical practice tools" in the spectrum (Council of Medical Specialty Societies March 2011).

The primary goal of practice guidelines is to improve the safety and quality of care, and to generate a uniform and evidence-based methodology for treating clinical problems. Certainly, such guidelines serve the interests of efficiency, and should reflect a standard of prudent, reasonable, and scientifically relevant patient management. Clinical practice guidelines "are intended to present a synthesis of current evidence and recommendations performed by expert clinicians and may affect the practice of a large number of physicians" (Choudhry, Stelfox, and Detsky 2002, p. 612).

Clinical practice guidelines are far-reaching, and may affect the management of scores of patients. Indeed, this is their intent. The credibility and influence of these guidelines are amplified by the imprimatur of the drafting organization or society. They often serve as a basis for medical decision-making, medical education, quality assurance and improvement initiatives, third-party reimbursement, and medical malpractice litigation. The accuracy and independence of guidelines are therefore paramount, and they create a "standard of care" which can act as a benchmark for physician conduct. The legal community, in particular, may embrace such guidelines as an element of the tort of negligence, positing that a failure to practice according to a given guideline reflects a deviation from accepted care. Problems with guideline content therefore negatively impact patients but also practitioners.

Given the fiduciary role of the individual physician in patient management and decision-making, it is easy to extend the role of fiduciary to professional societies in their role of formulating and endorsing clinical practice guidelines. Under this view, a professional organization is a moral aggregator which should place the interests of the benefactors of clinical practice guidelines above all other interests. Medical societies act through individuals. The physicians who sit on clinical practice guideline committees must therefore address and assiduously avoid conflicts of interest.

The past decades have been punctuated by outside scrutiny of medical societies promulgating clinical practice guidelines for failing in their duty of undistracted loyalty to patient care. In 2004, for example, the American Heart Association and the American College of Cardiology were criticized because seven of the nine panel members authoring the clinical practice guidelines for statin usage had various financial arrangements with the manufacturers. Ten years later, similar criticisms were leveled at new cholesterol management guidelines.

> The process by which these latest guidelines were developed gives rise to further skepticism. The group that wrote the recommendations was not sufficiently free of conflicts of interest; several of the experts on the panel have recent or current financial ties to drug makers. In addition, both the American Heart Association and the American College of Cardiology, while nonprofit entities, are heavily supported by drug companies. The American people deserve to have important medical guidelines developed by doctors and scientists on whom they can confidently rely to make judgments free from influence, conscious or unconscious, by the industries that stand to gain or lose.
>
> (Abramson and Redberg 2013)

Such distrust of clinical practice guidelines creates several potential and mutually related harms. First, an atmosphere of taint arising out of suspected conflict of interest can potentially undermine the entire panoply of practice guidelines, leading to a failure by physicians to trust and follow those that are well-established and well-tested. Second, patients themselves may feel threatened when they learn that their treatment might be linked to special interests (physician and industry gain) versus their interests. And, finally, as previously noted, wariness or cynicism regarding the generation of practice guidelines can demean on a wholesale basis the medical profession in general.

VI Clinical Practice Guidelines and the Scope of the Conflict of Interest Problem

In 2002, Choudry et al. from the University of Toronto were among the first to examine the magnitude of the ties between the pharmaceutical industry and authors of clinical practice guidelines. The study found that 87% of the 100 guideline authors (37 guidelines examined in total) had some form of interaction with the pharmaceutical industry, and that 38% of guideline authors had served as employees or consultants for industry. On average, clinical guideline authors reported interactions with 10.5 different pharmaceutical companies, and received funding from a mean of 6.7 companies. In total, 59% of authors had relationships with companies whose products were specific to the guideline under consideration. Two additional findings from the Toronto study merit attention. First, the majority (42 of 44) of the clinical practice guidelines failed to offer *any* conflict of interest declarations concerning the authors, while 11 of the 44 guidelines simply disclosed that "a pharmaceutical company had sponsored the creation and writing process" (Choudhry, Stelfox, and Detsky 2002, p. 615). Second, 7% of the authors believed that their relationship with industry influenced the guideline recommendations. Based upon these findings, Choudry et al. noted a "need for appropriate disclosure of financial conflicts of interest for authors of CPGs and a formal process for discussing these conflicts prior to CPG development" (Choudhry, Stelfox, and Detsky 2002, p. 612).

Other studies highlight similar statistics with respect to conflicts of interest. Mendelson et al. examined conflicts of interest in 17 American College of Cardiology/American Heart Association Guidelines formulated through 2008. Using disclosure lists, these authors noted that 56% of the 498 participants in clinical practice guideline development reported a conflict of interest. However, these authors noted that "a large percentage of individuals with guideline experience reported no disclosures, suggesting that there is a substantial pool of potential guideline writers and reviewers without COIs" (Mendelson et al. 2011, p. 577).

VII Managing Conflicts of Interest

Conflict of interest policies are crafted to protect the integrity, credibility, independence, and reliability of clinical practice guidelines. "The anchoring authority of the guideline process is the belief that guidelines are evidence based, not opinion based, and therefore their conclusions flow directly from the conclusions of studies" (Sniderman and Furberg 2009, p. 429). Procedural safeguards, therefore, form the basis for securing the authority of guidelines, and fall into three broad categories. Disclosure is a foundational element of conflict of interest management, and provides a veneer of transparency to the guideline formulation process. Disclosure, however, presupposes that the disclosed information has informational value which is useful to a decision-making process—that is, to practice according to the guideline or not. Disclosures which merely accompany an established clinical practice guideline are of questionable value, as the guideline has already been afforded the authority and endorsement of the originating society. Limitation or elimination of industry relationships are simply different points on the spectrum of "cure" for conflicts of interest. The potential downside of either is the forced choice between industry relationships versus participation in guideline formulation.

The American College of Cardiology considers guideline and clinical document development critical to its mission, and has designed policies "to ensure that authors disclose all relationships with industry and other entities to eliminate the possibility of undue bias" (Brindis and Harrington 2010, p. 901). The American College of Cardiology requires annual disclosure of relationships with industry on the Electronic Disclosure Database (Brindis and Harrington 2010). The College's *Principles for Relationships with Industry* require "full disclosure of all relevant RWI [relationships with industry] prior to appointment to a writing committee, covering the 12 months prior to participation" (American College of Cardiology 2013). Further, the College parses the level of the financial relationship with industry into (1) no monetary reimbursement versus modest (less than $10,000) versus significant (greater than or equal to $10,000) and (2) type (speaker, consultant, researcher, *et cetera*) (American College of Cardiology 2013). The College mandates that the Chair of the Committee developing the guideline, plus greater than 50% of the committee members, must have no relevant relationships with industry, and any relationships that otherwise exist on the committee must be disclosed in the publication of the clinical document.

The policies of the American College of Cardiology are similar to those set forth in the *Code for Interactions with Industries* of the Council of Medical Specialty Societies in 2011. The Council is comprised of 45 Member Organizations, including the American College of Cardiology, but, notably, not the American Heart Association (https://cmss.org/membership/societies/, accessed 9/16/21). In addition to policies governing conflict of interest management among guideline committee writers, the *Code* addresses the management of interactions between professional societies and industry in relation to guideline development (see Table 10.2). The American College of Cardiology and the Council of Medical Specialty Societies policies also mirror the Institute of Medicine report, "Guidelines We Can Trust" (see Table 10.3) (Lo and Field 2009).

VIII Discussion

The fundamental question posed in conflicts of interest is whether an "agent" (the physician, professional society, or clinical practice guideline committee member) can serve two "masters" or "principals" (industry and the patient), and reconcile real or apparent competing interests (self-interest versus patient welfare). This is the classic agency problem from economics. Relevant data with respect to the material impact of conflicts of interest on clinical practice guidelines remain lacking. While there is an accepted view that conflicts of interests portend bias or undue influence (subconscious or overt), such concerns remain unsupported in practice due to lack of data.

It is clear, however, that medical societies crafting and disseminating clinical practice guidelines are increasingly sensitized to the conflict of interest issue. A society drafting guidelines, particularly those pertaining to pharmaceutical or medical device usage, is positioned as a "learned intermediary" between the manufacturer and physicians (and their patients) relying on the guidelines. Ideologically, such positioning alone demands the strictest attention to conflicts of interest in order to maintain medicine's professional standing and public trust.

Disclosure remains the cornerstone for *managing* conflicts of interests relating to clinical practice guidelines. *Management* should not be confused with *resolution*, however. While disclosure is a useful metric for *identifying* a conflict of interest, the more crucial consideration is whether disclosure actually protects against bias and overt or subliminal influence. As Steven Nissen has observed:

> Proponents of the current system have also argued that disclosure of these relationships is sufficient to ensure the independence and scientific integrity of the CPG document. While sunlight is always a good disinfectant, there is nothing about disclosure that inherently guarantees scientific independence of the CPG document. The deliberations in writing CPGs take place in secret. In fact, current policies of professional societies forbid participants in

Table 10.2 Council of Medical Subspecialty Societies' Principles for Medical Specialty
Societies Developing Clinical Practice Guidelines

7.1.	Societies will base Clinical Practice Guidelines on scientific evidence.
7.2.	Societies will follow a transparent Guideline development process that is not subject to Company influence. For Guidelines and Guideline Updates published after adoption of the Code, Societies will publish a description of their Guideline development process, including their process for identifying and managing conflicts of interest, in Society Journals or on Society websites.
7.3.	Societies will not permit direct Company support of the development of Clinical Practice Guidelines or Guideline Updates.
7.4.	Societies will not permit direct Company support for the initial printing, publication, and distribution of Clinical Practice Guidelines or Guideline Updates. After initial development, printing, publication and distribution is complete, it is permissible for Societies to accept Company support for the Society's further distribution of the Guideline or Guideline Update, translation of the Guideline or Guideline Update, or repurposing of the Guideline content.
7.5.	Societies will require all Guideline development panel members to disclose relevant relationships prior to panel deliberations, and to update their disclosure throughout the Guideline development process.
7.6.	Societies will develop procedures for determining whether financial or other relationships between Guideline development panel members and Companies constitute conflicts of interest relevant to the subject matter of the guideline, as well as management strategies that minimize the risk of actual and perceived bias if panel members do have conflicts.
7.7.	Societies will require that a majority of Guideline development panel members are free of conflicts of interest relevant to the subject matter of the Guideline.
7.8.	Societies will require the panel chair (or at least one chair if there are co-chairs) to be free of conflicts of interest relevant to the subject matter of the Guideline, and to remain free of such conflicts of interest for at least one year after Guideline publication.
7.9.	Societies will require that Guideline recommendations be subject to multiple levels of review, including rigorous peer-review by a range of experts. Societies will not select as reviewers individuals employed by or engaged to represent a Company.
7.10.	Societies' Guideline recommendations will be reviewed and approved before submission for publication by at least one Society body beyond the Guideline development panel, such as a committee or the Board of Directors.
7.11.	Guideline manuscripts will be subject to independent editorial review by a journal or other publication where they are first published.
7.12.	Societies will publish Guideline development panel members' disclosure information in connection with each Guideline and may choose to identify abstentions from voting.
7.13.	Societies will require all Guideline contributors, including expert advisors or reviewers who are not officially part of a Guideline development panel, to disclose financial or other substantive relationships that may constitute conflicts of interest.
7.14.	Societies will recommend that Guideline development panel members decline offers from affected Companies to speak about the Guideline on behalf of the Company for a reasonable period after publication.
7.15.	Societies will not permit Guideline development panel members or staff to discuss a Guideline's development with Company employees or representatives, will not accept unpublished data from Companies, and will not permit Companies to review Guidelines in draft form.

Table 10.3 Institute of Medicine Standards for Developing Trustworthy Clinical Practice Guidelines

1.1:	The process by which a CPG is developed and funded should be detailed explicitly and be publicly accessible.
2.1:	Prior to selection of the CPG group, individuals being considered for membership should declare all interests and activities potentially resulting in COI with development group activity, by written disclosure to those convening the guideline development group. Disclosure should reflect all current and planned commercial, noncommercial, intellectual, institutional, and patient/public noncommercial, intellectual, institutional, and patient/public activities pertinent to the potential scope of the CPG.
2.2a:	All COI of each GDG member should be reported and discussed by the prospective development group prior to the onset of his or her work.
2.2b:	Each panel member should explain how his or her COI could influence the CPG development process or specific recommendations.
2.3:	Members of the GDG should divest themselves of financial investments they or their family members have in, and not participate in marketing activities or advisory boards of, entities whose interests could be affected by CPG recommendations.
2.4a:	Whenever possible, GDG members should not have COI.
2.4b:	In some circumstance, a GDG may not be able to perform its work without members who have COI, such as relevant clinical specialists who receive a substantial portion of their income from services pertinent to the CPG.
2.4c:	Members with COI should represent not more than a minority of the guideline development group.
2.4d:	The chair or co-chairs should not be a person(s) with COI.
2.4e:	Funders should have no role in CPG development.

Abbreviations
COI   conflict of interest
CPG   clinical practice guideline
GDG   guideline development group

writing groups from disclosing the internal deliberations of the CPG committee. A preliminary version of CPG is not posted for public comment. Accordingly, we will never know the extent to which financial relationships affected the internal discussion and deliberations leading to the final CPG recommendations. For CPGs to be truly independent and respected, even the appearance of impropriety must be avoided.

(Nissen 2011, pp. 584–585)

Complete elimination or divestiture of *all* industry relationships on the part of all individuals would certainly be antiseptic, although potentially untenable in reality. Draconian measures may disincentivize those who productively interact with industry from participation on clinical practice guideline committees. However, there are ways to achieve greater levels of divestiture, or of ensuring that individuals without conflicts are favored or empowered in guideline development processes. The American College of Cardiology and Institute on

Medicine policies on guideline committee composition could be extended (e.g., 75% of committee members without conflicts). To ensure expertise on guideline committees, professional societies could "train" individuals without conflicts in the art of guideline writing. These individuals could be given limited access to information from industry that might be important for guideline development, without concurrently receiving any money (Mendelson, Meltzer, Campbell, Caplan and Kirkpatrick 2011).

Across-the-board disassociations of societies from industry would jeopardize the financial viability these organizations and is, therefore, unlikely to gain any traction among professional societies and organizations. But societies could, theoretically, do more to separate out the guideline production and oversight process. Rather than taking guideline production costs from the general budget (which includes industry money), guideline development expenditures could be earmarked from membership dues. The society could require not only that the guidelines committee members be relatively free from conflicts of interest, but also those who choose the guidelines committee members and anyone tasked with reviewing and approving the guideline. The Council of Medical Subspecialty Societies recommends multiple other means for societies to mitigate the impact or appearance of conflict in relations with industry, from forbidding society endorsements of specific products (e.g., American Heart Association and Quaker Oats), to limiting product advertising at scientific sessions (Council of Medical Specialty Societies 2015).

IX Conclusion

Professional societies in cardiology are playing an increasingly prominent and important role in the education of clinicians and the development of practice standards in the form of clinical practice guidelines. Yet these professional societies and their constituent members maintain extensive ties to the pharmaceutical and device industries, creating conflicts of interest. These societies share the fiduciary responsibilities of their individual members in areas implicating patient care and welfare, including eschewing self-interest and self-dealing.

Conflicts of interest arise when industry relationships appear to compromise professionalism, objectivity, scientific integrity, and reliability. In particular, the generation of clinical practice guidelines with their wide-ranging impacts on clinical care, quality assurance, pay for performance, education and legal proceedings, obligates professional societies to hold to the strictest standards of conflict of interest disclosure and resolution. Disclosure has become the "gold standard" for managing conflicts of interest in the context of guideline formulation, along with limitations of industry ties among guideline committee members. Such policies invest the guideline formulation process with a level of protection and reliability, but the adequacy of these measures to address the important issue of conflicts of interest remains a topic of debate.

Notes

1 *Patient Protection and Affordable Care Act §6002* (Transparency Reports and Reporting of Physician Ownership or Investment Interests) (2010); *see also* Department of Health and Human Services, Centers for Medicare & Medicaid Services. 78 Fed. Reg. 27, 9458 (Final Rule February 8, 2013) (codified at 42 CFR Parts 402 and 403).

2 CMS.gov. *Centers for Medicare & Medicaid*. http://www.cms.gov/Regulations-and-Guidance/Legislation/National-Physician-Payment-Transparency-Program/Public-Access-to-Data.html. Accessed April 28, 2014.

References

Abramson, J.D., and R.F. Redberg. 2013. Don't give more patients statins. *New York Times* November 13. www.nytimes.com/2013/11/14/opinion/dont-give-more-patients-statins.html.

American College of Cardiology. 2013. *Principles for relationships with industry*. http://www.cardiosource.org/~/media/Files/ACC/About/2013/05/Principles%20for%20Relationships%20with%20Industry%20130520.ashx. Accessed February 20, 2014.

Beauchamp, T.L., L. Walters, J.P. Kahn, and A.C. Mastroianni. 2014. Ethical theory and bioethics. In: *Contemporary Issues in Bioethics*, 8th edition, Beauchamp, T., L. Walters, J.P. Kahn, and A.C. Mastroianni (eds). New York: Wadsworth Cengage Learning.

Brindis, R., and R. Harrington. 2010. President's page: The ACC reconfirms commitment to transparent relationships with industry, *Journal of the American College of Cardiology* 56 (11): 900–902.

Brody, H. 2007. *Hooked: Ethics, the medical profession, and the pharmaceutical industry*. New York: Rowman & Littlefield Publishers, Inc.

Cadet, J.V. 2011. Cardiac societies scrutinized for industry conflicts: Fair? *Cardiovascular Business*. http://www.cardiovascularbusiness.com/topics/healthcare-economics/cardiac-societies-scrutinized-industry-conflicts-fair. Accessed January 12, 2014.

Carlisle, J.R. 2004. Ethics and bioethics. In: *Legal medicine* (pp. 165–174), Sanbar, S.S., M.H. Firesone, F. Buckner, and A. Gibofsky et al., (eds). Philadelphia: Mosby.

Cassel, C.K., and D.B. Reuben. 2011. Specialization, subspecialization, and subsubspecialization in internal medicine, *New England Journal of Medicine* 364(12): 1169–1173.

Centers for Medicare & Medicaid. http://www.cms.gov/Regulations-and-Guidance/Legislation/National-Physician-Payment-Transparency-Program/Public-Access-to-Data.html. Accessed April 28, 2014.

Choudhry, N.K., H.T. Stelfox, and A.S. Detsky. 2002. Relationships between authors of clinical practice guidelines and the pharmaceutical industry, *JAMA* 287(5): 612–617.

Council of Medical Specialty Societies. 2011. *Code for interactions with companies*. http://www.cmss.org/uploadedFiles/Site/CMSS_Policies/CMSS%20Code%20for%20Interactions%20with%20Companies%20Approved%20Revised%20Version%203-19-11CLEAN.pdf. Accessed January 15, 2014.

DeMott, D.A. 2006. Breach of fiduciary duty: On justifiable expectations of loyalty and their consequences, *Arizona Law Review* 48(4): 925–956.

Furrow, B.R., and P.B. Molinoff. 2009. Health law and bioethics. In: *The Penn Center guide to bioethics*, Ravistsky, V., A. Fiester, and A.L. Caplan (eds). Dordrecht: Springer Publishing Company.

Fye, W.B. 1996. *American cardiology: The history of a specialty and its college*. Baltimore: The Johns Hopkins University Press.

Grassley, C.E. 2013a. *Disclosure of drug company payments to doctors.* http://www.grassley.senate. gov/about/disclosure-drug-company-payments-doctors. Accessed March 4, 2014.

Grassley, C.E. 2013b. *Physician Payments Sunshine Act regulations released.* http://www. grassley.senate.gov/news/news-releases/physician-payments-sunshine-act-regulations-released. Accessed March 5, 2014.

Hippocratic Oath. http://en.wikipedia.org/wiki/Hippocratic_Oath. Accessed January 10, 2014.

Institute of Medicine. 2011. *Clinical practice guidelines we can trust.* Washington, DC: The National Academies Press.

Kirkpatrick, J.N., M.B. Kadakia, and A. Vargas. 2012. Management of conflicts of interest in cardiovascular medicine. *Progress in Cardiovascular Diseases* 55(3): 258–265.

Lo, B., M.J. Field, (eds). 2009. *Committee on conflict of interest in medical research, education, and practice, Institute of Medicine: Conflict of interest in medical research, education, and practice.* Washington, DC: National Academies Press.

Mendelson, T.B., M. Meltzer, E.G. Campbell, A.L. Caplan, and J.N. Kirkpatrick. 2011. Conflicts of interest in cardiovascular clinical practice guidelines, *Archives of Internal Medicine* 171(6): 577–584.

Molinoff, P.B. 2009. Conflict of interest in American universities. In: *The Penn Center guide to bioethics* (pp. 281–291), Ravistsky, V., A. Fiester, and A.L. Caplan (eds). Dordrecht: Springer Publishing Company.

Nissen, S.E. 2011. Can we trust cardiovascular practice guidelines? *Archives of Internal Medicine* 171 (6): 584–585.

Norris, S.L., H.K. Holmer, and L.A. Ogden et al. 2011. Conflict of interest in clinical practice guideline development: A systematic review, *PlosOne* 6(10): 1–6.

Norris, S.L., H.K. Holmer, and L.A. Ogden et al. 2012. Conflict of interest disclosures for clinical practice guidelines in the national guideline clearinghouse, *PlosOne* 7(11): 1–8.

Parmley, W.W., E.R. Passamani, and B. Lo. 1998. 29th Bethesda conference: Introduction. *Journal of the American College of Cardiology* 31(5): 922–925.

Patient Protection and Affordable Care Act §6002 (Transparency Reports and Reporting of Physician Ownership or Investment Interests) (2010); Department of Health and Human Services, Centers for Medicare & Medicaid Services. 78 Fed. Reg. 27, 9458 (Final Rule February 8, 2013) (codified at 42 C.F.R. Parts 402 and 403).

Pelligrino, E.D., and A.S. Relman. 1999. Professional medical associations: Ethical and practical guidelines, *JAMA* 282(10): 984–986.

Qaseem, A., F. Forland, F. Macbeth, G. Ollenschläger, and S. Phillips et al. 2012. Guidelines international network: Toward international standards for clinical practice guidelines, *Annals of Internal Medicine* 156(7): 525–531.

Relman, A.S. 1980. The new medical-industrial complex, *New England Journal of Medicine* 303(17): 963–970.

Relman, A.S. 2003. Your doctor's drug problem, *New York Times*, Nov. 18. https://www. nytimes.com/2003/11/18/opinion/your-doctor-s-drug-problem.html.

Royce, J. 1908. *The philosophy of loyalty.* New York: The MacMillan Company.

Sniderman, A.D., and C.D. Furberg. 2009. Why guideline-making requires reform, *JAMA* 301(4): 429–431.

Weber, T., and C. Ornstein. 2011. Medical groups shy about detailing industry financial support, *ProPublica* (May 5). http://www.propublica.org/article/medical-groups-shy-about-detailing-industry-financial-support/single. Accessed January 15, 2014.

11 Error, Malpractice, and Complication

A Practical Approach

David M. Zientek

I Introduction

The Institute of Medicine's landmark study, *To Err is Human*, estimated that as many as 98,000 patients die yearly from medical error and stimulated interest in preventing and responding to adverse events (Kohn, Corrigan and Donaldson 1999). While briefly touching on other forms of adverse events, the study primarily focused on preventable errors resulting from problems in the systems for delivering medical care rather than on individual caregivers. A systems approach de-emphasizes individual culpability so as to increase the willingness of caregivers to report error and to create greater awareness that restructuring delivery of care may reduce the likelihood of error. Nonetheless, concern has been raised that the pendulum has swung too far away from personal responsibility for untoward events leaving caregivers, institutions, and patients unsure of who is accountable for addressing errors (Pellegrino 2004; Wachter and Pronovost 2009; Bell Delbanco, Anderson-Shaw, McDonald, and Gallagher 2011). To help resolve this confusion it is important to recognize the spectrum of adverse events that may occur and define the moral response to each.

This chapter will consider three types of adverse events patients may suffer as a result of medical intervention, rather than the disease itself: preventable error, malpractice, and complication. Each will be defined, and in light of the case studies presented, an analysis of the moral accountability of the agents involved will demonstrate that ethical obligations to patients, families, and the healthcare system as a whole vary significantly depending on the type of adverse event.

II Defining Preventable Error, Malpractice, and Complication

The Institute of Medicine defined an adverse event as "an injury caused by medical management rather than the underlying condition of the patient" (Kohn, Corrigan and Donaldson 1999, p. 28). This may include several distinct types of event. A "preventable adverse event" was defined as one caused by error, either in the planning or the execution of a treatment plan, with a subset of these being "negligent adverse events" defined by certain legal criteria (Kohn,

DOI: 10.4324/9781003240273-16

Corrigan and Donaldson 1999). Adverse events also occur without any identifiable error or negligence. In determining the moral culpability and ethical obligations of each agent involved, it is helpful to separate adverse events into three categories: preventable error, malpractice, and complication (Zientek 2010).

Preventable error is the primary focus of the Institute of Medicine's study. In this type of error, a poorly designed system is in place to provide care to patients, such as failure to have and enforce standardized protocols to avoid infection of central lines in intensive care units. While individuals within that system may have some culpability for an adverse event, this type of error is one in which placing different caregivers in the same situation is likely to reproduce the error. Malpractice, on the other hand, is far more dependent on the individual, though institutional processes may contribute. Examples include physicians performing procedures not indicated for the patient's condition, or ignoring protocols to prevent harm, such as the "time out" to confirm the correct procedure is performed on the correct patient. This is a "negligent" error and is legally defined by three elements: the standard of care is not met, the patient suffers harm, and the harm results from failure to meet the accepted standard of care (Berlinger 2005). Finally, complications are separate from other adverse events. Complications are not preventable; rather, they occur with a given statistical frequency for any treatment given the state of medical knowledge at the time of the event. Informed consent should typically include disclosure of possible complications to the treatment or procedure. Here, neither the system nor the individual practitioner is, strictly speaking, morally culpable (Pellegrino 2004; Zientek 2010). The following cases illustrate these three different types of adverse event.

III Case Reports

Case 1:

Mrs. K was a 58-year-old patient admitted with uncontrolled hypertension. On her second hospital day, a weekend, her physician ordered 30 mg of extended release blood pressure medication nifedipine. Her nurse, a new graduate working on the medical floor, submitted the order to the pharmacy, but then noticed three 10 mg capsules of short acting nifedipine in the medication box left over from a prior patient. Unaware of the risk of a sudden drop in blood pressure with short acting, rather than the gradual onset of antihypertensive effect with the extended release medication, she administered what she believed was an equivalent dose. Shortly afterward, the patient developed profound hypotension and slow heart rates requiring transfer to the intensive care unit and a temporary pacemaker. On review of the chart, it became clear that the patient's acute decompensation was the result of the medication error. Mrs. K was informed of the error, recovered over the succeeding three days and was discharged without residual complication.

Case 2:

Dr. P is a highly respected cardiologist performing over half of the coronary stent and angioplasty procedures at his local hospital. Due to his high volume, he is often invited by device manufacturers to participate in research protocols and to be the first to use new technology. Nonetheless, several complaints have been filed with the State Medical Board, and lawsuits are pending in which patients' families allege malpractice relating to unnecessary procedures. Generally, angioplasty or stenting for stable patients is indicated for significant blockage of coronary arteries causing persistent chest pain despite adequate medical therapy, or blockages that supply a large portion of the heart muscle with objective evidence of reduced blood flow through the narrowing. An internal peer review by experienced cardiologists finds an unusually high percentage of Dr. P's diagnostic catheterization cases leading to coronary interventions. There appears to be a pattern of performing interventions on lesions of borderline significance with no objective evidence of poor blood flow or in patients with minimal symptoms. In several instances, complications resulted from the interventions, including coronary artery perforation requiring emergent surgery, and two patients dying from clots forming in stents with a resulting myocardial infarction. Despite these findings, the hospital has not taken disciplinary action due to fear of legal action by Dr. P against the hospital, and loss of his lucrative practice.

Case 3:

Dr. M performs an intracoronary stent procedure on a 69-year-old female with refractory angina pectoris despite maximal medical therapy. Approximately three hours later, the patient develops sudden left-sided weakness. Neurology consultation is obtained confirming a stroke and the patient treated appropriately. She has moderate improvement in weakness and is transferred to a rehabilitation facility. Review by the hospital peer review committee finds the indications and technique used for the procedure meet standard recommendations and no further action is taken.

IV Ethical Obligations in Responding to Adverse Events

In crafting a response to the different types of adverse events, ethical analysis leads to a series of steps common to each; however, the moral agents involved and the obligations for each step will vary by the nature of the event. These steps include: recognition that an event has occurred and immediate action to minimize harm to the patient, notifying the patient or surrogate of the adverse event, investigation of the cause of the event, apology or expression of sympathy, and, if indicated, compensation or restitution. The sequence of these steps may vary depending on circumstances and several may be concurrently undertaken. A summary of the steps for each type of adverse event is provided in Table 11.1.

Recognition and Amelioration of Adverse Event: The fundamental obligation underlying appropriate response to any error or complication is acting for the good of the patient regardless of the impact on practitioner or institutional reputation or financial interest. Beneficence and nonmaleficence require minimizing and, if possible, correcting harm to the patient from an adverse event. For example, if the wrong medication is given, actions to minimize the risk of harm or allergic reaction, and appropriate monitoring must be immediately instituted. For this to happen, the event must first be recognized and brought to the attention of appropriate clinical and administrative personnel. While straightforward with an obvious injury such as stroke following cardiac catheterization, in other instances, such as infection of a central line, recognition and reporting of an event may not be so clear.

Studies suggest that physicians, nurses, and other healthcare professionals frequently recognize error, poor judgment or incompetence in systems or colleagues, but rarely confront the person or report findings to administrators (Maxfield, Grenny, McMillan, Patterson and Switzler 2008). These professionals cite fear of reprisal, belief that change is not possible, or uncertainty about who bears responsibility for reporting an event as reasons for failing to act (Maxfield,

Table 11.1 Flow Chart

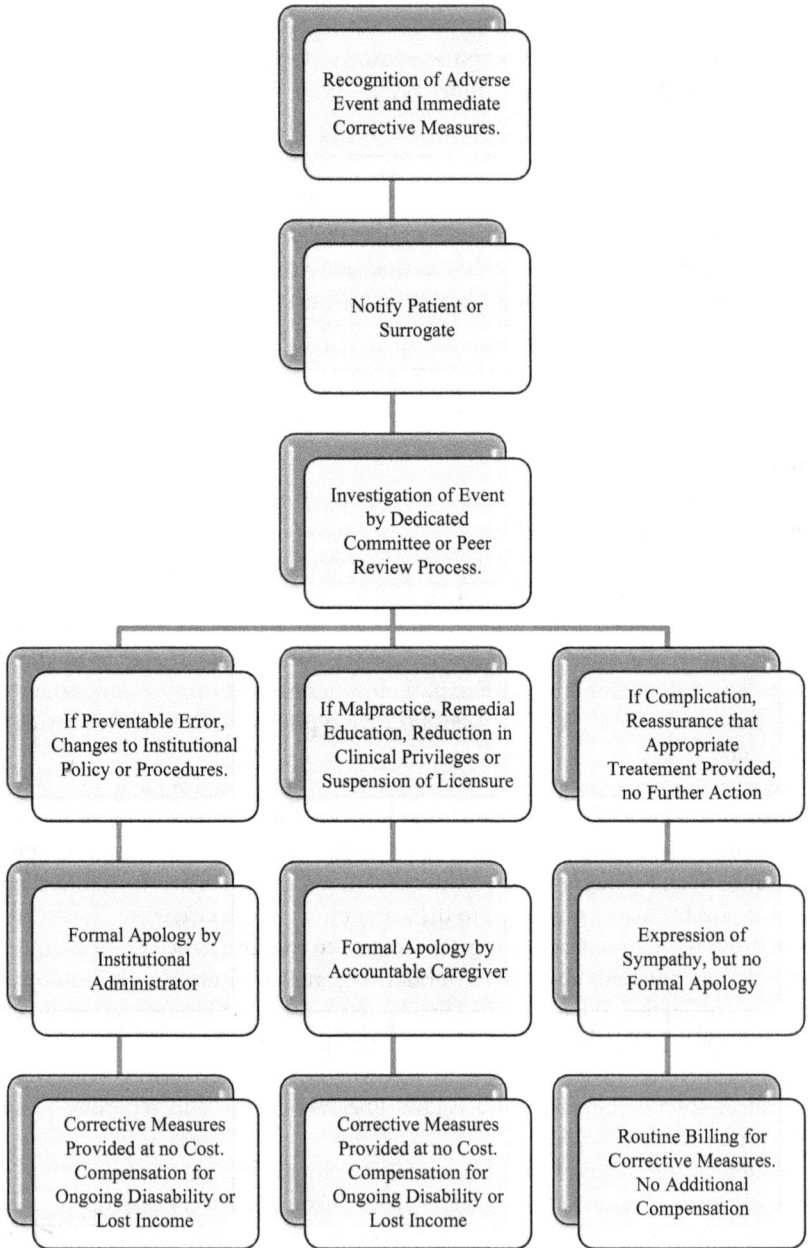

Grenny, McMillan, Patterson and Switzler 2008). The nurse who administers the wrong medication, even if significant blame is with a system that provides insufficient supervision or unreliable methods for dispensing medications, may be reluctant to come forward and report the error. In addition, providers may question the importance of reporting "near misses" in which the wrong medication or procedure was almost given or performed; yet, it is these cases which may allow for changes in process preventing error in the future. Finally, the physician who commits malpractice by failing to follow the standard of care may be the only one aware of the event, especially in an outpatient setting. Unless the event causes catastrophic harm, the physician may be reluctant to report the occurrence for fear of disciplinary action or liability.

Overcoming these obstacles remains a significant challenge. With regard to preventable error, in which systems play a major role, it is crucial for organizations to foster a culture in which recognition and reporting of error is seen as integral to performance at all levels. The custodial worker witnessing a physician going from patient to patient without washing hands must feel comfortable confronting the physician or reporting to an administrator without fear of retribution and with confidence that action will be taken (Maxfield, Grenny, McMillan, Patterson and Switzler 2008). In the case of malpractice or complication, in which individual clinicians have a greater role than the institution, it may be more difficult to instill this culture. However, in the academic setting, and perhaps increasingly as hospitals and physicians form integrated systems, the culture may have a significant influence on the physician's willingness to recognize and report events. For physicians in solo or other private practice settings, the increasing emphasis on reporting of adverse events in professional codes of ethics and medical training will hopefully foster such a culture throughout the profession (see, e.g., Snyder and Leffler 2005; Council on Ethical and Judicial Affairs 2007).

Notification of Patient or Surrogate: Once an adverse event is recognized and remedial action instituted, the next step will be notification of the patient or surrogate of the event. One underlying ethical principle is respect for the patient's autonomous self-determination. To participate in informed consent for procedures, especially if required to correct injury caused by error, malpractice or complication, the patient must be fully aware of their medical condition and the cause of injury. In addition, many ethicists see honesty and truth telling as fundamental obligations of professionals and crucial to the effectiveness of the healing relationship. Thus, patients must be given accurate information on the adverse event to decide if they have sufficient confidence in their caregivers or if they wish to seek out alternate providers.

Immediately after an adverse event, before an investigation, it may not be possible fully to explain the event to the patient. For preventable error, it may not be clear exactly what combination of systems and individuals accounted for the event. As a result, many institutions with disclosure programs notify the patient or surrogate that an adverse event has occurred, is being investigated, and further meetings will be arranged as information becomes available (DeVita 2001;

University of Pittsburg Medical Center-Presbyterian Hospital 2001; Massachusetts Coalition for the Prevention of Medical Errors 2006).The person notifying the patient in the case of preventable error will most often be the attending physician, though if a system problem appears highly likely, it may be appropriate for an administrator to provide this information. In the case of harm resulting from failure to follow the standard of care, or complication, the attending physician should provide notification. If the reason for the occurrence is clear, it may be appropriate at this time to provide an apology; however, if the cause is not clear, or for considerations of liability, it may be appropriate to notify the patient of the occurrence only pending review.

Investigation of the Event: After a caregiver or institution becomes aware of an adverse event and the patient is notified, formal review should be undertaken. The moral imperative is to determine if changes in the way care is delivered, in the case of preventable error or complications, or education, supervision, or change in privileges for practitioners, in the case of malpractice, can prevent future harm to patients. This is also the primary argument for reporting and investigating the "near miss." Some also argue that institutions should have ongoing review of physician performance and health, as done in the airline industry, preemptively to identify educational gaps or health issues that may impact patient care (Leape and Fromson 2006). It is at this stage that accountability should be determined. For issues determined to result from faulty systems, "collective accountability" may be most appropriate with both appropriate administrative personnel and the involved clinicians empowered and held accountable for correcting flaws in the system (Bell, Delbanco, Anderson-Shaw, McDonald and Gallagher 2011). If review suggests an individual is primarily accountable, recommendations for corrective action or punishment should be determined.

Before an adverse event occurs, institutions should have some mechanism for review in place.This may be a committee expressly for reviewing error, or alternately a peer review, risk management, or ethics committee could serve this purpose (Massachusetts Coalition for the Prevention of Medical Errors 2006). When it appears most likely that an event is the result of a system error, a larger multidisciplinary committee might be most appropriate, whereas in the case of likely malpractice or complication, a peer review committee or morbidity and mortality conference may be the most appropriate venue. Despite the fact that a complication occurs when a treatment has been undertaken for the correct indication and performed correctly, it is beneficial to review these occurrences to confirm this is the case. After completion of the review, findings should be presented to the patient. A key element in such presentations will be balancing the confidentiality conferred upon peer review with regard to legal discovery and essential to encouraging caregivers honestly to disclose and discuss events, while recognizing the obligation to apologize in the next step of the process. The physician in private practice who is involved in an event in the outpatient setting may have a challenge reviewing the case. The reflective solo practice physician might approach a local institution's peer review committee, members of a group practice, or other practitioners to review any occurrence.

Apology or Expression of Sympathy: After review, a determination will need to be made that the event represents avoidable error, malpractice, or complication. Surveys indicate that in order to preserve a trusting relationship, patients want to know what can be done to prevent errors in the future, and desire apology and emotional support from caregivers (Gallagher, Waterman, Ebers, Fraser and Levison 2003; Lazare 2006). According to Lazare, an apology consists of four parts: acknowledging the injury to the patient while identifying the responsible party, an explanation of why an error occurred, an "expression of remorse, shame, forbearance, and humility," and some form of reparation (Lazare 2006, p. 1402). In this context, forbearance means a commitment not to repeat the error (Lazare 2006). I will consider reparation as a separate step.

Many raise the concern that providing an apology to patients may increase liability and distrust of the healthcare system. Traditionally, caregivers are advised to avoid disclosing error or apologizing for fear of litigation; yet it may be precisely the failure to communicate in this setting that gives the appearance of attempting to conceal error, increasing distrust of caregivers and encouraging legal action to discover what actually transpired (May and Aulisio 2001; Mazor, Simon, Yood, Martinson, Gunter, Reed et al. 2004; Berlinger 2005; Clinton and Obama 2006). This may have several adverse consequences. First, reluctance honestly to apologize for and confront error or malpractice prevents open discussion of root causes and may perpetuate the error (May and Aulisio 2001). In addition, if it is found that error or malpractice is likely and was concealed, patients may be less likely to settle a case and juries more likely to return punitive damages (Robbennolt 2003; Mazor, Simon, Yood, Martinson, Gunter, Reed et al. 2004). Preliminary studies at the University of Michigan and the Veterans Affairs Hospital of Lexington, Kentucky, where error disclosure and apology policies have been implemented, suggest no increase in legal fees, claims, or liability costs (see Robbennolt 2003; Berlinger 2005; Clinton and Obama 2006; Gallagher, Studdert and Levinson 2007; Taft 2007). Indeed, if it is widely known that a healthcare system carefully reviews cases and offers compensation where error or malpractice is determined, the legal community will be unlikely to pursue action when the institution does not offer compensation.

Using Lazare's framework, if it is determined that an adverse event resulted from preventable error, the apology should occur at the time the findings of the investigation into the event are presented to the patient or surrogate. Given that preventable error has an element of a flawed system, this type of adverse event is best viewed in terms of "collective accountability" and it is most appropriate that an administrative representative of the institution present the apology (Lazare 2006). If a particular individual had a major role in the event, it may be appropriate to identify that person as accountable and have them participate in the apology; however, in most instances the collective approach would protect individuals from being singled out, encouraging them to participate in reporting and identifying the causes of an error. A detailed description of how the system failed, and plans to correct this flaw should be presented. Preliminary plans for compensation, as outlined in the next section, may also be provided at this time.

With malpractice, apology may be a more challenging step. As defined, malpractice involves individuals and it is appropriate for the responsible caregiver to provide the apology; however, there may be significant conflict between an institution and an individual practitioner. Most successful disclosure programs reported to date have been at academic or Veterans Affairs institutions where the institution and caregivers are likely to share liability coverage, and caregivers are often employees of the institution with aligned interests (see Robbennolt 2003; Berlinger 2005; Clinton and Obama 2006; Gallagher, Studdert and Levinson 2007). In a community hospital or private practice, it is more likely the clinician and institution will have separate liability insurers. Physicians may have provisions in malpractice policies invalidating coverage if they admit error without approval from the insurer, though some have argued that such clauses would not be enforceable if error is honestly disclosed to a patient (Banja 2005; Taft 2007). While some private malpractice carriers have undertaken innovative approaches to encouraging disclosure and compensation, the majority of private practitioners will have to negotiate a course between the professional obligation to apologize to patients and potential conflict with malpractice carriers.

For true complications, an expression of sympathy rather than apology is indicated. Here, there is no culpable individual or system, and hence no corrective measures to prevent future complication. Since adverse events are often equated with error or malpractice by patients, presentation of the result of an investigation, perhaps by an outside reviewer, will enhance the patient's acceptance of the event as an unavoidable complication. The profession does have an ongoing obligation for research to improve technology and reduce complication.

Compensation for Adverse Events: One concern with disclosure is that caregivers or institutions will see apology as sufficient for discharging their duty to patients harmed by error or malpractice. Justice demands more of the profession. As noted, Lazare includes reparation as an element of apology (2006). Berlinger, influenced by the Judeo-Christian tradition, warns against expecting "cheap grace"; to heal relationships between patient, family and caregivers, justice demands some form of penance or an attempt to correct the wrong before forgiveness can be entertained (2005). While the goals of malpractice litigation are to deter substandard care and compensate patients when harmed, the current system does a poor job distinguishing negligent from systemic error or even complication. The high cost of litigation may deter some deserving patients from pursuing damages and significantly reduce the compensation actually accruing to the patient (May and Aulisio 2001; Hoffman 2005).

For either preventable error or malpractice, justice is served by not charging patients or insurance for the error or corrective procedures. Beyond forgiving charges, in cases of death, ongoing disability, or loss of income, additional compensation may be indicated. The Michigan and Lexington Veterans hospital disclosure programs offer compensation when investigation determines error has occurred, and patients are invited to have an outside attorney review any proposed settlement for fairness (Robbennolt 2003; Berlinger 2005).

Once again, the approach is more difficult for the clinician in private practice. While it is appropriate for caregivers involved in malpractice to forego payment and compensate the patient; if they were not part of an academic or governmental institution, they will likely have to negotiate with malpractice carriers to carry out this obligation. As integrated healthcare delivery systems become more common, alignment of clinician and institutional liability may be more common. Some private insurers such as COPIC, a Colorado malpractice carrier, have policies to encourage disclosure of error providing up to $30,000 for patient out-of-pocket health expenses when error does not cause death or is not clearly negligent (Gallagher, Studdert and Levinson 2007). While patients do not give up the right to sue, litigation has been infrequent and few suits lead to compensation (Gallagher, Studdert and Levinson 2007). For malpractice, compensation may also require "penance" beyond financial payments. The accountable practitioner may, after review by an appropriate organization, be required to undergo further training, relinquish some privileges, or in truly egregious instances forfeit medical licensure.

It should be noted that while the primary focus of a response to adverse events is the injured patient, involved caregivers also suffer. It is rare that an adverse event results from malevolent intentions, but rather is committed by otherwise good and competent providers (Kohn, Corrigan and Donaldson 1999; May and Aulisio 2001). Denham argues that the involved caregiver is a "second victim" subject to shame and psychological distress (2007). After error or malpractice, the involved clinician should be treated with respect, recognizing their intent to help patients. Opportunities to learn from errors and psychological counseling, along with assurance that the caregiver will not be ostracized or terminated for good faith participation in the review of a case, are important obligations of the institution.

A complication is very different with regard to compensation. With no culpability for error or malpractice, the institution and caregivers can legitimately charge for the procedure and corrective action. It may be appropriate in cases of financial hardship to provide corrective care at no cost; however, it should be made clear that this is not an admission of culpable error (Zientek 2010). It is now possible to review the cases presented earlier.

V Case Review

Case 1 is an example of preventable error. While an individual nurse gave the incorrect medication, the system, by providing insufficient supervision and staffing on a weekend for an inexperienced nurse and failing to remove unused medications from patient care areas, made this event far more likely. Recognition of the error and appropriate action was instituted promptly, and the patient honestly informed of the error; however, this case occurred before the recent interest in systems error. While an ad hoc group changed policy to return unused medication to the pharmacy, a formal process for review of error should be put in place to review not only pharmacy issues, but also staffing, and the corrective measures that should have been provided to the patient at no cost. While the physician did notify the patient, an apology from an institutional administrator should have been provided along with explanation of measures to prevent future error. It is notable that given honest disclosure of the error, no legal action was taken by the patient.

Case 2 presents an instance of malpractice. Here, the physician repeatedly performed procedures outside the standard of care in which coronary lesions of equivocal significance were treated without objective evidence of ischemia and several patients were harmed. While there is a system component, with the institution reluctant to pursue corrective action due to the physician's status and fear of legal action, the clinician is ultimately culpable for making these decisions. Ideally, the physician faced with complaints to the medical board and lawsuits should honestly review cases to determine if the standard of care was met. If not, the physician should come forward with an apology to harmed patients and work with malpractice carriers to compensate patients for healthcare and injuries. If the physician is unsure how to proceed, or the institution identifies the problem before the practitioner comes forward, it may be most appropriate to have a peer review make recommendations with regard to apology, compensation, and the need for further training or restriction in privileges.

Finally, case 3 is an example of an unavoidable complication. In this case, appropriate corrective action was taken after prompt recognition of the injury to the patient. It would be ideal to have such a case considered by a peer review committee to confirm the standard of care was met and reassure the patient that this is the case. An expression of sympathy, but not a formal apology, is called for, and in general, it is acceptable to bill for the procedure and subsequent care.

VI Conclusion

The Institute of Medicine's report on medical error stimulated interest in responding to and preventing adverse events using a systems approach. The report focused on de-emphasizing individual moral culpability in an effort to encourage disclosure and open discussion of adverse events with the goal of modifying systems of care to make recurring error less common. While this focus has benefits, it may overlook adverse events in which individual accountability is more appropriate and corrective actions should focus on improving individual performance, or alternatively, events in which no culpable error occurs and hence no corrective measures are needed.

When an adverse event occurs, moral obligations toward patients on the part of healthcare institutions and providers underlie a five-step process in responding to the event. While these steps are common to the three types of event that may be distinguished, the responsible moral agents and their ethical responsibilities vary depending on the type of event. Understanding the differences between these events is essential to crafting an appropriate response.

References

American Medical Association, Council on Ethical and Judicial Affairs. 2007. *Code of medical ethics*. Chicago, IL: American Medical Association.

Banja, J.D. 2005. Does medical error disclosure violate the medical malpractice insurance cooperation clause? In: *Advances in patient safety: From research to implementation (Volume 3: Implementation issues)*, Henriksen, K., J.B. Battles, E.S. Marks. et al. (eds). Rockville, MD: Agency for Healthcare Research and Quality.

Bell, S.K., T. Delbanco, L. Anderson-Shaw, T.B. McDonald, and T.H. Gallagher. 2011. Accountability for medical error: Moving beyond blame to advocacy, *Chest* 140(2): 519–526.

Berlinger, N. 2005. *After harm: Medical error and the ethics of forgiveness*. Baltimore, MD: The Johns Hopkins University Press.

Clinton, H.R. and B. Obama. 2006. Making patient safety the centerpiece of medical liability reform, *The New England Journal of Medicine* 354(21): 2205–2208.

Denham, C.R. 2007. Trust: The 5 rights of the second victim, *Journal of Patient Safety* 3(2): 107–119.

DeVita, M.A. 2001. Honestly, do we need a policy on truth? *Kennedy Institute of Ethics Journal* 11(2): 157–164.

Gallagher, T.H., D. Studdert, and W. Levinson. 2007. Disclosing harmful medical errors to patients, *The New England Journal of Medicine* 356(26): 2713–2719.

Gallagher, T.H., A. Waterman, A.G. Ebers, V.J. Fraser, and W. Levison. 2003. Patients' and physicians' attitudes regarding the disclosure of medical errors, *The Journal of the American Medical Association* 289(8): 1001–1007.

Hoffman, D.N. 2005. The medical malpractice insurance crisis, again, *The Hastings Center Report* 35(2): 15–19.

Kohn, L.T., J.M. Corrigan, and M.S. Donaldson (eds). 1999. *To err is human: Building a safer health system*. Washington, DC: National Academy Press.

Lazare, A. 2006. Apology in medical practice: An emerging clinical skill, *The Journal of the American Medical Association* 296(11): 1401–1404.

Leape, L.L., and J.A. Fromson. 2006. Problem doctors: Is there a system-level solution? *Annals of Internal Medicine* 144(11):107–115.

Massachusetts Coalition for the Prevention of Medical Errors. 2006. When things go wrong: Responding to adverse events. A consensus statement of the Harvard hospitals. http://psnet.ahrq.gov/resource.aspx?resourceID=3474. (Accessed December 03, 2012.)

Maxfield, D., J. Grenny, R. McMillan, K. Patterson, and A. Switzler. 2008. *Silence kills: The seven crucial conversations for healthcare*. http://www.silencekills.com. (Accessed December 3, 2012.)

May, T., and M.P. Aulisio. 2001. Medical malpractice, mistake prevention, and compensation, *Kennedy Institute of Ethics Journal* 11(2): 135–146.

Mazor, K.M., S.R. Simon, R.A. Yood, B.C. Martinson, M.J. Gunter, and G.W. Reed et al. 2004. Health plan members' views about disclosure of medical errors, *Annals of Internal Medicine* 140(6): 409–418.

Pellegrino, E.D. 2004. Prevention of medical error: Where professional and organizational ethics meet. In: *Accountability: Patient safety and policy reform*, Sharpe, V.A. (ed). Washington, DC: Georgetown University Press.

Robbennolt, J.K. 2003. Apologies and legal settlement: An empirical examination, *Michigan Law Review* 102(460): 460–515.

Snyder, L., and C. Leffler for the Ethics and Human Rights Committee, and American College of Physicians. 2005. Ethics manual, fifth edition, *Annals of Internal Medicine* 142(7): 560–582.

Taft, L. 2007. Disclosure danger: The overlooked case of the cooperation clause, *Harvard Health Policy Review* 8(2): 46–53.

University of Pittsburg Medical Center-Presbyterian Hospital. 2001. Guidelines for disclosure and discussion of conditions and events with patients, families, and guardians, *Kennedy Institute of Ethics Journal* 11(2): 165–168.

Wachter, R.M., and P.J. Pronovost. 2009. Balancing "no blame" with accountability in patient safety, *The New England Journal of Medicine* 361(14):1401–1406.

Zientek, D.M. 2010. Medical error, malpractice and complications: A moral geography, *HEC Forum* 22(2): 145–157.

12 Ethical Practice in Cardiovascular Nursing

Joy Penticuff and Angela Clark

I Introduction

For the purposes of this chapter, we define ethical nursing practice as *nurses' ability to meet their ethical obligations to patients* as articulated in the *American Nurses Association Code of Ethics for Nurses* (ANA 2015a). This definition does not limit solely to the nurse's own actions the obligation to prevent harm and to do good. Consistent with the *ANA Code*, the definition also includes *the nurse's obligation to address harms arising from the actions of other healthcare professionals or from systems of care delivery*. Therefore, in exploring factors that may play a role in nurses' views of whether they are able to practice ethically, it is necessary to take into account nurses' ability to address aspects of their work environments that threaten patients' safety or best interests and the quality of healthcare patients are provided.

Characteristics of practice environments may support or hinder nursing moral agency when nurses attempt to make changes to ameliorate actual or potential harms to patients, thereby impacting nurses' ethical practice. Characteristics of practice environments also influence the quality of care that nurses can provide, thereby affecting patient outcomes, patient satisfaction, and the fulfillment nurses derive from their work. When nurses repeatedly find that they cannot meet their ethical obligations, moral distress may ensue, with serious consequences to the nurses themselves and to the quality of care they provide. Moral distress may cause some nurses to distance themselves from patients and other healthcare staff, or to leave nursing altogether. For other nurses, this distress becomes a catalyst, motivating them to address the aspects of practice environments that hinder ethical practice and to create environments that promote ethical practice.

To illustrate how the above factors can influence nurses' ethical practice, we present a hypothetical case of a patient with cardiovascular disease who develops a life-threatening post-surgical infection. The chapter then discusses current views of the moral agency of bedside nurses and describes organizational characteristics of hospital units that impact nurses' perceptions of their moral options. The nursing profession's fundamental goal of *caring for the needs of vulnerable others* is presented within the context of perceived limitations of moral options and resulting moral distress. The case depicts the emergence of promising new

DOI: 10.4324/9781003240273-17

strategies for addressing moral distress and supporting ethical nursing practice. The chapter concludes with application of the *American Nurses Association Code of Ethics with Interpretative Statements* (2015a) to the nursing care described in the hypothetical case, which follows.

II Case Study

Mr. C.: A Patient with a Post-CABG Complication

Medical Indications. Mr. C., a 69-year-old history professor, was admitted to Memorial Hospital experiencing angina and dyspnea. His outpatient diagnostic evaluation showed severe chronic aortic regurgitation, and his cardiologist, Dr. W., recommended an immediate aortic valve replacement (AVR) with coronary artery bypass grafting (CABG).

Contextual Features Surrounding the Case. Memorial Hospital is a 655-bed facility in a large urban area which treats patients of diverse social and economic status. The hospital provides a wide variety of specialized care, including extensive cardiovascular, neurology/neurosurgery services, and a renowned heart failure clinic. Their 62-bed critical care unit includes designated beds for non-surgical coronary care and for cardiovascular surgery. Within the past ten months, a sizable number of the unit's most experienced cardiovascular nurses have reached retirement age and as they have left the unit, their vacancies have been filled by nurses who are less experienced and are unfamiliar with the unit's policies and procedures. The unit has a culture of ongoing high-quality in-service nursing education, and the new nurses are in the process of being oriented to care for patients with acute cardiovascular problems.

Medical Indications. Admission data included normal vital signs with body mass index (BMI) in the obese range and complaints of shortness of breath and palpitations. Medical history included rheumatic fever as a child when living in India and a myocardial infarction about two years ago. Other pertinent history includes Type 2 diabetes mellitus with fair control (recent hemoglobin A1C 7%; 154 mg/dL); treatment for situational depression nine years ago during a divorce; and hypertension which is long standing but in reasonable control.

Nursing Perspective. Mr. C. was experiencing a significant amount of dyspnea and chest pain when he was admitted to the pre-surgical coronary care unit. His wife accompanied him throughout his admission and was by his side as he was shown to his hospital room. Mr. C. had been informed by his cardiologist, Dr. W., that he was being admitted to the hospital because he needed heart surgery and he appeared somewhat anxious as he changed out of his street clothes and into the hospital gown.

Patient Preferences. As part of the standard admission procedure at Memorial Hospital, Mr. C. had been asked by the admissions clerk whether he had any Advance Directives: A Living Will, a Durable Power of Attorney for Healthcare Decisions, or any other directives related to his medical care. Mr. C. stated that he had a Living Will and had designated his wife as his Durable Power of Attorney for Healthcare.

Medical Indications. Surgery was performed by two board-certified cardiovascular surgeons using a bioprosthetic aortic valve for replacement. A median sternotomy was done for AVR with CABG surgery. A saphenous vein graft along with one internal thoracic mammary artery was used.

Nursing Perspective. Two experienced critical care RNs admitted Mr. C. to the critical care unit for recovery and a Cardiovascular Clinical Nurse Specialist (Advanced Practice RN) assessed the patient. There were no immediate complications detected. Due to nursing staff shortages, a new nurse being oriented to the unit was assigned to monitor Mr. C.'s vital signs and to provide nursing care under the supervision of the Clinical Nurse Specialist.

The critical care unit policies allowed open visitation so Mr. C.'s wife and two adult children (son and daughter) took turns at the bedside. They seemed very intimidated by the critical care environment and asked few questions. Mr. C.'s wife appeared overwhelmed and fearful of the level of acuity and technology in use—multiple intravenous pumps, a ventilator, various monitoring devices with alarms and constantly changing physiologic readings.

Medical Indications. In approximately nine hours, Mr. C. was extubated. Chest tube drainage was excessive for the first 12 hours and vasopressors were continued with hemodynamic monitoring. Mr. C.'s recovery trajectory over the next few days was fairly typical. On post-op day two, he appeared stabilized and was communicating clearly with his family and nurses. He remained in the critical care unit for two more days for treatment of new onset symptomatic intermittent atrial fibrillation which was treated pharmacologically. His sternal wound was assessed daily for redness, dehiscence, pain or purulent discharge (Lemaignen et al. 2015). Leg wounds for vein harvesting were assessed per protocol. His blood glucose was high and treated with short-acting insulin doses. On post-op day five, Mr. C. was transferred out of critical care to a regular nursing unit, where he complained of chills and headache but was afebrile.

Nursing Perspective. Mrs. C. asked when her husband could be discharged and said that two other relatives with the same surgery had been hospitalized for only five days. Mr. C. began telling his family and the medical team that he didn't feel like going home and was worried that something wasn't right. He stated that he felt worse each day. His family took turns sitting with him and also seemed anxious.

Medical Indications. In the evening of post-op day eight Mr. C. spiked a temperature of 102 degrees and blood cultures were done. His sternal wound was tender and red and delayed healing was evident, so a stat wound culture was done also. The nurse notified the on-call physician for the Cardiovascular Surgery group and learned that a Cardiovascular Clinical Nurse Specialist (CNS), Ms. B., was making evening rounds. Ms. B. notified one of the cardiovascular surgeons and they discussed options. Empiric antibiotic therapy was initiated pending culture results. By the next day, the wound was dehiscing at the bottom and thick, serosanguinous drainage was noted. Dr. W. ordered additional site care by the Wound Care team. Consults were initiated with an Infectious Disease physician group who saw the patient, reviewed the cultures, and ordered target antibiotics to cover methicillin-resistant staphylococcus aureus (MRSA). Cardiac ECHO testing revealed that the new heart valve was working perfectly.

Nursing Perspective. Over the next few days, the wound completely opened up. Family members were horrified, upset, and angry. Mrs. C. remained constantly at her husband's bedside and said she wasn't going home until he was discharged. Isolation precautions were put in place which further frightened the family. Communication between the family and the cardiovascular surgeon group was tense, because these physicians seemed not to appreciate the patient's distress over the infected sternal wound. Dr. W. told the patient and family that the heart valve surgery was a success. In response to Mrs. C.'s questions about the open sternal wound, he said that a referral had been made to the Infectious Disease physician group and that they would treat the wound infection. He did not mention the prognostic implications of the deep sternal wound infected with MRSA.

A myriad of emotions was expressed by the nurses taking care of Mr. C., including frustration, anger, sadness, defensiveness, and empathy. Two charge nurses held a brief meeting with the unit head nurse to explore what else they might be able to do for Mr. C. and his family. The nurses validated that the Social Worker and Case Manager were already seeing the family, yet neither the nurses nor the social worker felt that their actions were being effective in relieving the distress of the patient and his family. They felt powerless to alter the poor prognosis of the sternal wound MRSA infection.

Medical Indications. Dr. W. called in a Plastic Surgery physician group to evaluate Mr. C. and the diagnosis of a Type 2 deep sternal wound infection (DSWI) was made. These infections typically occur during the second to fourth week after surgery and present with osteomyelitis, purulent drainage, cellulitis, and mediastinal suppuration (Singh et al. 2011)—all of which were present in Mr. C.

Nursing Perspective. During the assessment by the Plastic Surgery physician, Dr. G., the nurse noted that Mr. C. was crying, as was his wife. He was now requiring additional medication in order to sleep at night, more pain medications, and an anti-depressant was added to the regimen. Mr. C.'s son began to argue with Dr. G. and asked the nurse to call in the cardiovascular surgeon, Dr. W., to talk with the family. The son demanded of Dr. W., "What's going on here? Can't you just sew that thing back up and let us get out of here?" The nurse spent as much time as possible trying to comfort the family, but her patient load of six patients that day left insufficient time for the kind of conversation that might have helped the family gain a realistic understanding of Mr. C.'s medical condition. The nurses caring for Mr. C. and interacting with his wife and children knew that a deep sternal wound infected with MRSA could develop into a life-threatening situation; they also knew that this possibility had not been presented to the patient or to his family.

Moral distress was becoming visible in the nursing staff who felt frustrated and helpless. It was an awareness that something was very wrong with the management of this patient and with the communication with the family.

The nurse caring for Mr. C. contacted the Social Worker and asked her to increase the number of visits to the family and also inquired whether the family wanted to talk to any clergy. Mrs. C. refused and said "just the surgeon please."

Dr. W. arrived about nine hours later; the son had gone home, and Mrs. C. was sleeping. He apologized and said he had been in a lengthy surgery all day and couldn't leave. This seemed to help the patient and his wife to some extent. He explained the process of referrals and that the goal was the best medical care possible for the patient.

Medical Indications. Mr. C. was taken back to surgery the next morning. Mediastinal widening was seen on imaging. A deep cavity was debrided with pockets of purulent drainage seen. Osteomyelitis was diagnosed and antibiotics were adjusted. Mr. C. was moved back to ICU, put in an isolation room, and the family was allowed open visitation. Additional blood cultures revealed early sepsis.

Unlike a superficial infection, deep sternal wound infections represent one of the worst complications that can occur after cardiac surgery including a sternotomy. Though the incidence is estimated to be between 1–5% after a median sternotomy, the mortality can range from 10 to 47% (Gummert et al. 2002; Losanoff et al. 2002; Singh et al. 2011).

Nursing Perspective. The family seemed not to understand the reasons for the patient's worsening trajectory and continued to ask about setting up home health. Mr. C. was despondent, in pain, febrile, not sleeping well despite medication, and repeatedly asked to go home. Throughout this time he remained conscious.

Medical Indications. His sepsis state progressed, as indicated by lab work analysis and his vital signs. Despite adjustments in antibiotics, little wound healing occurred. The hospital epidemiologist reported that no cluster or outbreak of infections in the two units where the patient had received care had occurred (Bryan and Yarbrough 2013).

Nursing Perspective. The Clinical Nurse Specialist called a 20-minute team conference focused on Mr. C. that included the unit nurse leaders, Social Worker, Hospital Epidemiologist, Pharmacist, and the Case Manager. No physician was able to attend, even though surgery, infectious disease, and plastics team members were invited. The family was not included at this point.

Content at the conference included technical facts about the wound infection and prevention efforts in place for preventing hospital-acquired infections. Several of the more experienced nurses raised the question of whether there might have been breaks in these prevention procedures. The Clinical Nurse Specialist said that it was possible that any of a number of factors might have contributed to Mr. C.'s MRSA infection. Admission nasal swabs had shown that a high number of the patients admitted to the hospital were already carrying MRSA. A large number of professionals from other specialty areas of the hospital had come into the unit to examine Mr. C. Another factor was that with the retirement of many of the unit's most experienced nurses, nurses with less experience and less familiarity with the unit's procedures had by necessity been assigned to Mr. C.'s care. Any one of these factors may have resulted in this infection. All present agreed that priority should be given to stepping up the full orientation of the unit's less experienced nurses, especially regarding healthcare-associated infection prevention procedures, and the Clinical Nurse Specialist committed to taking responsibility to make that happen. Additionally, the unit manager, who holds a Master's degree in nursing leadership, said he would contact the infection control department and request a consult to assure that the unit's infection control procedures were consistent with the latest evidence-based research from the Centers for Disease Control.

Toward the end of the meeting, some of the bedside nurses spoke of the angst they were experiencing because of uncertainty about the patient's future, his pain and suffering, and concerns that the family was either in denial or did not understand the prognostic implications of drug-resistant infection and sepsis. The majority of nurses caring for Mr. C. viewed the ongoing medical treatment as futile in achieving the goal of patient recovery and discharge home.

At the conclusion of the meeting, all present were in agreement that it was imperative that the medical staff discuss with Mr. C. and his family the possibility that successful closure and healing of the sternal wound were unlikely and that Mr. C. might not survive his medical condition. The Clinical Nurse Specialist and Social Worker committed to arranging a meeting in which all of the key nurses and physicians involved in Mr. C.'s care would be present. Because of the unit's history of a lack of multidisciplinary collaboration, another conclusion was that a request should be made to the nursing supervisor for allocation of special resources so that this multidisciplinary, high-stakes meeting could be in the format of a Unit-Based Ethics Conversation (UBEC) facilitated by one of the hospital's clinical ethicists.

III Moral Agency of Bedside Nurses

Twenty years ago, Chambliss (1996) conducted an 11-year sociological study of nurses in hospital settings. Obviously, a lot has changed in nursing and in healthcare systems since his study, but some of his findings remain valid. He described large, multispecialty acute care hospitals as steeply hierarchical institutions, and this remains true today. He concluded that bedside nurses in the closing years of the 1990s had very little influence on patient treatment beyond what they themselves did in providing nursing care.

The past twenty years have seen profound changes within both the profession of nursing and the healthcare system. These changes have produced increased recognition of the fundamental necessity of good nursing care to ensure good patient outcomes. The nursing shortage, especially the shortage of highly experienced critical care nurses, has focused attention on the crucial role nurses play in keeping patients safe and in supporting good patient outcomes.

Likewise, the increasing educational preparation of nurses, the incorporation of Master's-prepared Clinical Nurse Specialists and Advance Practice nurses into critical care settings and into primary care clinics, the expanding educational preparation of nurse administrators in organizational leadership, and the increasing research, theory development, and health policy influences of academic nurses in major universities and of nurse administrators in large healthcare systems have had strongly beneficial effects on the moral agency of bedside nurses. Still, some of Chambliss' findings are as true today as they were twenty years ago. Among these are that:

- The majority of nurses who practice in critical care settings are hospital employees and are, therefore, required to comply with policies and procedures within the hierarchical structure of complex healthcare organizations.
- Nurses' roles and limited power within these organizations impede the contribution of their understanding of what would improve patients' well-being and outcomes in collaborative decision-making with physicians, administrators, and other members of the healthcare team.
- Nurses carry out crucial routines to support patients, to help them recover, to save their lives, and to ease the dying process, but these vital tasks often are unnoticed and nurses' important work remains largely undervalued.
- For the most part, the ethical problems nurses face are inseparable from the organizational settings in which they arise.

Chambliss (1996, p. 88) notes, "In many ways, the ethics of nursing points to a broader ethics of organizational life." He states further,

> Ethical difficulties are not indications of unintended flaws in the system but are instead expressions of that system in its most basic features. In particular, ethical problems are an expression of interest group conflict played out in the hospital.
>
> (1996, p. 11)

This view was echoed 12 years later by Barsky (2008), who defined an ethical conflict as a "crisis in interaction in which each party becomes wrapped in self-interest, fails to see other sides, and feels victimized, hurt, or disempowered" (p. 166). Conflict emerges "when patients, surrogates, or clinicians perceive that their goals related to care and outcomes are being thwarted by the incompatible goals of others" (Edelstein et al. 2009, p. 342).

Edelstein et al. (2009) note that ethical conflicts usually begin as disagreements about an issue, or as a perception of unfairness in the process of dealing with an issue, or as an emotional response to a situation. There may be disagreements about the medical plan of care or disputes with a policy, or concerns about fair patient or staff treatment. Nurses, in particular, have moral concerns about patient suffering (Peter and Liaschenko 2004; Penticuff 2008). A commonality in ethical conflicts is that they frequently arise in the care of seriously ill patients toward the end of life. In these situations, ethical conflicts tend to be complex and emotionally charged.

Meth et al. (2009) and Swetz, Crowley, Hook, and Mueller (2007) view ethical conflicts as usually resulting from multiple overlapping root causes that complicate the disagreements that occur. Ethical discord is exacerbated by poor communication in which some members of the patients' multidisciplinary healthcare team do not speak up and others are not willing to listen or to consider alternative perspectives. Differences in power dynamics play a large role in many of these multidisciplinary team conflicts (Dubler and Liebman 2011). Schlairet (2009) notes that system processes to facilitate good communication often are missing in conflict situations, and that, without adequate communication, moral differences usually become more entrenched.

IV Nursing Care

Despite the fact that nurses work within organizational settings that often limit their ability to practice ethically, it seems just as true today as it was when, twenty years ago, Chambliss noted, "*Caring* is the ideal and figures centrally in the stories nurses tell of their own best work" (Chambliss 1996, p. 63). It remains true that the profession of nursing holds *caring for the needs of vulnerable others* as a primary aspirational goal (ANA 2015a, 2015b).

An aspect of nursing *caring* that is on the one hand obvious, and on the other hand overlooked, is that for nurses to take into account each patient's unique responses to illness and to treatment, the nurse must be physically close (Peter and Liaschenko 2004). Very often the nurse is within arm's length of the patient in providing nursing care. Touching, close observation, and dialogue combine in the process of nursing care in a manner that allows the nurse to live up to the ideal of *caring*: to meet the patient's most important needs (Penticuff 1997). Each nurse does good by ameliorating—as one can—the patient's pain, suffering, anxiety, and vulnerability. All of these nursing actions have a notion of caring embedded in them (Benner and Wrubel 1989). Thus, the essential grounding of caring is the experience of using one's knowledge, skills, judgment, and compassion to meet the needs of individual patients who are experiencing perhaps the most intense adversity of their lives (Penticuff 1997). This is the foundation of nurses' understanding of what it takes to meet their ethical obligations to patients.

Caring within arm's length (Penticuff 1997) exposes nurses to patient situations that demand ethical action. The patient looks to the nurse for help, and if the nurse cannot or does not help, if the nurse believes that she or he is unable to meet the ethical obligations to do what is good and to avoid what is harmful for patients, the nurse's inner sense of fulfilling ethical obligations erodes and moral distress may ensue (Thomas and McCullough 2015).

The concept of moral distress, formulated by Jameton (1984) in the early 1980s and further explicated by Wilkinson (1987/88), describes what nurses feel when they are unable to act according to their moral judgment. The American Association of Critical Care Nurses (AACN 2008; see also AACN 2004) defined moral distress as occurring when nurses know the appropriate action to take but are unable to act upon it and/or act in a manner contrary to their personal and professional values, undermining their integrity and authenticity. The constraints to action that hinder nursing ethical practice may be institutional, procedural, or social, threatening the nurse's ability to exercise moral integrity and do the right thing (*ANA Code of Ethics* 2015a).

Moral distress has been associated with negative consequences for both people and systems. At the individual level, moral distress can cause burnout, lack of empathy, and job dissatisfaction, while at the organizational level it may lead to reduced quality of care, increased staff turnover, and poor patient outcomes (Pauly et al. 2012; Burston and Tuckett 2013; McCarthy and Gastmans 2015; Oh and Gastmans 2015; Whitehead et al. 2015; Henrich et al. 2017).

V Organizational Characteristics and Ethical Nursing Practice

The work of Atabay et al. (2015), Lawrence (2011), Hamric (2012) and Hamric and Blackhall (2007) identified several factors that increase the likelihood that practice environments will engender moral distress. These include increased patient acuity, nurse staffing shortages, lack of intra- and interdisciplinary collaboration, and an unsafe or inadequate moral climate. McCauley (2005) found that issues contributing to moral distress include workload, incompetence of self or others leading to inadequate care, witnessing unnecessary suffering, moral compromise, and negative provider judgments about patients and/or their families.

In the vast majority of large hospitals, bedside patient care is carried out by multiple nurses whose expertise and commitment to high-quality care may vary. Many hospitals do not have sufficient nursing staff; nurses with experience and expertise in critical care are in especially short supply. Nurses also may vary in the extent of their affiliation with the multidisciplinary care team and their affirmation of the ethical climate of a specific nursing unit. Some nurses are full-time core staff, some "float" through multiple units, some are "travelers" who spend limited time in any one city or hospital. A pervasive organizational problem in many hospitals, large and small, is that this hodge-podge of nurses cannot be viewed as reliably familiar with unit procedures or reliably committed to the values of core nursing staff.

In 2005, AACN identified six essential standards for establishing and sustaining healthy critical care work environments: skilled communication, true collaboration, effective decision-making, appropriate staffing, meaningful recognition, and authentic leadership (AACN 2005). Following the publication of these standards, three landmark organizational research studies, known as the *Critical Care Nurse Work Environment Studies*, were conducted under the auspices of AACN by Ulrich and her colleagues (2006, 2009, and 2014). Findings from these studies have shown consistent relationships between healthy work environments for nurses and improved patient and nurse satisfaction, ultimately leading to improved patient outcomes. Improved work environments and reduced ratios of patients to nurses have been associated with increased care quality and patient satisfaction (Aiken et al. 2012). Patient satisfaction has been shown to be associated with better patient outcomes, such as lower 30-day hospital readmission rates (Boulding et al. 2011).

In fiscal year 2013, hospital reimbursement by Medicare became linked to patient satisfaction and quality scores (US Department of Health and Human Services 2012). Therefore, research findings that nurse work satisfaction has a significant effect on patient satisfaction with nursing care and overall patient satisfaction are especially important (Sengin 2003).

VI AACN Findings Related to Ethical Nursing Practice

In addition to findings about improved patient outcomes, the *Critical Care Nurse Work Environment Studies* have consistently demonstrated the impact of work environment factors on nurses' perception of their ability to meet their ethical obligations to patients. Of particular interest are the findings about critical care nurses' levels of moral distress across the three studies. The reported incidence of moral distress decreased from 2006 to 2008, but increased from 2008 to 2013 ($P < .05$). In 2013, 23.3% of the respondents said they experience moral distress frequently, while 9.4% said they experience it very frequently (Table 12.1).

A large body of research on healthy critical care work environments has consistently found that appropriate staffing and creating opportunities for all members of the multidisciplinary team to discuss, learn from, and resolve morally distressing situations are major strategies for addressing nurses' and other healthcare professionals' moral distress.

VII Strategies to Support Ethical Nursing Practice

Within the past few years, nursing ethicists have called for the profession to respond to moral distress by using it as a catalyst for positive action and a means by which to support ethical practice (Rushton 2016; Rushton et al. 2016; Rushton, Schoonover-Shoffner and Kennedy 2017). Aburn et al. (2016) and Musto et al. (2015) have described a counterbalance to moral distress: the concept of moral resilience. Moral resilience reflects an individual's capacity to sustain or restore her or his integrity in response to moral complexity, confusion, distress, or setbacks.

Table 12.1 Percentage of Respondents Who Reported Experiencing Moral Distress

	2006	2008	2013
Very frequently	6.8	5.6	9.4
Frequently	19.4	17.6	23.3
Occasionally	45.6	45.3	42.8
Very rarely	28.2	31.5	24.5

Because of rounding, percentages may not total 100. All changes from 2008 to 2013 are significant at $P < .05$.

VIII Combatting Moral Distress and Building Moral Resilience

As noted in the case study, the nurses decided to combat their moral distress by taking action. They arranged a Unit-Based Ethics Conversation (UBEC) to address their ethical concerns about Mr. C.'s care. The UBEC program is one of a number of unit-level interventions that are being employed in critical care units across the country and internationally to develop moral resilience and combat moral distress of nurses and other healthcare professionals. The UBEC aims to create an environment allowing nurses, physicians, and others to engage in open dialogue on ethical questions. The program is particularly effective when, from the start, participation includes all of the key multidisciplinary team members: the nurses providing bedside care, nursing managers, the patient's Social Worker and Case Manager, and, of course, the key physicians involved in the patient's treatment. In Mr. C.'s case, the UBEC was implemented with the inclusion of a Clinical Ethicist skilled in facilitating collaborative decision-making and familiar with the process of bioethical mediation (Dubler and Liebman 2011).

This high-stakes meeting was scheduled with the help of the Director of Memorial Hospital's Ethics Committee, a highly respected nurse whose credentials included a Master's degree in healthcare ethics and a doctorate in nursing practice (DNP). Because of this director's involvement in extending the invitation, all of the physicians invited to the meeting appreciated its importance and made arrangements to attend.

The UBEC meeting was held the following evening and all who had been invited participated. After introductions all around, Dr. W. told everyone present that he truly appreciated the hard work of all of the team members caring for Mr. C. The topic of the necessity of informing Mr. C. and his family of the poor prognosis associated with MRSA was introduced by the Clinical Ethicist. All the physicians present agreed that this needed to be done and Dr. W. took responsibility for informing the patient.

The nurse manager of the unit told the group that one of the Advanced Practice Nurses from the hospital's oncology unit had been trained in Buckman's protocol for breaking bad news (Buckman 1992) and had just finished a clinical ethics residency at another major hospital in the city (Grace et al. 2014). Dr. W. asked whether this nurse might be available to assist him in the ensuing difficult conversation with Mr. C. and his family. The participants were pleased to learn that nursing administration had arranged for this Clinical Nurse Specialist to be available across hospital units to support professionals when difficult conversations were necessary. Dr. W. took the business card the unit manager offered and said he would contact the Clinical Nurse Specialist immediately after the meeting. Another important outcome from this meeting was that the physicians agreed that a series of UBEC meetings could be helpful in increasing collaboration in the unit and addressing ethical issues and made individual commitments to attend. Meetings were then scheduled for one evening each month over the next six months.

After this initial UBEC meeting, participants talked about the relief they felt and how much they looked forward to the six future meetings. Helft et al. (2009) reported that implementation of UBECs in a Pediatric ICU decreased the level of moral distress of the multidisciplinary team and increased their collaboration, both in instances of ethical issues and in efforts to improve the quality of routine care.

This initial UBEC was the first of a number of changes that the multidisciplinary team embarked on. They went on to implement multidisciplinary daily patient conferences, and enlisted the support of the community members of Memorial's Hospital Board in challenging hospital administration to provide safe RN-patient ratios and an appropriate nursing staff skill-mix. Nursing administration collaborated with bedside nurses to establish a department of evidence-based nursing practice and to develop a career ladder that gave meaningful recognition and reward for clinical and professional excellence. The Clinical Nurse Specialists across the hospital collaborated with bedside nurses and key physicians to establish standing nursing orders and multidisciplinary walking rounds. The department of evidence-based practice structured surveys and collected baseline and post-intervention data to assess the effectiveness of these changes in improving multidisciplinary communication and in decreasing the likelihood of ethical conflict.

IX Application of the *ANA Code of Ethics* (2015)

This part of the chapter is based on the *Interpretive Statements* accompanying the *ANA Code of Ethics* (2015a) as explicated by Winland-Brown, Lachman and Swanson (2015), and Lachman, Swanson, and Windland-Brown (2015) in their work applying the *Code* to clinical practice. The following discussion applies relevant portions of the *Code* to the case of Mr. C.

The *Code* and its *Interpretative Statements* emphasize that to promote Mr. C.'s health fully, the nurses should encourage an honest dialogue between Mr. C. and Dr. W. The *Code* also includes obligations that nurses must respect the patient's "right to self-determination." Mr. C. had the capacity to understand his diagnosis and to participate in the decisions for his treatment. From the case situation, his wife should be included in these discussions and Mr. C. may want his daughter and son to be involved in the decision-making process as well. The *Code* states that "patients have a moral and legal right to determine what will be done with and to their person" (2015a, p. 2). The physician, patient, and family need to know the diagnosis and prognosis in order to make informed decisions about treatment. Whether treatment is aimed toward cure of the infection, or is aimed at palliation, Mr. C. and his family need to engage in an advance care planning conversation with Dr. W. The nurse's obligation is to assure that the patient has accurate, complete, and understandable information on which to base his decisions.

The *ANA Code* states that the nurse's primary commitment is to the patient. This provision focuses on the nurse's obligation to assure the primacy of the patient's interests regardless of conflicts that arise between clinicians or patient and family. This requires that nurses caring for Mr. C. have a primary commitment to Mr. C. and his family. His nurses need to provide opportunities for Mr. C. and his family to participate in his care, including honest discussions about available resources and treatment options. Another aspect of this provision involves "conflict of interest for nurses." Mr. C.'s case illustrates several possible conflicts: between physician and nurses, physician and patient, physician and family members, and nurses and family members. Nurses promote Mr. C.'s best interests when they speak up and raise questions about his understanding of his prognosis, thus supporting interprofessional collaboration with physicians. Nurses must address conflicting expectations from patients, families, and physicians, as well as conflicts arising between their own professional and personal values.

The third interpretive statement relates to "collaboration." "Nurses are responsible for articulating, representing, and preserving the scope of nursing practice, and the unique contributions of nursing to patient care" (2015a, p. 6). This collaboration "requires mutual trust, recognition, respect, transparency, shared decision-making and open communication among all who share concern and responsibility for health outcomes" (2015a, p. 6). If nurses are reluctant to open a dialogue with the physician concerning a patient's possible lack of understanding of diagnosis or prognosis, other professionals can be used: other healthcare colleagues, leaders, and the hospital ethics committee. Throughout the process of collaboration, the desired outcome is always a demonstrated commitment to the patient.

The possibility that the unit's procedures for preventing healthcare-associated infections may have been violated by nurses or other members of the healthcare team, or the possibility that these procedures are not up to date is addressed by the Code's *Interpretive Statements* of nurses' "professional responsibility in promoting a culture of safety." Clinical nurses have the ethical obligation to know and disseminate the most recent research findings to support best practices. Professional nurses have an obligation to develop practice standards that support ethical practice and nursing's body of knowledge. Nurse managers and executives must support the autonomy of nurses in executing these standards to maintain quality patient care.

The nurse is responsible for reporting any errors or near-misses to the appropriate authority, ensuring disclosure of the errors to patients, and establishing processes to investigate these errors to prevent recurrence. The nurse also must not remain silent in the event of an error. Breaks in technique that increased the probability of Mr. C.'s hospital-acquired MRSA infection must be addressed by the nursing staff. This obligation is reinforced by the *Interpretative Statement*, obligating nurses to protect patient health and safety by acting on questionable practice. "Reporting questionable practice, even when done appropriately, may present substantial risk to the nurse; however, such risk does not eliminate the obligation to address threats to patient safety" (2015a, p. 13). The nurses caring for Mr. C. are obligated to report breaks in preventive procedures by any multidisciplinary team members, even his physicians.

The third *Interpretative Statement* focuses on "responsibility for nursing judgments, decisions, and actions." This Statement emphasizes the need to provide safeguards for patients, nurses, colleagues, and the environment, and nurses' responsibility to "bring forward difficult issues related to patient care and/or institutional constraints upon ethical practice for discussion and review" (2015a, p. 16). The 2015 revision of the *Code* places a duty on nurse executives for safeguarding nurses' access to organizational committees and institutional boards, as well as inclusion in decision-making processes relevant to patient care ethics, quality, and safety. Nurses who participate on these committees and boards "are obligated to actively engage in, and contribute to, the decisions that are made" (2015a, p. 16). The nurse administrator's provision of resources needed to implement the initial UBEC meeting and the subsequent ones was consistent with obligations articulated in the Code.

The Code's *Interpretive Statements* note that "employer policies do not relieve the nurse of responsibility for making assignment or delegation decisions" (2015a, p. 17). The nurse manager's assignment of inexperienced nurses to care for Mr. C., including their participation in his wound-dressing changes, violates this aspect of the *Code*, even though the manager was dealing with a lack of nurses properly prepared to perform this task safely for M. C.

The Code's *Interpretive Statements* maintain that nurse administrators "must respond to concerns and act to resolve the concern in a way that preserves the integrity of the nurses" (2015a, p. 21). This was carried out by the implementation of the UBECs. This fourth interpretative statement also addresses the concept of conscientious objection. This means refusing to participate in a decision or action the nurse believes may endanger a patient, family, or community, or nursing practice itself because it violates the nurse's moral standards. Nurses must understand that these acts of moral courage do not insulate them from formal or informal consequences (Lachman, Swanson, and Windland-Brown 2015). Any erosion of the ethical environment could result in moral distress for nurses. Therefore, nurses have an obligation to express their conscientious objection to the appropriate authority.

The *Code* states that the nurse, through individual and collective effort, establishes, maintains, and improves the ethical environment of the work setting and conditions of employment that are conducive to safe, quality health care. "Nurses in all roles must create a culture of excellence and maintain practice environments that support nurses and others in the fulfillment of their ethical obligations" (2015a, p. 24). The Code's *Interpretative Statements* emphasize that "nurses are responsible for contributing to a moral environment that demands respectful interactions among colleagues, mutual peer support, and open identification of difficult issues..." (2015a, p. 24). "The workplace must be a morally good environment to ensure safe, quality patient care and professional satisfaction for nurses and to minimize and address moral distress, strain, and dissonance" (2015a, p. 24). Again, the nurses caring for Mr. C. carried out this ethical obligation by transforming their ethical distress into action that supported important changes to the unit's ethical environment.

Finally, the Code's *Interpretative Statements* address the "articulation and assertion of values" and asserts the need for professional nursing organizations to provide a unified voice for the profession. Various professional organizations of nursing "communicate to the public the values that nursing considers central to the promotion or restoration of health, the prevention of illness or injury, and the alleviation of suffering" (2015a, p. 35). By acting in unity, nurses can have a noteworthy impact on health policies. The "integrity of the profession" is based on the knowledge and observance of essential documents, such as the *Code* (ANA 2015a) and *Nursing: Scope and Standards of Practice* (ANA 2015b). These documents support the covenant between the nursing profession and society. This promise also is supported by defined educational requirements for entry into practice, augmented utilization of advanced practice nurses, increased focus on certification, and nursing's commitment to evidence-based practice (Lachman, Swanson, and Windland-Brown 2015).

X Conclusion

This chapter has described a hypothetical case illustrating nurses' moral agency, organizational characteristics, moral distress, and strategies for resolving moral distress and improving ethical nursing practice. The chapter ends with application of Nursing's *Code of Ethics* and its accompanying *Interpretative Statements* (2015a) to clarify ethical nursing practice.

References

Aburn, G., M. Gott, and K. Hoare. 2016. What is resilience? An integrative review of the empirical literature, *Journal of Advanced Nursing* 72(5): 980–1000.

Aiken, L.H., W. Sermeus, K. Van den Heede, D.M. Sloane, R. Busse, M. McKee, and C. Tishelman. 2012. Patient safety, satisfaction, and quality of hospital care: cross sectional surveys of nurses and patients in 12 countries in Europe and the United States, *BMJ*, *344*: e1717.

American Association of Critical-Care Nurses, Ethics Work Group. 2004. *The 4A's to rise above moral distress.* http://www.aacn.org/WD/Practice/Docs/4As_to_Rise_Above_ Moral_Distress.pdf.

American Association of Critical-Care Nurses. 2005. *AACN standards for establishing and sustaining healthy work environments: A journey to excellence.* http://www.aacn.org/WD/ HWE/Docs/HWEStandards.pdf.

American Association of Critical-Care Nurses. 2008. *Position Paper: Moral Distress.* http:// www.aacn.org/wd/hwe/content/resources.

American Nurses Association. 2015a. *Code of ethics for nurses with interpretive statements.* http://www.nursingworld.org/codeofethics.

American Nurses Association. 2015b. Nursing: Scope and Standards of Practice, third edition. American Nursing Association.

Atabay, G., B.G. Çangarli, and s,. Penbek. 2015. Impact of ethical climate on moral distress revisited: Multidimensional view, *Nursing Ethics* 22(1): 103–116.

Barsky, A. 2008. A conflict resolution approach to teaching ethical decision making: Bridging conflicting values. *Journal of Jewish Communal Service* 83(2): 164–169.

Benner, P., and J. Wrubel. 1989. *The primacy of caring: Stress and coping in health and illness.* New York: Addison-Wesley Publishing Company.

Boulding, W., S.W. Glickman, M.P. Manary, K.A. Schulman, and R. Staelin. 2011. Relationship between patient satisfaction with inpatient care and hospital readmission within 30 days, *The American Journal of Managed Care* 17(1): 41–48.

Bryan, C.S., and W.M. Yarbrough. 2013. Preventing deep wound infection after coronary artery bypass grafting: A review. *Texas Heart Institute* 40(2): 125–139.

Buckman, R. 1992. *How to break bad news: A guide for health care professionals.* Baltimore: The Johns Hopkins University Press.

Burston, A.S., and A.G. Tuckett. 2013. Moral distress in nursing: Contributing factors, outcomes and interventions, *Nursing Ethics* 20(3): 312–324.

Chambliss, D.F. 1996. *Beyond caring: Hospitals, nurses, and the social organization of ethics.* Chicago: University of Chicago Press.

Dubler, N.N., and C.B. Liebman. 2011. *Bioethics mediation: A guide to shaping shared solutions,* revised and expanded edition. Nashville: Vanderbilt University Press.

Edelstein, L.M., E.G. DeRenzo, E. Waetzig, C. Zelizer, and N.O. Mokwunye. 2009. Communication and conflict management training for clinical bioethics committees, *HEC Forum* 21(4): 341–349.

Grace, P.J., E. Robinson, M. Jurchak, A.A. Zollfrank, and S.M. Lee. 2014. Clinical ethics residency for nurses: An education model to decrease moral distress and strengthen nurse retention in acute care, *Journal of Nursing Administration* 44(12): 640–646.

Gummert, J.F., M.J. Barten, and C. Hands et al. 2002. Mediastinitis and cardiac surgery — An updated risk factor analysis in 10,373 consecutive adult patients, *Thoracic Cardiovascular Surgery* 50(2): 87–91.

Hamric, A.B. 2012. Empirical research on moral distress: Issues, challenges, and opportunities, *HEC Forum* 24(1): 39–49.

Hamric, A.B., and L.J. Blackhall. 2007. Nurse-physician perspectives on the care of dying patients in intensive care units: Collaboration, moral distress, and ethical climate, *Critical Care Medicine* 35(2): 422–429.

Henrich, N.J., P.M. Dodek, E. Gladstone, L. Alden, S.P. Keenan, S. Reynolds, and P. Rodney. 2017. Consequences of moral distress in the intensive care unit: A qualitative study, *American Journal of Critical Care* 26(4): e48–e57.

Helft, P.R., P.D. Bledsoe, M. Hancock, and L.D. Wocial. 2009. Facilitated ethics conversations: A novel program for managing moral distress in bedside nursing staff. *JONA'S Healthcare Law, Ethics and Regulation,* 11(1): 27–33.

Jameton, A. 1984. *Nursing practice: The ethical issues.* Englewood Cliffs, NJ: Prentice-Hall.

Lachman, V.D., E.O. Swanson, and J. Windland-Brown. 2015. The new 'code of ethics for nurses with interpretive statements': Practical clinical application, part II. *MEDSURG Nursing,* 24(5): 363–366, 368.

Lawrence, L.A. 2011. Work engagement, moral distress, education level, and critical reflective practice in intensive care nurses, *Nursing Forum* 46(4): 256–268.

Lemaignen, A., G. Birgand, W. Ghodhbane, and S. Alkhoder et al. 2015. Sternal wound infection after cardiac surgery: Incidence and risk factors according to clinical presentation. *Clinical Microbiology and Infection* 21(7): 674.e11–e18.

Losanoff, J.E., B.W. Richman, and J.W. Jones. 2002. Disruption and infection of median sternotomy: A comprehensive review, *European Journal of Cardio-Thoracic Surgery* 21(5): 831–839.

McCarthy, J. and C. Gastmans. 2015. Moral distress: A review of the argument-based nursing ethics literature, *Nursing Ethics* 22(1): 131–152.

McCauley, K. 2005. President's note: All we needed was the glue, *AACN News,* May 22:2.

Meth, N.D., B. Lawless, and L. Hawryluck. 2009. Conflicts in the ICU: Perspectives of administrators and clinicians, *Intensive Care Medicine* 35(12): 2068.

Musto, L.C., P.A. Rodney, and R. Vanderheide. 2015. Toward interventions to address moral distress: Navigating structure and agency, *Nursing Ethics* 22(1): 91–102.

Oh, Y. and C. Gastmans. 2015. Moral distress experienced by nurses: A quantitative literature review, *Nursing Ethics* 22(1): 15–31.

Pauly, B.M., C. Carcoe, and J. Storch. 2012. Framing the issues: Moral distress in health care. *HEC Forum* 24(1): 1–11.

Penticuff, J.H. 1997 Nursing perspectives in bioethics. In: *Japanese and Western bioethics* (pp. 49–60), K. Hoshino (ed). Dordrecht: Kluwer Academic Publishers.

Penticuff, J.H. 2008. Suffering, compassion, and ethics: Reflections on neonatal nursing. In: *Nursing and health care ethics: A legacy and a vision* (pp. 283–292), Pinch, E., and A.M. Haddad (eds). Silver Spring MD: American Nurses Association.

Peter, E., and J. Liaschenko. 2004. Perils of proximity: A spatiotemporal analysis of moral distress and moral ambiguity. *Nursing Inquiry* 11(4): 218–225.

Rushton, C.H. 2016. Moral resilience: A capacity for navigating moral distress in critical care, *AACN Advanced Critical Care* 27(1): 111–119.

Rushton, C.H., M. Caldwell, and M. Kurtz. 2016. CE: Moral distress: A catalyst in building moral resilience, *The American Journal of Nursing*, 116(7): 40–49.

Rushton, C.H., K. Schoonover-Shoffner, and M.S. Kennedy. 2017. A collaborative state of the science initiative: Transforming moral distress into moral resilience in nursing. *American The Journal of Nursing February* 117(2): S2–S6.

Schlairet, M.C. 2009. Bioethics mediation: The role and importance of nursing advocacy, *Nursing Outlook* 57(4): 185–193.

Sengin, K.K. 2003. Work-related attributes of RN job satisfaction in acute care hospitals, *Journal of Nursing Administration* 33(6): 317–320.

Singh, K., A. Anderson, and G. Harper. 2011. Overview and management of sternal wound infection, *Seminars in Plastic Surgery* 25(1): 25–33.

Swetz, K.M., M.E. Crowley, C.C. Hook, and P.S. Mueller. 2007. Report of 255 clinical ethics consultations and review of the literature, *Mayo Clinic Proceedings* 82(6): 686–691.

Thomas, T.A., and L.B. McCullough. 2015. A philosophical taxonomy of ethically significant moral distress, *Journal of Medicine and Philosophy* 40(1): 102–120.

Ulrich, B.T., R. Lavandero, D. Woods, and S. Early. 2014. Critical care nurse work environments 2013: A Status Report. *Critical Care Nurse* 34(4): 64–79.

Ulrich, B.T., R. Lavandero, and K.A. Hart et al. 2009. Critical care nurses' work environments 2008: A follow-up report, *Critical Care Nurse* 29(2): 93–102.

Ulrich, B.T., R. Lavandero, K.A. Hart, D. Woods, J. Leggett, and D. Taylor. 2006. Critical care nurses' work environments: A baseline status report, *Critical Care Nurse* 26(5): 46–55.

US Department of Health and Human Services. 2012. HCAHPS: Patients' perspectives of care survey 2012. https://www.cms.gov/Medicare/Quality-Initiatives-Patient-Assessment-Instruments/HospitalQualityInits/HospitalHCAHPS.html.

Whitehead, P.B., R.K. Herbertson, A.B. Hamric, E.G. Epstein, and J.M. Fisher. 2015. Moral distress among healthcare professionals: Report of an institution-wide survey, *Journal of Nursing Scholarship* 47(2): 117–125.

Wilkinson, J.M. 1987/88. Moral distress in nursing practice: Experience and effect, *Nursing Forum* 23(1): 16–29.

Winland-Brown, J., V.D. Lachman, and E.O. Swanson. 2015. The new code of ethics for nurses with interpretative statements (2015): Practical Clinical Application, Part I. *MEDSURG Nursing* 24(4): 268–271.

Part V

Cardiovascular Medical Research

13 Ethics in Cardiovascular Research

Ana S. Iltis and Douglas E. Lemley

I Historical and Contemporary Context for Human Research Ethics

The desire to know truly, to do good and avoid harm, and to use resources efficiently all drive human research. Without research, that is, without systematic investigations to understand disease processes, physiology, and the effects of drugs, devices, surgeries, and other interventions, patients may be exposed to ineffective, unsafe, or unnecessary treatments.[1] There is a long list of examples of untested beliefs that shaped treatment and ultimately proved to be useless at best, and harmful or fatal at worst. For example, premature infants briefly were exposed to high concentrations of oxygen during the late 1940s for treatment of cyanosis and respiratory distress, resulting in an increased incidence of subsequent infantile blindness due to retrolental fibroplasia (Cohen 1998). In 1961 Beecher described earlier efforts to treat angina pectoris through ligation of the internal mammary arteries. This procedure, initially popularized in 1939, was thought to shunt extracardiac blood flow to the coronary arteries. It remained in clinical use for the next 20 years. Canine studies, however, demonstrated no reproducible evidence that it was effective. By 1958 evidence began to accumulate that ligation of the mammary arteries was of no greater human clinical benefit than a sham operation (Adams 1958). The benefits were due, Beecher argues, to the psychological power of the placebo effect, meaning that patients routinely were exposed to surgical risks when the surgery itself provided no true physiological benefit (Beecher 1961). Paradoxically, direct grafting of the left internal mammary artery to the left anterior descending artery came to be thought of as the "gold standard" of coronary artery revascularization (Karthik and Fabri 2006).

There are many examples of ongoing disagreements among health care professionals about which among the practices considered standard of care are best. These disagreements (sometimes) can be resolved through well-designed research studies. Yet many studies require that clinicians enroll patients into research. Patients expect their physicians to make decisions based on what they believe is best for them. When enrolled in research studies, interventions might be randomly assigned, participants might receive a placebo, and participants might undergo procedures or tests solely or primarily for the purpose of

DOI: 10.4324/9781003240273-19

gathering data meant to benefit others. This tension between the goals and duties associated with clinical care and research is one of the primary concerns that has shaped the research regulatory system and the research ethics literature. Conflation of these not always equivalent ends constitutes the "therapeutic misconception". It continues to vex clinicians, researchers, regulators, and scholars.

The standard of care in modern cardiology perhaps faced no greater challenge than the failed hypothesis of the Cardiac Arrhythmia Suppression Trial (CAST) of the 1980s. CAST put to the test the seemingly rational assumption that the administration of anti-arrhythmic agents to asymptomatic or mildly symptomatic post-myocardial infarction (MI) patients who experienced ventricular premature complexes (VPCs) would diminish their risk of subsequent arrhythmic death (Pratt and Moye 1990). Prior research had established VPCs as a risk factor for sudden death post-MI independent of left ventricular function (Bigger et al. 1984). CAST's precursor investigation, the Cardiac Arrhythmia Pilot Study (CAPS) also had demonstrated the adequate suppression of VPCs within the target population by the study drugs encainide, flecainide, and moricizine (CAPS Investigators 1986, 1988). Nevertheless, the long-term ability of anti-arrhythmic therapy to reduce the incidence of sudden death had yet to be proven.[2]

CAST was designed to evaluate the effectiveness of three of the same anti-arrhythmic pharmaceuticals that had been used in CAPS (i.e., encainide, flecainide, and moricizine) over a five-year period of subject recruitment and observation (1987–1992). This particularly careful investigation had taken the uncommon precautionary step of starting with an open-label titration period meant to identify those individuals who responded favorably to at least one of the three study drugs. Only then were these pre-screened individuals randomized to treatment with a proven effective agent or placebo (The CAST Investigators 1989). As further evidence of its commitment to subject safety, CAST also had adopted the more routine oversight afforded by periodic submission of its data to an independent Data Safety and Monitoring Board (DSMB). To the great consternation of CAST investigators, its DSMB in April, 1989 uncovered incontrovertible evidence that "the number of deaths from arrhythmia …, deaths from a non-arrhythmic cardiac event, and total mortality were higher among patients assigned to encainide or flecainide" (CAST 1989, p. 409). These two Class IC anti-arrhythmic agents immediately were removed from further study, although investigation of moricizine continued (CAST-II) (CAST 1989; Echt et al. 1991). Unfortunately CAST-II came to a similarly dreadful outcome prompting its premature discontinuation in 1991 (CAST-II Investigators 1992; Pratt and Moye 1995).

With refutation of the heretofore clinically accepted suppression hypothesis, "the common practice of using anti-arrhythmic drugs to suppress asymptomatic arrhythmias in patients after acute [MI was] curtailed" (Pratt and Moye 1995, p. 245). Revelation of the unexpected adverse results of CAST and CAST-II could well have been delayed even longer in the absence of rigorous adherence to established scientific methods of clinical investigation and independent oversight of research.

In recent years, comparative effectiveness research (CER) has gained significant attention. CER is "designed to inform health-care decisions by providing evidence on the effectiveness, benefits, and harms of different treatment options. The evidence is generated from research studies that compare drugs, medical devices, tests, surgeries, or ways to deliver health care" (AHRQ n.d.).

One might expect that CER studies comparing different standard practices would be far less controversial than studies of new interventions since participants are getting one among several of the accepted routine treatments. However, some CER studies have generated significant discussion regarding the ethical conduct of research. For example, the Surfactant, Positive Pressure, and Pulse Oximetry Randomized Trial (SUPPORT) study group compared outcomes for preterm infants whose oxygen saturation was maintained at the low end of the standard of care (85–89%) with outcomes in infants maintained at the high end of the standard (91–95%) (SUPPORT 2010). One key concern regarding SUPPORT is what risks should have been anticipated and disclosed to parents. Given the uncertainty that existed over whether infants maintained at lower oxygen saturation levels were less likely to develop retinopathy of prematurity (i.e., retrolental fibroplasia), but more likely to die or experience neurological injury, some have argued that the possibility of death as a study risk should have been disclosed (Macklin et al. 2013, 2014; Merz 2014; OHRP 2013a, 2013b). Others disagree (Drazen et al. 2013; Hudson et al. 2013; Magnus and Caplan 2013; Wilfond et al. 2013).

Should investigators have anticipated the *possibility* that infants in one group might be at greater risk for death than infants in the other group and, if so, should they have told parents of this possibility? Jon Merz has argued that if investigators saw no possibility of there being a difference in outcomes such as the low oxygen group doing worse in terms of death, then the study would not have been justified. The oxygen rates simply should have been kept low across the board to reduce the incidence of blindness (Merz 2014). A second concern is whether the claim that infants in the study all received standard of care interventions was accurate. Study participants' treatment deviated from the treatment they typically would have received in their particular neonatal intensive care unit (NICU) in a number of ways, including the use of pulse oximeters that were designed to mask the participants' assigned group. Moreover, it is not clear that any of the participating research sites routinely used the lower target range of 85–89%. A national survey of NICU directors performed prior to SUPPORT in 2001 had documented the absence of any set standard of care regarding administration of oxygen to premature infants.

Of the 120 institutions reporting an oxygen saturation target range, (a) none had an upper limit lower than 92% and a substantial minority had an upper limit of 94%, and (b) a substantial majority had a lower limit of 86% or higher (Macklin and Shepherd 2013; Anderson et al. 2004, p. 11). In other words, restricting oxygen saturation to a maximum of 89% was not an *established* standard even though the 85–89% range falls within the *accepted* standard of 85–95%. CER is important and holds great promise, but investigators should be careful not to assume that (1) a study involves merely minimal risk or no additional risk simply because a study compares different standard practices or (2) that what they label "standard of care" in fact is standard.

Many commentators refer to the Nuremberg Code as the basis of contemporary research ethics regulation and oversight. The Code consists of ten principles to be followed when using humans in research (1949: 181–82). Although the Nuremberg Code often is cited and remains influential, it did not lead to significant changes in US research practices. In 1966 Henry Beecher described 22 studies he believed were unethical (1966). His *New England Journal of Medicine* paper similarly remains highly cited and relevant, but it did not lead to changes in US research practices. It was public revelations of the United States Public Health Service (USPHS) Tuskegee Syphilis Study, in which poor African-American sharecroppers in Alabama who had syphilis were observed for decades without adequate information about why they were being studied, and therefore without their informed consent. Even after penicillin was found to be safe and effective for treating the disease during World War II and thereafter became widely available in the United States, the study subjects never were told about or experienced its beneficial effects. Researchers intentionally withheld treatment and prevented them from seeking treatment elsewhere (Jones 1981). The study continued until 1973. Revelations of the study prompted the US Congress to pass the National Research Act in 1974. This statute established the National Commission for the Protection of Research Subjects of Biomedical and Behavioral Research to identify principles and guidelines that ought to be followed in the ethical pursuit of human research.

The National Commission produced a series of reports over the next several years, such as reports on research on fetuses (1975), prisoners (1976), and children (1977), as well as the *Belmont Report* (1979), its most widely known and cited publication. The Commission recommend that three ethical principles govern human research, and these remain highly influential:

1. **Respect for Persons**: The judgments of autonomous persons, those "capable of deliberation about personal goals and of acting under the direction of such deliberation," must be respected. Special protections are owed to those who are not autonomous and thus are not capable of self-determination (B.1). This principle leads to the obligation to obtain informed consent. Valid informed consent requires investigators to disclose sufficient information about the study and to disclose it in a manner and context in which potential subjects can understand it. The request for consent must be done in a way that allows people to make voluntary decisions that are free from coercion and undue influence (C.1).

2. **Beneficence**: Beneficence requires that researchers "(1) do not harm and (2) maximize possible benefits and minimize possible harms" (B.2). In practice, this means that research risks must be reasonable in relation to the anticipated benefits to subjects or society, research risks are minimized, and potential benefits maximized (C.2).

3. **Justice**: The principle of justice calls for the fair distribution of research benefits and burdens. Researchers must avoid denying persons benefits to which they are entitled and imposing undue burdens on persons (B.3). This leads to the requirement that there be fair procedures and outcomes in the selection of research subjects. No one population should be unduly burdened by participation in research, nor should one population be offered the opportunity to participate in potentially beneficial research while others are denied the opportunity (C.3).

II Regulation of Research in the United States

In the United States the minimum conditions for the ethical conduct of human research established in the *Belmont Report* and in many of the National Commission's other reports are embodied in the federal regulations governing human research. These regulations govern much, not though not all, human research. The Food and Drug Administration (FDA) regulations appear at 21CFR50 (Code of Federal Regulations) and 21CFR56. The Department of Health and Human Services (DHHS) has its regulations at 45CFR46. Since 1991 16 other federal agencies, such as the Department of Defense, have shared the HHS regulations. The regulations for those 16 agencies appear in various places in the CFR, and are referred to as the Common Rule.[3] Many other countries have somewhat similar policies and regulations.

Regulations establish a minimum set of obligations that researchers, sponsors, and institutions must respect to be compliant. The ethical conduct of research requires not merely adherence but appropriate interpretation and application of the regulations as well as an appreciation for ethical obligations on which the regulations are silent. Eleven areas relevant to research ethics are based not only on these regulations and National Commission documents, but also upon guidance that has been provided from bodies such as the Office of Human Research Protections (OHRP), the Council for International Organization of Medical Sciences (CIOMS), the United Nations Educational, Scientific and Cultural Organization (UNESCO), and the World Medical Association.

A Research Oversight and Independent Review

Human research ordinarily requires independent review prior to initiating a study and at regular intervals during a study. This review is intended to ensure that the study meets the requirements set forth in the federal regulations governing human research so as to protect participants. Even studies that qualify as exempt (see 45CFR46.101.b) typically face some institutional process to verify such exemption. Independent review committees, typically called institutional review boards (IRBs) in the United States and research ethics boards (REBs) or research ethics committees (RECs) elsewhere, conduct the reviews. They have a number of responsibilities and must meet specific membership requirements (45CFR46.107).

The main requirements for IRB review and approval are found in the CFR (45CFR46.111 and 21CFR56). Research using certain populations may have additional IRB membership requirements related to their specific "at risk" characteristics. For example, in the case of prisoners, there must be someone on the board who can represent the unique interests of this special group (e.g., unsubstantiated offers of early parole). Additionally special requirements exist for pregnant women, embryos, fetuses and neonates, and children (45CFR46, Subparts B, C, and D).

Some research can be reviewed on an expedited basis (see 45CFR46.110), meaning that it does not require full board review and instead may be reviewed by the chair of the IRB or by another designated, experienced reviewer (45CFR46.110). Research that qualifies for expedited review includes protocols posing only minimal risk to participants, and that can be classified into one of nine categories specified by the Secretary of DHHS, e.g., collection of biological specimens through noninvasive measures and collection of limited amounts of blood.[4]

IRBs may be able to influence very little regarding protocols they review. IRBs typically are institution-specific bodies. However, they often review protocols that cannot be changed substantially because they are part of industry-sponsored or multi-center trials. An IRB might determine that the risks to participants could be reduced further, for instance, but requiring such a change from the local investigator is a *de facto* rejection of the protocol because he or she is powerless to change it. Thus, IRB members either accept what they deem a flawed study, perhaps requiring minor changes in a consent form, or they reject the study.

Imagine a study for a new medication for hypertension.[5] An investigator proposes a placebo-controlled study that will recruit people whose blood pressure, without medication, is at least 160/100. All participants will be taken off of their current medication for hypertension and will go through a two-week wash-out period. They will be randomized, one-half to the study drug and one-half to placebo. The study will last six weeks. Numerous IRB members argue that it is not safe to leave hypertension untreated, especially for as many as eight weeks (for those in the placebo arm). They know that this is an industry-sponsored study, the investigator submitting it is one of many across the country conducting the study, and the investigator will be unable to change the study design to improve participant safety. The IRB can reject the study, or approve it perhaps with changes to the warnings in the consent form or some other small factor.

Numerous authors have argued that the oversight system is deeply flawed and perhaps, in at least some cases, no oversight should be required. Complaints include: (1) IRBs sometimes judge the same studies or same types of studies differently (Hirshon et al. 2002; Stark et al. 2010); (2) IRBs infringe on academic freedom (Gunsalus et al. 2006); (3) oversight requirements hinder research and stifle potentially life-saving creativity (Whitney and Schneider 2011); and (4) IRBs make informed consent documents harder to read (Schneider 2010).

Despite these criticisms, there are important reasons to have an oversight system in place, including the need to protect the integrity of the research system and the public's trust in the research system (London 2012).

B Research Design

Investigators have a number of ethical obligations associated with study design. Protocols must be designed so as to minimize risks and maximize potential benefits to participants and society. The research risks also must be reasonable in relation to the anticipated benefits. While this sounds straightforward, it is not always so. Questions including which risks should be considered research risks and how the overall risk of participation should be assessed, have generated a substantive literature (see, for example Weijer and Miller 2004; Emanuel and Miller 2001; Miller and Brody 2003; Wendler and Miller 2007). A central disagreement concerns whether each component of a study, including the interventions done for therapeutic *versus* nontherapeutic purposes, should be evaluated separately (component analysis or dual track assessment) or as a whole (net risks test).

Review of research involving special populations, including children, requires additional considerations of risk and potential benefit. For example, a study involving children designated as posing only minimal risk need not offer participants a prospect of direct benefit, but such potentiality ordinarily must exist for a study involving more than minimal risk (45CFR46.404 and 405). Investigators and IRBs perceive risk differently and assign risk labels differently (Shah et al. 2004). Additionally, studies that pose only a minor increase over minimal risk and promise to yield critical information about the subjects' disorder or condition, may be approved although no prospect of direct benefit exists (45CFR46.406). Such studies raise numerous questions, including how we are to judge that the risk posed represents only a minor increase over minimal risk and why only children with a particular disorder or condition may be exposed to more than minimal risk without the prospect of direct benefit (Iltis 2007).

Obligations regarding minimizing risk and maximizing potential benefit raise a number of challenging questions. Given the obligation to minimize risks and maximize potential benefits, when may investigators justifiably claim that they have done so? To what extent may resource limitations justify failing to minimize risk? When may investigators justifiably claim that a study poses the prospect of direct benefit to participants? A significant concern is what Nancy King has called "benefit creep," the exaggeration or even fabrication of potential benefit to subjects (King 2000). Benefit creep poses special problems in pediatric research that may only be permissible if there is a prospect of direct benefit to participants. Study "hype" is well-documented in phase one studies that are aimed only at assessing safety (see, e.g., King 2000; Harmon 2010).[6]

In some cases scholars have argued that it would be unethical to conduct a phase one study, and that research should instead begin at the phase two stage, where participants have a better chance of receiving therapeutic benefit (Coutelle and Ashcroft 2012). However, such a practice would raise serious concerns about safety. Bypassing the safety testing done in a phase one study and providing doses expected to be therapeutic could expose participants to even greater risk. Suggestions to skip phase one also might reflect a larger concern with trying to increase the potential for direct benefit to participants. A number of proposals have been made to design studies to increase the possibility of direct benefit to participants, to speed up the time needed to conduct a study, and so on (see, e.g., Horn 2007; Groeneveld et al. 2007; Reingold et al. 2011; Fitzpatrick et al. 2006).

Some discussions of ethical research design and appropriate risk–benefit relationship focus heavily on the importance of equipoise. Despite numerous accounts of equipoise, the concept generally refers to genuine uncertainty among a relevant group of clinicians regarding the superiority of one intervention over another (Freedman 1987; Fried 1974). Genuine uncertainty is supposed to help justify the enrollment of patients because clinicians can rest assured that they are not knowingly asking their patients to accept an inferior intervention since they really do not know which is best. Of course, this does not justify other risks participants might face because of study participation, but it should address the worry that by randomly assigning an intervention the physician intentionally is withholding the best known treatment.

Study design also must include a plan for monitoring safety and responding to new information about possible risks (45CFR46.111). Sometimes such data safety monitory plans are simple, e.g., a local medical monitor reviews data periodically. In other cases they involve independent DSMBs that review data and adverse events, and periodically assess the permissibility of continuing a study. They might recommend early termination if, for example, the risks are too high or the data clearly demonstrate that one arm of the study is superior – or inferior (e.g., CAST) – to the other. Nevertheless the integrity and reliability of DSMBs has been questioned (Drazen and Wood 2010). Decisions about terminating a study early involve numerous, competing considerations. For example, a study that ends early because of participant safety concerns may be weaker scientifically than one carried out over a longer period of time.

Hence, studies must address scientifically or socially valuable questions and their design must be scientifically valid (Emanuel et al. 2000). Participants should not be exposed to research risks or burdens if a study is unlikely to yield useful, generalizable information. One must accept that knowledge gained is itself a study benefit, and that an awareness of new or different kinds of knowledge can be valuable to gain (see Kimmelman 2007).

Scientific validity is essential for the ethical conduct of research because, as often is said, bad science is bad ethics. A study that exposes people to research risks and burdens but cannot achieve the end of providing generalizable knowledge is unethical. Concerns regarding scientific validity include not only basic questions about the statistical plan and research methods, but also successfully recruiting the necessary number of participants and timely completion of the study. Unless a study yields an extraordinary level of direct benefit to participants, any study that cannot be completed, cannot yield useful data contributing to generalizable knowledge, or has an unfavorable risk-benefit profile should raise concerns about the justification for beginning it in the first place (Iltis 2005; Scott and Magnus 2014).

C Research Population Selection

The USPHS/Tuskegee study as well as many other studies, such as those reported by Beecher (1966), involved populations that were prone to being taken advantage of because they were in some sense marginalized, e.g., elderly hospitalized patients, prisoners, the poor, and children, including those with intellectual disabilities. Such over-use of vulnerable populations raised concerns about the need for special protections for persons who might be easy to exploit.

Participant populations necessarily will be limited in some way and include only certain categories when the conditions under investigation affect only members of particular groups. But insofar as a wide range of persons are affected, the expectation is that participant populations should be diverse. The obligation here is not to achieve statistically proportionate representation but rather to ensure that no group is targeted for recruitment because they seem to be easy targets or are deemed expendable. The *Belmont Report* describes the obligation this way:

> Against this historical background [of abuses in biomedical research], it can be seen how conceptions of justice are relevant to research involving human subjects. For example, the selection of research subjects needs to be scrutinized in order to determine whether some classes (*e.g.,* welfare patients, particular racial and ethnic minorities, or persons confined to institutions) are being systematically selected simply because of their easy availability, their compromised position, or their manipulability, rather than for reasons directly related to the problem being studied.
>
> (1979: B.3)

Researchers should take care to identify an appropriate study population, to justify their inclusion and exclusion criteria, and to develop a plan to recruit a diverse study population.

Although much of the concern regarding participant selection has focused on the need to avoid over-including vulnerable people, exclusion and under-representation also pose problems. Excluded or poorly represented populations might be unable to enjoy the benefits of research because findings may not be generalizable to them. These concerns drove the literature concerning gender and medical research and the need to include women and evaluate gender differences in clinical research (Holdcroft 2007; Merkatz et al. 1993; NIH 1994; Rochon et al. 1998; Simon 2005). There has been special concern regarding the under-representation or exclusion of females from studies of cardiovascular disease which affects significant numbers of women (Harris and Douglas 2000).

Despite the admirable intentions to establish just subject representation in clinical research as outlined in the *Belmont Report*, concerns over the role of race in research did not end with Tuskegee. BiDil was approved by the FDA in 2005 specifically for the treatment of congestive heart failure (CHF) in African Americans. Although this action could be conceived as a positive step toward social and distributive justice, in reality at its core this landmark approval afforded its physician/scientist developers and pharmaceutical executives a means of extending the drug's patent life as well as the promise of greater corporate gain: "BiDil became an ethnic drug through the intervention of law and commerce as much as through medical [mis]understanding of biological differences that correlate with racial groups" (Kahn 2004, p. 3).

BiDil arose as a reformulation of two previously existing, and generically available vasodilators, hydralazine and isosorbide dinitrate (H-I). It was first studied in its generic form during the 1980s in two separate trials, each utilizing a mixed race population of male study subjects. Vasodilator Heart Failure Trial (V-HeFT) I investigated the effect of adding H-I *vs.* placebo or prazosin in combination with existing digoxin and diuretic therapy of chronic CHF. Reduced mortality in the H-I treated group was of no more than "borderline statistical significance" (Cohn et al. 1986). However, in 1987 Dr. Cohn submitted a methods patent[7] to the Patent and Trademark Office (PTO) for the combined use of hydralazine and isosorbide as a distinct intervention for the treatment of chronic CHF[8] (Sankar & Kahn 2005). Subsequently, V-HeFT II evaluated chronic CHF treatment by using standard digoxin and diuretic treatment in combination with H-I *vs.* enalapril, an angiotensin converting enzyme (ACE) inhibitor. Two-year survival in the H-I group was virtually unchanged since V-HeFT I, but also statistically significantly inferior to that now achieved with enalapril (Cohn et al. 1991). Thereafter, "ACE inhibitors became a new first-line therapy for treating heart failure" (Sankar & Kahn 2005, p. 456 citing Cohn et al. 1991).

Nevertheless commercial interest in the now-patented method of H-I combination therapy persisted. Heart failure was thought to be exacerbated in the absence of sufficient blood levels of nitric oxide (NO); isosorbide functions as a NO "donor", and hydralazine is an anti-oxidant that may enhance nitrate efficacy (Bauer and Fung 1991; Münzel et al. 1996; Franciosa et al. 2002). Cohn licensed his patent to Medco, a relatively small North Carolina pharmaceutical company. He and Medco reformulated hydralazine (37.5 mg) and isosorbide dinitrate (20 mg) into a single tablet fixed combination drug that became officially trademarked as BiDil® in 1995.[9] Medco conducted bioequivalence studies, and submitted a new drug application (NDA) to the FDA in 1997. However, due to inadequate *statistical* strength of its documentation of efficacy as based upon old data from the V-HeFT I and II trials BiDil at that time was rejected by the FDA's Cardiovascular and Renal Drugs Advisory Committee. Thereafter Medco allowed its lease of intellectual property rights to BiDil to revert back to Dr. Cohn (Kahn 2004; Sankar & Kahn 2005).

Neither V-HeFT I nor II demonstrated a substantially statistically significant difference in survival favorable to H-I (i.e., BiDil) within a male mixed-race population. However, retrospective analysis of those studies' data that had been derived from a subset of African American men was suggestive of benefit within this specific subject population (Carson et al. 1999).[10] Cohn then relicensed his intellectual property rights for BiDil to a Massachusetts biotechnology company, NitroMed, that specialized in the development of NO-related medications. He and Carson in 2000 jointly obtained a *race-specific* methods patent from the PTO to use BiDil for treatment of CHF in African American patients.[11] The following year NitroMed approached the FDA with an amended NDA for *race-specific* approval of BiDil (Kahn 2004; Sankar & Kahn 2005). "Thus was BiDil reborn as an 'ethnic' drug" (Kahn 2004, p. 18).

Heavily relying upon Carson's 1999 *post hoc* data analysis the single race African American Vasodilator Heart Trial (A-HeFT) thereafter was conducted among 1050 "self-identified" black male and female subjects (Taylor et al. 2004). BiDil vs. placebo now was investigated as an adjunct to then current CHF therapy including β-blockers and neurohormonal inhibitors. Despite the previously reported relative inefficacy of ACE inhibitor treatment of black patients (Exner et al. 2001),[12] approximately 70% of participants in each arm of the trial were in fact receiving ACE inhibitors (Kahn 2007; Taylor et al. 2004). The study was halted prematurely when routine DSMB review detected a 43% survival advantage within the BiDil-treated subjects (Kahn 2007; Sankar & Kahn 2005; Taylor et al. 2004; Temple & Stockbridge 2007).

"BiDil [became] the FDA's first approval of a racially targeted drug" in June, 2005 (Yu et al. 2009, p. 57). In the process, the mere alteration of Cohn's method patent to a race-specific indication extended its longevity from 2007 to 2020. For an additional thirteen years BiDil could be free from market competition from a *single-pill* generic equivalent (Sankar & Kahn 2005). Conveniently for NitroMed, physicians also were free to use BiDil "off label" for the treatment of CHF in non-black patients. Paradoxically the combined use of BiDil's generic components, hydralazine and isosorbide dinitrate, remained approved for use in *all* races when used as *two separate drugs* (Bibbins-Domingo and Fernandez 2007). Ironically, BiDil's significantly higher price came to be viewed as exploitative of the very people for whom it had been approved (Saul 2005; Sankar & Kahn 2005; Yu et al. 2009).

Superficially this "discovery" would appear to have been a great advantage for many medically underserved African American patients. Indeed, "BiDil [gained] cultural capital by being characterized as a means to redress an important health disparity …" (Kahn 2004, p. 33) Nevertheless BiDil's approval also was met with substantial controversy. Criticism of the FDA's favorable decision has been centered upon both the poor scientific quality of A-HeFT[13] as well as the substantial ethical conflicts of interest it has raised (Kahn 2004; Bibbins-Domingo and Fernandez 2007; Ellison et al. 2008).

Aside from the not so subtle "statistical mischief" employed in the research and development of this "ethnic" drug,[14] perhaps the most egregious lapse of scientific and ethical judgment was the misrepresentation of race as a purely biological entity. Granted the 1990s was a time of greater awareness of the need for representation of minorities in clinical research. The National Institutes of Health (NIH) Revitalization Act of 1993 was passed with this specific intent.[15] In 1997

President Clinton issued a public apology for the federal government's role in the abhorrent treatment of African Americans throughout the 40-year duration of the Tuskegee Syphilis Study.[16] Nonetheless the concept of "race-as-biology" had long since been discredited by the time the A-HeFT report was published in 2004 (Goodman 2000). It is convenient to use a patient's race as a proxy for his unknown genetic traits, but the color of one's skin and his genome are not synonymous. As medical conditions typically are multifactorial with multiple, diverse manifestations, race or ethnicity entails not only one's biology, but also the inseparable sociocultural, environmental, and economic facets of individual lives (Darity Jr. et al. 2010; Lee et al. 2001). "[I]t is … a mistake to uncritically accept old racial classifications when we study medical treatments. The task is to determine how the social meaning of race can affect biological outcomes …" (Duster 2001).

It is important to note that both Cohn's original method patent application for H-I combined therapy in 1987, and BiDil's initially rejected NDA in 1997 were related to the treatment of CHF – period; no racial specification was asserted. Not until that rejection and Medco's subsequent release of intellectual rights to BiDil was the V-HeFT I/II data retrospectively analyzed and interpreted by its authors as an indication for race-based use of the drug. Kahn (2004, p. 35) summarizes well the conflation of social with biological categories in BiDil's evolution into an ethnic drug:

> Hydralazine and isosorbide dinitrate do not address the social issues of heart failure, only the individual biological ones … Cohn's and Carson's [2000] patent is not for a method of treatment that merely correlates with a social group – it specifies a chemical therapy for 'African Americans'. That is, it specifies African Americans as a biological group, and it has received the approval of the federal government [i.e., FDA and PTO] for this classification.

The "logic of race" ties BiDil to Tuskegee. As syphilis previously was hypothesized to be a different disease in black and white people, so too now has been CHF. Each circumstance was marred by

> the willingness [of physicians, researchers, and the federal government] to allow for an unknown factor (assumed to be biological) to explain what is claimed as racial differences … Tuskegee was invoked in spirit to remember the disparities as well as the failures and betrayals in American medicine for African Americans.
>
> (Reverby 2008, pp. 478, 480)

D Informed Consent

The ethical conduct of research requires that, in most cases, investigators obtain informed consent from research participants (or their legal surrogates) (see 45CFR46.116) and to document their informed consent with a signature (see 45CFR46.117). In some cases, investigators may forego the standard documentation of informed consent, or even proceed without obtaining informed consent (45CFR46.116 and 117). While the informed consent requirement is simple on paper, satisfying the ethical obligation raises numerous questions and concerns, including who may give consent and when investigators may be confident that they have fulfilled their obligation.

"Informed consent" is not merely another form to be completed; it is a process of communication. Ordinarily to give informed consent a potential research participant must be legally competent and have decisional capacity, study information must be disclosed so that the person can understand and appreciate the information, and the individual must be able to make and communicate a free and voluntary informed decision (Beauchamp and Childress 2009; Berg et al. 2001; Faden and Beauchamp 1986).

1 Competence and Capacity

The terms "competence" and "capacity" are used in different ways and sometimes they are used interchangeably. To give informed consent to research participation a person must have the legal authority to do so (e.g., a young child may not give consent because the child is not recognized legally as a competent decision-maker) and have the mental capacity to make decisions. Decision-making capacity typically requires the ability to understand and appreciate information, and to reason and deliberate so as to make choices (Buchanan and Brock 1989; Grisso and Appelbaum 1998). Views about when investigators should assess decisional capacity prior to obtaining informed consent vary, particularly in light of evidence that biases or other factors may lead investigators and IRB members to assume that members of some groups lack capacity despite evidence to the contrary (Luebbert et al. 2008; Tait et al. 2011). Investigators may outline in their protocols plans for assessing decisional capacity. If participants are likely to lose their decision-making capacity during the course of a study, as might be the case when participants have early signs of dementia, they may be asked to appoint someone to assume decision-making responsibility on their behalf when they no longer are able to make their own competent decisions.

The obligation to show respect for persons (National Commission 1979) or respect for autonomy (Beauchamp and Childress 1979), from which the obligation to obtain informed consent is derived, is not limited to respecting existing decisional capacity but, in some cases, to fostering such capacity (Beauchamp and Childress 2009). Investigators should be familiar with techniques that might help to foster decision-making capacity for research participation such as the use of interactive questions during the informed consent process (Palmer et al. 2008).

Depending on the circumstances and abilities of the children involved, investigators also may be obligated or encouraged to obtain the *assent* of a participant who is a minor (see subpart B of 45CFR46). Some scholars have argued that some adolescents have decision-making capacity comparable to that of some adults who are allowed to make their own decisions (Oberman 1996; Society for Adolescent Medicine 2003; Weithorn 1983; Weithorn and Campbell 1982). Although much of the literature has focused on using the so-called mature minor doctrine to allow adolescents broad authority over health care decisions, it is logical that some would extend this authority to the research setting. There are both empirical and normative debates about the permissibility of recognizing adolescents as being in authority over clinical or research participation decisions (Cherry 2013; Iltis 2013; Steinberg 2013).

2 Disclosure

The CFR specifies categories of information that must be disclosed to potential research participants as part of the informed consent process (45CFR46.116, 21CFR50.25), and consent forms are to be written in lay language that potential participants can understand. Investigators must tell people that they are being asked to participate in research, the type of study, the study's purpose, what they will be asked to do in the study, approximately how many people will be enrolled, the research risks and potential benefits, the possibility that there may be unforeseeable risks, the discomforts and burdens associated with participation, compensation and costs associated with participation, what will happen if they are injured as a result of their participation, and who to contact if they have questions regarding the study itself or their rights. Participants must be permitted to withdraw from a study, and they must be told that they have this right. They also should be told what kind of updates they will receive during a study, such as new risk information that might affect their willingness to continue participation within that study. Investigators and IRBs make judgments about how to apply these requirements in particular studies such as whether a particular risk is too remote to disclose at the outset, or whether a risk is characterized appropriately as a research risk or merely a risk of having a condition or receiving standard treatment. These questions have taken on new significance in the face of greater emphasis on CER and learning health care systems models (IOM 2007; Solomon and Bonham 2013; Faden et al. 2013; Grady and Wendler 2013).

Failure to disclose risk information known at the start of a study, or that emerges during the course of study can be serious. The investigation into the death Jesse Gelsinger, an 18-year-old man who died while taking part in a gene transfer study at the University of Pennsylvania in 1999, revealed that important risk information had been omitted from the consent form Gelsinger signed. Most notably, prior animal testing of mice and monkeys exposed to high doses of the same virus used as a vector in the current study had experienced serious liver inflammation (i.e., acute hepatitis), and some had died. The consent form approved by the University of Pennsylvania appears to have included information about known animal deaths, but the consent form the investigators gave Gelsinger did not (Wilson 2010).

The case of Ellen Roche at Johns Hopkins University involved a failure to communicate risk information that became available during the study. The investigator failed to tell Roche, a healthy volunteer in a study designed to improve understanding of the pathophysiology of asthma, and the IRB that a previous participant had developed respiratory problems after inhaling hexamethonium during the course of study (Savulescu and Spriggs 2002). Investigators changed the inhalant slightly in an effort to avoid the problem also without notifying the IRB. Roche experienced respiratory failure, was hospitalized in the ICU, and died (Lo 2010, p. 35).

Incidental findings raise numerous questions about the obligations of investigators and the rights and interests of study participants. Incidental findings are those "concerning an individual research participant that has potential health or reproductive importance and is discovered in the course of conducting research but is beyond the aims of the study" (Wolf et al. 2008, p. 219). As part of the informed consent process potential participants should be told how incidental findings will be handled. Much of the literature currently points to the concept of "actionability," although that specific term not always is used. A number of authors have argued that information that is deemed "actionable" may or should be reported, whereas "non-actionable" information does not have to be disclosed or should not be disclosed (see, for example, Ravitsky and Wilfond 2006; Wolf et al. 2008).

Questions regarding the return of individual study results to participants have emerged in recent years, particularly in the context of research involving genetic testing and screening. The National Bioethics Advisory Commission explored the issue in its report on research on human biological samples (1999). Developing and disclosing a plan for return or non-return of results is important. Discussion of returning results includes concerns over the validity and reliability of the information, the significance of the information, and the actionability of the information (i.e., Is there anything you can do about it?) (Wolf 2012). Much has been made, for example, about the return of results of genetic testing wherein researchers do not know what, if anything the information means for a person's health. Guidelines from professional working groups emphasize these factors (Lomax and Shepard 2013; Wolf et al. 2008).

3 Understanding and Appreciation

To facilitate understanding and appreciation of research information consent forms must be written in lay language, information must be offered in formats that foster understanding and appreciation, and investigators must be willing and able to answer questions. However, the obligation of investigators to ensure that participants actually have achieved these goals is debated (see Palmer 2008; Anderson and Iltis 2008). Major barriers to understanding and appreciation of information include the advanced language used and the complex nature of some of the information (Anderson and Iltis 2008; Hochhauser 1999; Iltis 2006).

The therapeutic misconception may reflect a failure to understand and appreciate research information adequately (Appelbaum et al. 1982). Appelbaum and his colleagues identified the therapeutic misconception among research participants enrolled in psychiatric studies (1982, 1987), and it has since been widely documented in numerous research settings (e.g., Daugherty et al. 2000; Yoder et al. 1997). The therapeutic misconception as originally defined referred to a failure to appreciate "the possibility that there may be a major disadvantage to participating in clinical research that stems from the nature of the research process itself" (Appelbaum et al. 1987). Much of the literature now uses the term in broader ways to describe cases in which research participants mistakenly believe that they will benefit directly from their research participation (see Hochhauser 2002), or to describe situations in which people participate in research to obtain therapeutic benefit (see Dresser 2002). The therapeutic misconception also describes cases in which people fail to understand the true purpose of research mistakenly believing it to be merely an extension of their clinical care, or to see research as a way to access better, cutting-edge treatment. Others distinguish among the related notions of therapeutic misestimation, namely situations in which "the research subject underestimates risk, overestimates benefit, or both" and therapeutic optimism, namely situations in which "the research subject hopes for the best personal outcome" (Horn and Grady 2003, p. 12). The loose use of the term 'therapeutic misconception' has led to calls for greater clarity (Henderson et al. 2007).

4 Free and Voluntary Consent

Ordinarily investigators are required to obtain free and voluntary informed consent from research participants or their legally authorized representatives. They must minimize the possibility of coercion or undue influence (45CFR46.116). Coercion is likely to be rare if we understand it as the *Belmont Report* describes; "[C]oercion occurs when an overt threat of harm is intentionally presented by one person to another in order to obtain compliance" (National Commission 1979 C.1). Undue influence, however, is harder to identify in actual practice. It "occurs through an offer of excessive, unwanted, inappropriate, or improper reward or other overture in order to obtain compliance" (National Commission 1979 C.1). The obligation to minimize undue influence and coercion often leads to restrictions (e.g., Dickert and Grady 1999; Grady 2001) or prohibitions (e.g., McNeil 1997; Reame 2001) on payments to research participants. (Payments refers to cash, gift cards, or other equivalent potential inducements that neither reimburse nor compensate a research participant for expenses incurred.) Although not everyone argues that payments should be very modest or non-existent (e.g., Savulescu 2001; Zink 2001; Iltis 2009), many do. They worry that offers of money or offers of too much money will be irresistible or leave people unwilling to consider the research risks (e.g., Ackerman 1989; Levine 1986; Macklin 1981). Recent findings suggest that subjects motivated to participate by a financial offer have significantly better understanding of research information than participants who are motivated primarily by another goal (Stunkel et al. 2010). Although not definitive this information challenges the assumption that any connection exists between payment offered, and reduced understanding or appreciation of important research information.

E Privacy and Confidentiality

Investigators must protect the privacy and confidentiality of research participants, and protocols must explain how this will be done. These obligations generally are understood as extensions of the duty to respect persons or autonomy. Privacy refers to "the right to be left alone" (Warren and Brandeis 1890), or to be free from exposure to or intrusion by others (Moskop et al. 2005). Confidentiality refers to protecting information disclosed or discovered during the health care encounter from disclosure to parties who are not entitled to the information (Moskop et al. 2005). Investigators must take appropriate measures to protect information that could be linked to participants, and ordinarily must conform to Health Insurance Portability and Accountability Act (HIPAA) regulations. Special concerns may emerge when information discovered during the course of a study could be important for family members (e.g., genetic information) or have public health implications (such as human immunodeficiency virus (HIV) positive status). Investigators conducting research in areas where they are likely to discover sensitive information should be particularly careful to disclose to potential participants how such information will be handled. Anticipating and planning for how to manage sensitive information, and disclosing this plan to potential participants are critical steps.

F Special Populations

The National Institutes of Health (NIH) regulations require special protections for children, pregnant women, fetuses, neonates, and prisoners (see subparts B, C and D of 45CFR46). Other populations, such as the intellectually disabled, and the educationally or economically disadvantaged, require additional protections as well, but the Common Rule does not specify requirements for these other circumstances.

Additionally, just as inclusion in research poses risks to participants, exclusion poses risks of harm as well. The lack of safety, efficacy, and dosing information for drugs used to treat conditions that affect women and children poses a health threat to these populations. Awareness of this problem has led to increased efforts to include these populations in research.

Pediatric clinical trials may be particularly challenging to design and perform. In addition to the stricter safety mandates they must follow, the altered pathophysiology and smaller size of children relative to adults introduces a more heterogeneous population of subjects to study. (The common pediatric maxim, "Children are not small adults," is quite true.) Additionally, the rarity of many acquired and congenital disorders of children impairs recruitment and usually necessitates multicenter trials to acquire statistically meaningful numbers of subjects. As dosage reductions are required for medications used in children, the size of medical devices also must be reduced for pediatric application. All of these factors greatly increase the cost of pediatric research, and decrease commercial incentives for its performance. Consequently, the majority of medications and medical devices used in children have been done so "off-label." In an era of expanding "evidence-based medicine" such practices have become increasing unacceptable (Bates et al. 2012). "Post-marketing surveillance … [of] both drug and device safety assessment [is] crucial in the pediatric population …" (Bates et al. 2012, p. 481).

Numerous efforts over the past two decades have sought to encourage pharmaceutical companies to pursue the research necessary to label their products appropriately for pediatric use. For example, the 2002 Best Pharmaceuticals for Children Act, signed into law by President Bush in January 2002 (PL 107–109), provided additional mechanisms to request and fund research for both on-patent and off-patent pharmaceutical products in children. Manufacturers were offered financial incentives upon completion of such FDA-requested studies. Similarly, the Pediatric Research Equity Act (PREA, PL 108–155), passed by Congress in December 2003, gave the FDA the authority to require pediatric research to be performed for NDAs or supplemental marketing applications in order to determine appropriate dosing, establish safety, and identify side effects in children. Additionally, pediatric pharmaceutical studies now were required for all medications approved prior to PREA upon the introduction of any new dosage form, route of administration, or indication for use. These changes have had some effect:

> Since the passage of these statutes, many cardiovascular drugs … including several antihypertensive and lipid-lowering … as well as antiarrhythmic, antithrombotic, and heart failure medications … have been successfully studied, resulting in [new pharmaceutical] labelling for children.[17]
>
> (Bates et al. 2012, p. 483)

The NIH Revitalization Act of 1993 (PL 103-43) mandated greater inclusion of women as well as minorities in clinical research. It was preceded by the NIH's Office of Research on Women's Health in 1990. Advocacy for women as research subjects and patients was further advanced by the establishment of the FDA's Office of Women's Health (OWH) in 1994 (Elahi et al. 2016). Pregnant women have been particularly subject to exclusion from clinical drug trials due to unknown potential adverse fetal effects. A large, retrospective cohort study, funded in part by OWH (Li et al. 2011), failed to verify previously reported congenital cardiovascular malformations of fetuses exposed to ACE inhibitors during the first trimester (Cooper et al. 2006). Rather Li et al. reported that the ingestion of neither ACE inhibitors nor other anti-hypertensives was associated with a greater incidence of congenital heart defects in comparison with hypertensive control subjects.[18] OWH-funded post-marketing research also has established relatively excessive female cardiotoxicity to certain non-cardiovascular drugs in comparison with men, prompting their withdrawal from the market (General Accounting Office 2001).

G Stored Data and Biological Samples

With the ability to store large amounts of data and biological samples comes the ability to pursue research on identifiable, living human beings long after the data/samples were collected, raising many ethical questions (Kapp 2008; Meslin and Quaid 2004). Researchers are keen to use such stored information. When should investigators be required to obtain informed consent for the use of those samples? What constitutes valid consent for the use of those samples in the future? Although we might be tempted to dismiss the importance of informed consent for research on stored samples or to suggest that it is less important because there no longer is any direct interaction with participants, respect for participants and an interest in maintaining trust in the research enterprise suggest otherwise.

Litigation surrounding the use of stored samples from members of the Havasupai community demonstrates how important it can be for people to understand and agree on how their stored samples may be used. Members of the Havasupai tribe agreed to donate blood for what they believed was a diabetes study based on their discussions with investigators. The consent form stated that the samples were being taken for research on "the causes of behavioral/medical disorders" (de Melo-Martín and Wolf 2010). Their samples eventually were used for a variety of investigations, including studies on schizophrenia, inbreeding, and evolutionary genetics and migration patterns (de Melo-Martín and Wolf 2010). Members of the tribe objected to these other types of research, arguing that they could stigmatize the Havasupai. In some cases they were offensive because they contradicted the tribe's account of its origins. The tribe filed a suit against Arizona State University where the research was conducted. Eventually the university settled, agreeing to return their blood samples, pay financial compensation, apologize formally, and collaborate with the tribe to address health and social needs (de Melo-Martín and Wolf 2010).

The consent form used in the Havasupai study requested broad permission to use the samples to study behavioral/medical problems. Broad (sometimes called "blanket") consent, without any limits as to the kinds of conditions studied or the timeframe over which the sample will be used, raises concerns (de Melo-Martín and Wolf 2010). Alternatives include requiring consent for each use (which can be burdensome and make it impossible to pursue some research), and asking for separate consent for different categories of studies. The use of stored samples for genetic research also raises special concerns (Clayton et al. 1995; McGuire and Beskow 2010).

H Ancillary Care

Ancillary care refers to attention that "is not required to make a study scientifically valid, to ensure a trial's safety, or to redress research injuries" (Belsky and Richardson 2004). Examples include treatment of conditions such as infections, congenital heart defects, and dehydration and malnutrition that may be discovered during the course of conducting a study. Ancillary care issues are especially important in resource-poor settings where participants' needs may range from basic nutrition to complex health problems where no other treatment resources are likely to be available. Consider the case reported by Dickert and Wendler

(2009). A study involving children with severe malaria was planned in Mali to assess the relationship between this malady and pulmonary hypertension. The study involved a blood draw and an echocardiogram. The investigators expected that many participants would have untreated malaria as well as dehydration, infections, sickle cell disease, and other conditions. But they also knew that they might find rare conditions such as congenital heart defects and cancers of the blood which might not be treatable in resource-poor Mali. Anticipating this probability investigators included in their study budget sufficient funds to treat malaria, and plans to refer participants into the Malian health system for certain other treatable conditions. This allowed the investigators to meet most needs discovered incidentally during the course of the study. They met other needs by giving their time, effort, blood, or own their funds. There was one exception, a ventricular septal defect that could not be treated in Mali. Investigators connected that participant with clinicians in Mali who appealed for treatment in Europe. Whether or not the investigators had an obligation to meet those needs, an important motivation for many investigators is to meet as many needs as possible not only among their research participants but also among persons who are in close proximity to their participants (Taylor et al. 2011).

A number of models have been proposed to determine what and why ancillary care obligations exist (Belsky and Richardson 2004; Dickert and Wendler 2009; Participants 2008; Richardson 2004, 2008). Despite disagreement about the extent to which investigators must provide ancillary care many contributors to the literature recognize that investigators have a relationship with research participants, and that this relationship gives rise to obligations that do not apply to strangers. Investigators should anticipate and plan for being confronted by ancillary care needs. In some cases this may involve including funds in a study budget to address certain types of needs identified in the course of a study. However, too much emphasis on ancillary care obligations of researchers might undermine the understanding of researchers' primary goals and obligations, and could overwhelm researchers to the detriment of the research. It also could discourage research in areas where there is likely to be great need.

I Post-trial Access

Do investigators or sponsors have obligations to subjects and communities in which research was conducted after a study ends? If so, what are those obligations? In some settings, such as developed nations, this question might refer to ongoing access to unapproved drugs or devices that appear to be helping a person, or to a drug that the person cannot afford or is not covered by third-party payers. In poor communities where access to a drug, device, or intervention will be prohibitively expensive must investigators make it available? If so, should the intervention be made available to the participants, or to everyone in the community who needs it? For how long must post-trial access be provided by investigators/sponsors? How should the community be defined? Investigators often are required to establish and share plans for what will happen when a trial ends.

Among the reasons offered for requiring post-trial access to treatment include: (1) Compensation for the fact that participants exposed themselves to research risks and might have been harmed in the process; (2) Reciprocity: participants give of themselves for the study and post-trial access is a way of giving back; and (3) Justice: post-trial access is a form of counteracting the background of extraordinary poverty in which many people find themselves; and fulfilling the requirements set forth in the Declaration of Helsinki (Millum 2011; Usharani and Naqvi 2013; Zong 2008). This internationally recognized document stipulates,

> In advance of a clinical trial, sponsors, researchers and host country governments should make provisions for post-trial access for all participants who still need an intervention identified as beneficial in the trial. This information must also be disclosed to participants during the informed consent process.
> (2013, #34)

Such claims about ongoing post-trial obligations are controversial and raise numerous concerns (Grady 2005). If the obligation to provide post-trial access exists, who bears the obligation? Is it the obligation of sponsors, researchers, or others? If sponsors or researchers have the obligation to provide ongoing access, how long do they have this obligation, and why? Imposing such an obligation could discourage research in resource-poor countries, including research on serious conditions that affect their populations (Frankish 2003). On the other hand, if post-trial access is guaranteed it could be seen as a form of undue inducement to participate in research (Hutt 1998).

J Conflicts of Interest

Attention to individual investigator conflicts of interest (COI) in research has focused on financial conflicts of interest; yet other COIs are relevant as well, including institutional COIs and interests of investigators related to prestige or future funding. The primary concern is that COIs may interfere with data integrity or subject safety, i.e., investigators may falsely withhold information or alter their data. Ten years after Jesse Gelsinger's death, the Institute of Medicine published the report of its committee for the evaluation of COI in medical research. Recommendation 4.1 seemingly speaks to the very issue of that landmark case:

> Academic medical centers and other research institutions should establish a policy that individuals generally may not conduct research with human participants if they have a significant financial interest in an existing or potential product or a company that could be affected by the outcome of the research.
> (Lo and Field 2009)

Unfortunately, evidence of the pharmaceutical industry's apparent ability to cloud clinical judgment is not difficult to find. An advisory committee of the FDA convened in 2005 to discuss the potential for adverse cardiovascular side effects associated with the use of the COX-2 class of anti-inflammatory drugs (U.S. Food and Drug Administration 2005; Boumil and Berman 2010). Three of these agents (Vioxx, Celebrex and Bextra) that remained on the market after their meeting subsequently were in fact proven to be triggers for significant cardiovascular morbidity and mortality. Thereafter the Center for Science in the Public Interest examined the industry relationships of that committee's members. Ten of the 32 individuals had direct affiliations with the manufacturers of the specific drugs in question, and 17 additional members had ties to other drug companies (Center for Science in the Public Interest 2005; Boumil and Berman 2010). A *New York Times* article suggested that "had the 10 advisory committee members with the industry affiliations been excluded, the drugs would not have been recommended [to remain] on the market" (cited in Harris and Berenson 2005; Boumil and Berman 2010).

Although some have called for abolishing conflicts of interest (e.g., Angell 2005), many others hold that it would be impossible and perhaps imprudent to attempt to do so. They emphasize the importance of reducing and managing COIs (e.g., Goldner 2000). Institutions have developed a range of practices focusing on disclosure and management to address COIs. Many of these are not data-driven practices; we do not know whether they achieve the goals of managing COIs. In fact, there are reasons to suspect that they do not (see Cain et al. 2005; Sah 2012). In particular, disclosure of conflicts may have the opposite effect because disclosure can lead individuals "to feel morally licensed" to act on their biases (Cain et al. 2005, p. 1).

K *Community-Engaged Research*

Traditionally, researchers, often connected to large companies or to academic medical centers, have identified research questions, designed and carried out studies, analyzed data, and (sometimes) reported their results.[19] However, by the 1990s the pharmaceutical industry started to withdraw from its partnership with academic medical centers. A shift of clinical interest toward prevention and treatment of chronic diseases had occurred. Adequate trials now required larger numbers of more diverse subjects, a longer period of evaluation, and multicenter distribution. Growing discussion of the importance of community engagement in research continues.

Community engagement can mean many different things from a single consultation with community members to community-based participatory research wherein researchers and community members function as equal partners throughout the entire research process (Israel et al. 1998). Reasons to engage communities include demonstrating respect for the community and its members, promoting justice, improving the quality and value of the research, and improving health in communities (CTSA Community Engagement Committees 2009; Dresser 2001; Michener et al. 2012; Ross et al. 2010).

Community engagement can occur at any and all stages of research from identifying research questions, designing studies, applying for funding to data collection analysis and interpretation; and dissemination of results. Community-engaged research, particularly those models that call for greater community involvement such as community-based participatory research, require a shift in how researchers and institutions think about research. Therefore, investigators who work in this environment must develop appropriate skills and knowledge to collaborate successfully with their communities (Rosenthal et al. 2009). Challenges include determining appropriately what counts as a community, and what risks might accrue to people who are seen as members of a community because of the group's participation in research (Ross et al. 2010).

Research participants in community-engaged research may experience the same types of risk that are well-recognized in other human research, namely untoward physical, psychological, and socioeconomic outcomes. Persons perceived to be members of a community also face risks even if they do not participate in a study because, for example, they may experience stigma or socio-economic risks due to research conducted within or upon their community (Ross et al. 2010). Community engagement also might undermine the interests of community members whose interests are not well-represented by their community leaders who interact directly with researchers, and may influence restricted access to research participation (Ross et al. 2010).

Research in cardiovascular medicine and surgery is a prime candidate for community engagement. There is much to be learned about how best to prevent and manage disease in populations that goes beyond which medication, diet, and exercise regimen are most effective under *ideal* circumstances. Determining safety and efficacy of interventions as they are experienced in "real world" settings can be important to improving health, and identifying what *works base* may be learned only with community involvement. To engage communities successfully requires a commitment to approaching the entire research process differently as well as knowledge, skills, and multidisciplinary partners.

III Conclusion

This chapter has explored a range of ethical and regulatory obligations related to human research. The interpretation and application of even relatively clear and widely accepted obligations in new contexts routinely requires new and ongoing analyses. New questions sometimes call on us to explore the possibility that some of our long-standing regulatory or ethical requirements, or our interpretation of them might be misguided. The emerging practice of research ethics consultation speaks to the complexity of determining what ought to be done; how to apply rules, regulations, principles, and guidelines to new areas; and how to act in the face of uncertainty (Beskow et al. 2009; Cho et al. 2008; de Melo Martin et al. 2007).

Research ethics involves more than merely complying with legal and regulatory requirements. Much of this chapter has framed the ethical conduct of research around a discussion of IRBs and regulations, but investigators should remember that the regulations require thoughtful interpretation, judgment, and application by investigators and members of IRBs. Remember that the regulations remain silent on many important matters, and some existing regulations might be inappropriate and should be revised. These judgments drove the regulatory changes to the revised Common Rule published in January, 2017 (Federal Policy for the Protection of Human Subjects 2017).

Acknowledgements

We wish to thank the anonymous reviewers for their comments on this chapter.

Notes

1 The federal government defines research as "a systematic investigation, including research development, testing and evaluation, designed to develop or contribute to generalizable knowledge. Activities which meet this definition constitute research for purposes of this policy, whether or not they are conducted or supported under a program which is considered research for other purposes. For example, some demonstration and service programs may include research activities" (45CFR46.102.d). Human research involves human subjects, namely "living individual[s] about whom an investigator (whether professional or student) conducting research obtains (1) Data through intervention or interaction with the individual, or (2) Identifiable private information" (45CFR46.102.f).

2 See CAST Investigators, 1989 (ref. 16-24) and Echt et al. 1991 (ref. 5-15).

3 A table comparing the NIH and FDA human research regulations is available here: http://www.fda.gov/ScienceResearch/SpecialTopics/RunningClinicalTrials/EducationalMaterials/ucm112910.htm (accessed November 15, 2014).

4 Decision charts available from OHRP provide important guidance to investigators regarding research categories. These are available here: http://www.hhs.gov/ohrp/policy/checklists/decisioncharts.html (accessed October 7, 2014).

5 Some of the details have been changed, but I have reviewed such a proposal.

6 Such hyperbole exists outside of the research context as well. Consider Timothy Caulfield's discussion of stem cell interventions that promise a wide range of benefits to patients (2011).

7 A "methods" patent grants its holder a marketing monopoly of a combination of drugs for a specific purpose. Cohn could not qualify BiDil for a "combination of matter" patent because the combined product of its two generic drugs did not act differently than either drug used alone. See Sankar and Kahn 2005.

8 U.S. Patent #4,868,179; issued September 19, 1989. See Kahn 2004.

9 U.S. Trademark Registration #1896747; registered May 30, 1995. See Kahn 2004.

10 "The H-I combination appears to be particularly effective in prolonging survival in black patients and is as effective as enalapril in this subgroup. In contrast, enalapril shows its more favorable effect on survival, particularly in the white population … The uniquely favorable effect of [BiDil] in black patients suggests blacks … may have a greater deficiency of [NO] generation … Similarly, the apparent lesser efficacy of enalapril in this this subgroup suggests the renin-angiotensin system may not have as active a role in the black population …" See Carson et al. 1999, pp. 182, 186. Also refer to Kahn 2004; and Temple and Stockbridge 2007.

11 U.S. patent #6,465,463; issued October 15, 2002. See Kahn 2004.

12 Exner et al.'s 2001 conclusion was not universally accepted. Among others Kahn (Kahn (2004, p. 23) cites Daniel Dries et al. (2002), a co-author of Exner's paper « [E]nalapril appears to be equally efficacious in black and white patients." ('Efficacy of angiotensin-converting enzyme in reducing progression from asymptomatic left ventricular dysfunction in symptomatic heart failure in black and white patients …',

Journal of the American College of Cardiology, 40(2), p. 317.) Note, however, that Dries' work also is a *post hoc* analysis of an earlier study.

13 Note that the FDA rejected BiDil in 1997 on the basis of inadequate statistical validly of data derived from V-HeFT I and II. Yet A-HeFT, the single race study upon which the FDA issued its race-specific approval of BiDil eight years later, was derived from a *post hoc* analysis of subsets of the same data. Such analysis is prone toward both a loss of statistical power and covariate imbalances. Perhaps the rationale for A-HeFT was most undermined by the marked advances in CHF treatment that had been put into clinical practice since the V-HeFTs were published. See Ellison et al., 2008.

14 The underlying, and oft repeated premise that mortality from heart failure was twice as prevalent in the black vs. white population was based upon 1981 age-related data that failed to include the later onset of mortality in whites than blacks. Substantial narrowing of the mortality gap actually had occurred between 1980 and 1995. (See Kahn 2004, pp. 19–22; Carson et al. 1999. Citing Gillum (1987). 'Heart failure in the United States, 1970-1985', *American Heart Journal,* 113(4): 1043–45.) Additionally the *post hoc* manipulation of data subsets that characterized Carson and Cohn''s 1999 paper that justified A-HeFT was subject to both a loss of statistical power and faulty covariate imbalances. (See Ellison et al., 2008, pp. 2–4.)

15 Public Law 103-43, Subtitle B. Located at https://orwh.od.nih.gov/resources/pdf/NIH-Revitalization-Act_1993.pdf (Accessed January 9, 2017.)

16 'Remarks by the president in apology for study done in Tuskegee'. Located at http://clinton4nara.gov/textonly/New/Remarks/Fri/19970516-898.html (Accessed January 9, 2017.)

17 As pharmacodynamics and pharmacokinetics may change as a child matures, new pediatric drug labelling is specific to the age-range tested. "Most [Phase I] dose-response studies are performed in children aged 6 to 16 years …" See Bates, et al. (2012, p. 487).

18 Li et al. (2011) "mined" data from multiple sources to achieve a cohort of nearly a half million mother-infant pairs. Cooper et al. (2006) had a much smaller, although still substantial cohort of nearly 30,000 infants. Recall the potential risks of retrospective data review, particularly if smaller subsets are analyzed. Primary inspection of the referenced studies for the possibility of "statistical mischief" is beyond the scope of this chapter's focus of instruction.

19 There is evidence that significant amounts of research data never are reported despite the fact that participants were exposed to risks and burdens of research for the purpose of creating generalizable knowledge. On the under-reporting of research results, see Avorn 2006; Antes and Chalmers 2003; Wolford 2014.

References

Ackerman, T.F. 1989. An ethical framework for the practice of paying research subjects, *IRB: A Review of Human Subjects Research*, 11: 1–4.

Adams, R. 1958. Internal-Mammary-Artery ligation for coronary insufficiency, *New England Journal of Medicine*, 258(3): 113–15.

Agency for Healthcare Research and Quality. n.d. What is comparative effectiveness research? Online. Available: http://effectivehealthcare.ahrq.gov/index.cfm/what-is-comparative-effectiveness-research1/ (accessed October 1, 2014).

Anderson, C.G., W.E. Benitz and A. Madan. 2004. Retinopathy of prematurity and pulse oximetry: A national survey of recent practices, *Journal of Perinatology*, 24(3): 164–8.

Anderson, E.E. and A.S. Iltis. 2008. Assessing and improving research participants' understanding of risk: Potential lessons from the literature on physician-patient risk communication, *Journal of Empirical Research on Human Research Ethics: An International Journal*, 3(3): 27–37.

Angell, M. 2005. *The truth about the drug companies: How they deceive us and what to do about it*. New York: Random House Trade Paperbacks.

Antes, G. and I. Chalmers. 2003. Under-reporting of clinical trials is unethical, *Lancet*, 361: 978–9.

Appelbaum, P.S., L.H. Roth and C.W. Lidz. 1982. The therapeutic misconception: Informed consent in psychiatric research, *International Journal of Law and Psychiatry*, 5: 319–29.

Appelbaum, P.S., L.H. Roth, C.W. Lidz, P. Benson and W. Winslade. 1987. False hopes and best data: Consent to research and the therapeutic misconception, *Hastings Center Report*, 17(2): 20–4.

Avorn, J. 2006. Dangerous deception: Hiding the evidence of adverse drug effects, *New England Journal of Medicine*, 355: 2169–71.

Bates, K.F., V.L. Vetter, J.S. Li, S. Cummins, F. Aguel, C. Almond, A.M. Dubin, J. Elia, J. Finkle, E.A. Hausner, F. Joseph, A.M. Karkowsky, M. Killeen, J. Lemacks, L. Mathis, A.W. McMahon, E. Pinnow, I. Rodriguez, N.L. Stockbridge, M. Stockwell, M. Tassinari and M.W. Krucoff. 2012. Pediatric cardiovascular safety: Challenges in drug and device development and clinical application, *American Heart Journal*, 164(4): 481–92.

Bauer, J.A. and H. Fung. 1991. Concurrent hydralazine administration prevents nitroglycerin-induced hemodynamic tolerance in experimental hear failure, *Circulation*, 84: 35–9.

Beauchamp, T. and J. Childress. 1979. *Principles of biomedical ethics*. New York: Oxford University Press.

Beauchamp, T. and J. Childress. 2009. *Principles of biomedical ethics*. New York: Oxford University Press.

Beecher, H.K. 1961. Surgery as placebo: A quantitative study of bias, *Journal of the American Medical Association*, 176(13): 1102–7.

Beecher, H.K. 1966. Ethics and clinical research, *New England Journal of Medicine*, 274: 1254–60.

Belsky, L. and H.S. Richardson. 2004. Medical researchers' ancillary clinical care responsibilities, *British Medical Journal*, 328: 1494–6.

Berg, J., P. Appelbaum, L. Parker and C. Lidz (eds.) 2001. *Informed consent: Legal theory and clinical practice*, New York: Oxford University Press.

Beskow, L.M., C. Grady, A.S. Iltis, J.Z. Sadler and B.S. Wolfond. 2009. Points to consider: The research ethics consultation service and the IRB, *Hastings Center Report*, 31(6): 1–9.

Best Pharmaceuticals for Children Act. 2002. Public Law No. 107-109, 115 Stat. 1408.

Bibbins-Domingo, K. and A. Fernandez. 2007. BiDil for heart failure in black patients: Implications of the U.S. Food and Drug Administration approval, *Annals of Internal Medicine*, 146(1): 52–6.

Bigger, J.T., J.L. Fleiss, R. Kleiger, J.P. Miller, L.M. Rolnitzky and the Multicenter Post-Infarction Research Group. 1984. The relationships among ventricular arrhythmias, left ventricular dysfunction, and mortality in the 2 years after myocardial infarction, *Circulation*, 69(2): 250–8.

Boumil, M.M. and H.A. Berman. 2010. Revisiting the physician/industry alliance: The Bayh–Dole Act and conflict of interest management at academic medical centers, *Michigan State University Journal of Medicine and Law*, 15(1): 1–16.

Buchanan, A.E. and D.W. Brock. 1989. *Deciding for others: The ethics of surrogate decision making*. Cambridge: Cambridge University Press.

Cain, D.M., G. Loewenstein and D.A. Moore. 2005. The dirt on coming clean: Perverse effects of disclosing conflicts of interest, *Journal of Legal Studies*, 34(1): 1–25.

Cardiac Arrhythmia Pilot Study (CAPS) Investigators. 1986. The cardiac arrhythmia pilot study, *American Journal of Cardiology*, 57(1): 91–5.

Cardiac Arrhythmia Pilot Study (CAPS) Investigators. 1988. Effects of encainide, flecainide, imipramine and moricizine on ventricular arrhythmias during the year after acute myocardial infarction: The CAPS, *American Journal of Cardiology*, 61(8): 501–9.

Cardiac Arrhythmia Suppression Trial (CAST) Investigators. 1989. Preliminary report: Effect of encainamide and flecainide on mortality in a randomized trial of arrhythmia suppression after myocardial infarction, *New England Journal of Medicine*, 321(6): 406–12.

Cardiac Arrhythmia Suppression Trial II (CAST II) Investigators. 1992. Effect of the antiarrhythmic agent moricizine on survival after myocardial infarction, *New England Journal of Medicine*, 327(4): 227–33.

Carson, P., S. Ziesche, G. Johnson and J. Cohn for the Vasodilator-Heart Failure Trial Study Group. 1999. Racial differences in response to therapy for heart failure: Analysis of the vasodilator-heart failure trials, *Journal of Cardiac Failure*, 5(3): 178–87.

Caulfield, T. 2011. Blinded by science: Modern-day hucksters are cashing in on vulnerable patients, *The Walrus*, 8(7).

Center for Science in the Public interest. 2005. Conflicts of interest on COX-2 panel: Research from the CSPI's Integrity in Science Project February 25. Located at: <http://www.cspinet.org/new/200502251.html> (accessed March 4, 2016.)

Cherry, M.J. 2013. Ignoring the data and endangering children: Why the mature minor standard for medical decision making must be abandoned, *Journal of Medicine and Philosophy*, 38: 315–31.

Cho, M.K., S.L. Tobin, H.T. Greely, J. McCormick, A. Boyce and D. Magnus. 2008. Strangers at the benchside: Research ethics consultation, *American Journal of Bioethics*, 8(3): 4–13.

Clayton, E.W., K.K. Steinberg, M.J. Khoury, E. Thomson, L. Andrews, M.J. Ellis Khan, L.M. Kopelman and J.O. Weiss. 1995. Informed consent for genetic research on stored tissue samples, *Journal of the American Medical Association*, 274(22): 1786–92.

Clinical and Translational Science Aware (CTSA) Consortium Community Engagement Key Funstion Committee and CTSA Community Engagement Workshop Planning Committee. 2009. Researchers and their communities: The challenge of meaningful community engagement, Online. Available: <http://www.aecom.yu.edu/uploaded-Files/ICTR/CE%20Monograph.pdf?n=1851> (accessed November 13, 2014).

Cohen, P.J. 1998. The placebo is not dead: Three historical vignettes, *IRB: Ethics & Human Research*, 20(2–3): 6–8.

Cohn, J.N., D.G. Archibald, S. Ziesche, J.A. Franciosa, W.E. Harston, F.E. Tristani, W.B. Dunkman, W. Jacobs, G.S. Frances, K.H. Flohr, S. Goldman, F.R. Cobb, P.M. Shah, R. Saunders, R.D. Fletcher, H.S. Loeb, V.C. Hughes and B. Baker. 1986. Effect of vasodilator therapy on mortality in chronic congestive heart failure: Results of a Veterans Administration cooperative study, *New England Journal of Medicine*, 314(24): 1547–52.

Cohn, J.N., G. Johnson, S. Ziesche, F. Cobb, G. Francis, F. Tristani, R. Smith, B. Dunkman, H. Loeb, M. Wong, G. Bhat, S. Goldman, R.D. Fletcher, J. Doherty, C.V. Hughes, P. Carson, G. Cintron, R. Shabetai and C. Haakenson. 1991. A comparison of enalapril with hydralazine-isosorbide dinatrate ib the treatment of chronin congestive heart failure, *New England journal of Medicine*, 325(5): 303–10.

Cooper, W.O., S. Hernandez-Diaz, P.G. Arbogast, J.A. Dudley, S. Dyer, P.S. Gideon, K. Hall and W.A. Ray. 2006. Major congenital malformations after first-trimester exposure to ACE inhibitors, *New England Journal of Medicine*, 354(23): 2443–51.

Coutelle, C. and R. Ashcroft. 2012. Risks, benefits, and ethical, legal, and social considerations for translation of prenatal gene therapy to human application, in C. Coutelle and S.N. Waddington (eds.) *Prenatal gene therapy*. New York: Springer Verlag.

Darity, Jr., W., C. Royal and K. Whitfield. 2010. Race, genetics, and health: An introduction, *Review of Black Political Economy*, 37: 1–6.

Daugherty, C.K., D.M. Banik, et al. 2000. Quantitative analysis of ethical issues in phase I trials: A survey interview of 144 advanced cancer patients, *IRB*, 22(3): 6–14.

de Melo-Martín, I. and L.E. Wolf. 2010. The Havasupai Indian tribe case: Lessons for research involving stored biologic samples, *New England Journal of Medicine*, 363(3): 204–7.

de Melo-Martín, I., L.I. Palmer and J.J. Fins. 2007. Developing a research ethics consultation service to foster responsive and responsible clinical research, *Academic Medicine*, 82(9): 900–4.

Dickert, N. and C. Grady. 1999. What's the price of a research student? Approaches to payment for research participation, *New England Journal of Medicine*, 34: 198–202.

Dickert, N. and D. Wendler. 2009. Ancillary care obligations of medical researchers, *Journal of the American Medical Association*, 302(4): 424–28.

Drazen, J.M., C.G. Soloman and M.F. Greene. 2013. Informed consent and SUPPORT, *New England Journal of Medicine*, 368(20): 1929–31.

Drazen, J.M. and A.J. Wood. 2010. Don't mess with the DSMB, *New England Journal of Medicine*, 363(5): 477–8.

Dresser, R. 2001. *When science offers salvation: Patient advocacy and research ethics*. New York: Oxford University Press.

Dresser, R. 2002. The ubiquity and utility of the therapeutic misconception, *Social Philosophy and Policy*, 19(2): 271–94.

Dries, D.L., M.H. Strong, R.S. Cooper and M.H. Drazner. 2002. Efficacy of angiotensin-converting enzyme inhibition in reducing progression from asymptomatic left ventricular dysfunction to symptomatic heart failure in black and white patients, *Journal of the American College of Cardiology*, 40(2): 311–7.

Duster, T. 2001. Buried alive: The concept of race in science, *Chronicle of Higher Education*, 48(3): B11–2.

Echt, D.S., P.R. Liebson, B. Mitchell, R.W. Peters, D. Obias-Manno, A.H. Barker, D. Arensberg, A. Baker, L. Friedman, H.L. Greene, M.L. Huther, D.W. Richardson and the CAST Investigators. 1991. Mortality and morbidity in patients receiving encainide, flecainide, or placebo: The cardiac arrhythmia suppression trial, *New England Journal of Medicine*, 324(12): 781–8.

Elahi, M., N. Eshera, N. Bambata, H. Barr, B. Lyn-Cook, J. Beitz, M. Rios, D.R. Taylor, M. Lightfoote, N. Hanafi, L. DeJager, P. Wiesenfeld, P.E. Scott, E.O. Fadiran and M.B. Henderson. 2016. The Food and Drug Administration Office of Women's Health: Impact of science on regulatory policy: An update, *Journal of Women's Health*, 25(3): 222–34.

Ellison, G.T.H., J.S. Kaufman, R.F. Head, P.A. Martin and K.D. Kahn. 2008. Flaws in the U.S. Food and Drug Administration's rationale for supporting the development and approval of BiDil as a treatment for heart failure only in black patients, *Journal of Law, Medicine, & Ethics*, 36(3): 449–57.

Emanuel, E.J. and F.G. Miller. 2001. The ethics of placebo-controlled trials: A middle ground, *New England Journal of Medicine*, 345(12): 915–9.

Emanuel, E.J., D. Wendler and C. Grady. 2000. What makes clinical research ethical?, *Journal of the American Medical Association*, 283(20): 2701–11.

Exner, D.V., D.L. Dries, M.P. Domanski and J.N. Cohn. 2001. Lesser response to angio-tensin-converting-enzyme inhibitor therapy in black as compared with white patients with left ventricular dysfunction, *New England Journal of Medicine*, 344(18): 1351–7.

Faden, R. and T. Beauchamp. 1986. *A history and theory of informed consent*. New York: Oxford University Press.

Faden, R.R., N.E. Kass, S.N. Goodman, P. Pronovost, S. Tunis and T.L. Beauchamp. 2013. An ethical framework for a learning health care system: A departure from traditional research ethics and clinical ethics, *Hastings Center Report*, 134: S16–27.

Federal Policy for the Protection of Human Subjects. 2017. *Federal Register* 82, 12, January 19: 7149–7274.

Fitzpatrick, S., N. Downes and H. Korjonen-Close. 2006 *Clinical trial design*. Buckinghamshire: Institute of Clinical Research.

Franciosa, J.A., A.L. Taylor, J.N. Cohn, C.W. Yancy, S. Ziesche, A. Olukotun, E. Ofili, K. Ferdinand, J. Loscalzo and M. Worcel for the A-HeFT Investigators. 2002. African-American Heart Failure Trial (A-HeFT): Rationale, design, and methodology, *Journal of Cardiac Failure*, 8(3): 128–35.

Frankish, H. 2003. WMA postpones decision to amend Declaration of Helsinki, *Lancet*, 362: 963.

Freedman, B. 1987. Equipoise and the ethics of clinical research, *New England Journal of Medicine*, 317: 141–5.

Fried, C. 1974. *Medical experimentation: Personal integrity and social policy*. Amsterdam: North Holland.

General Accounting Office. 2001. Drug safety: Most drugs withdrawn in recent years had greater health risks for women. Located at: <http://www.gao.gov/assets/100/90642. pdf> (accessed January 12, 2017.)

Gillum, R.F. 1987. Heart failure in the United States, 1970–1985, *American Heart Journal*, 113(4): 1043–45.

Goldner, J.A. 2000. Dealing with conflicts of interest in biomedical research: IRB over-sight as the next best solution to the abolitionist approach, *Journal of Law, Medicine & Ethics*, 28: 379–404.

Goodman, A.H. 2000. Why genes don't count (for racial differences in health), *American Journal of Public Health*, 90(11): 1699–1702.

Grady, C. 2001. Monday for research participation: Does it jeopardize informed consent?, *American Journal of Bioethics*, 1(2): 40–4.

Grady, C. 2005. The challenge of assuring continued post-trial access to beneficial treat-ment, *Yale Journal of Health Policy, Law, and Ethics*, 1: 425–35.

Grady, C. and D. Wendler. 2013. Making the transition to a learning health care system, *Hastings Center Report*, 137: S32–3.

Grisso, T. and P.A. Appelbaum. 1998. *The assessment of decision-making capacity: A guide for physicians and other health professionals*. Oxford: Oxford University Press.

Groeneveld, G.J., M. Graf, I. van der Tweel, L.H. van den Berg and A.C. Ludolph. 2007. Alternative trial design in amyotrophic lateral sclerosis saves time and patients, *Amyotrophic Lateral Sclerosis*, 8(5): 266–9.

Gunsalus, C.K., E. Bruner, N. Burbules, L. Dash, M. Finkin, J. Goldberg, W. Greenough, G. Miller, M. Pratt, M. Iriye and D. Aronson. 2006. Improving the system for protecting human subjects: Counteracting IRB "mission creep", *The Illinois White Paper*, The Center for Advanced Study, U Illinois Law & Economics Research Paper No. LE06-016. Online. Available: <http://www.gunalus.net/IllinoisWhitePaperMissionCreep. pdf> (accessed November 18, 2014).

Harmon, A. 2010. New drugs stir debate on rules of clinical trials, *The New York Times*, September 18, A1. <https://www.nytimes.com/2010/09/19/health/research/19trial. html>.

Harris, D.J. and P.S. Douglas. 2000, Enrollment of women in cardiovascular clinical trials funded by the National Heart, Lung, and Blood Institute, *New England Journal of Medicine*, 343: 475–80.

Harris, G. and A. Berenson. 2005. 10 voters on panel backing pain pills had industry ties, *New York Times*, February 25, at A1. Located at: <http://www.nytimes. com/2005/02/25/politics/25fda.html> (accessed March 4, 2016.)

Henderson, G.E., L.R. Churchill, A.M. Davis, M.M. Easter, C. Grady, S. Joffe, N. Kass, N.M.P. King, C.W. Lidz, F.G. Miller, D.K. Nelson, J. Peppercorn, B.B. Rothschild, P. Sankar, B.S. Wilfond and C.R. Zimmer. 2007. Clinical trials and medical care: Defining the therapeutic misconception, *Public Library of Science Medicine*, 4(11): 1735–8.

Hirshon, J.M., S. Krugman, M. Witting, J. Furuno, R. Limcangco, A. Perisse and E. Rasch. 2002. Variability in institutional review board assessment of minimal-risk research, *Academic Emergency Medicine*, 9(12): 1417–20.

Hochhauser, M. 1999. Informed consent and patient's rights documents: A right, a rite, or a rewrite?, *Ethics & Behavior*, 9(1): 1–20.

Hochhauser, M. 2002. "Therapeutic misconception" and "recruiting doublespeak" in the informed consent process, *IRB: Ethics and Human Research*, 24: 11–2.

Holdcroft, A. 2007. Gender bias in research: How does it affect evidence based medicine? *Journal of the Royal Society of Medicine*, 100: 2–3.

Horn, S. 2007. A primer on alternative study designs for evidence-based practice: Harnessing natural variation for effectiveness research, Online. Available: <http:// www.isisicor.com/RecentProjPubs/Primer.htm> (accessed November 18, 2014).

Horn, S. and C. Grady. 2003. Misunderstanding in clinical research: Distinguishing therapeutic misconception, therapeutic misestimation, & therapeutic optimism, *IRB: Ethics and Human Research*, 25(1): 11–6.

Hudson, K.L., A.E. Guttmacher and F.S. Collins. 2013. In support of SUPPORT: A view from the NIH, *New England Journal of Medicine*, 368(25): 2349–51.

Hutt, L.E. 1998. A discussion of the ethical prospect of providing drug trial subjects with post-trial access to drug tested: A Canadian perspective, *Health Law Journal*, 6: 169–87.

Iltis, A.S. 2005. Stopping trials early for commercial reasons: The risk–benefit relationship as a moral compass, *Journal of Medical Ethics*, 31: 410–14.

Iltis, A.S. 2006. Lay concepts in informed consent to biomedical research: The capacity to understand and appreciate risk, *Bioethics*, 20(4): 180–90.

Iltis, A.S. 2007. Pediatric research posing a minor increase over minimal risk and no prospect of direct benefit: Challenging 45 CFR 46.406, *Accountability in Research*, 14: 19–34.

Iltis, A.S. 2009. Payments to normal healthy volunteers in phase 1 trials: Avoiding undue influence while distributing fairly the burdens of research participation, *Journal of Medicine and Philosophy*, 34: 68–90.

Iltis, A.S. 2013. Parents, adolescents, and consent for research participation, *Journal of Medicine and Philosophy*, 38: 332–46.

Institute of Medicine (IOM). 2007. *The learning healthcare system*. Washington, DC: National Academies Press.

Israel, B.A., A.J. Schulz, E. Parker and A. Becker. 1998. Review of community-based research: Assessing partnership approaches to improve public health, *Annual Review of Public Health*, 19: 173–202.

Jones, J. 1981 [1993]. *Bad blood: The Tuskegee syphilis experiment*. New York: The Free Press.

Kahn, J. 2004. How a drug became "ethnic": Law, commerce, and the production of racial categories in medicine, *Yale Journal of Health, Policy, Law, and Ethics*, 4(1): 1–46.

Kahn, J. 2007. Race in a bottle, *Scientific American*, August, pp. 40–5.

Kapp, M.B. 2008. Biobanking human biological materials, *Pharmaceutical Medicine*, 22(2): 75–84.

Karthik, S. and B.M. Fabri. 2006. Left internal mammary usage in coronary artery bypass grafting: A measure of quality control, *Annals of the Royal College of Surgeons of England*, 88: 367–9.

Kimmelman, J. 2007. The therapeutic misconception at 25: Treatment, research, and confusion, *Hastings Center Report*, 37(6): 36–42.

King, N.M.P. 2000. Defining and describing benefit appropriately in clinical trials, *Journal of Law Medicine & Ethics*, 28(4): 332–43.

Lee, S.S., J. Mountain and B.A. Koenig. 2001. The meanings of 'race' in the new genomics: Implications for health disparities research, *Yale Journal of Health Policy, Law, and Ethics*, 1: 33–75.

Levine, R.J. 1986. *Ethics and Regulation of Clinical Research*, 2nd ed. Baltimore, MD: Urban and Schwartzenberg.

Li, D., C. Yang, S. Andrade, V. Tavares and J.R. Ferber. 2011. Maternal exposure to angiotensin converting enzyme inhibitors in the first trimester and risk of malformations in offspring: A retrospective cohort study, *British Medical Journal*, 343: 887.

Lo, B. 2010. *Ethical issues in clinical research: A practical guide*. Philadelphia: LWWW.

Lo, B. and M.J. Field (eds.) 2009. Conflicts of interest in biomedical research *Conflict of interest in medical research, education, and practice*. Washington: National Academies Press, pp. 117–118.

Lomax, G.P. and K.A. Shepard. 2013. Return of results in translational iPS cell research: Considerations for donor informed consent, *Stem Cell Research & Therapy*, 4: 6–10.

London, A.J. 2012. A non-paternalistic model of research ethics and oversight: Assessing the benefits of prospective review, *Journal of Law, Medicine & Ethics*, 40(4): 930–44.

Luebbert, R., R.C. Tair, J.T. Chibnall and T.L. Deshields. 2008. IRB member judgments of decisional capacity, coercion, and risk in medical and psychiatric studies, *Journal of Empirical Research on Human Research Ethics*, 3(1): 15–24.

Macklin, R. 1981. On paying money to research subjects, *IRB: A Review of Human Subjects Research*, 3: 1–6.

Macklin, R. and L. Shepherd. 2013. Informed consent and standard of care: What must be disclosed, *American Journal of Bioethics*, 13(12): 9–13.

Macklin, R., L. Shepherd and A. Dreger. 2014. The OHRP and SUPPORT – Another view *New England Journal of Medicine*, e3: 1–3.

Macklin, R., L. Shepherd, A. Dreger, A. Asch, F. Baylis, H. Brody, L.R. Churchill, C.H. Coleman, E. Cowan, J. Dolgin, J. Downie, R. Dresser, C. Elliott, M.C. Epright, E.K. Feder, L.H. Glantz, M.A. Grodin, W. Hoffman, B. Hoffmaster, D. Hunter, A.S. Iltis, J.D. Kahn, N.M. King, R. Kraft, R. Kukla, L. Leavitt, S.E. Lederer, T. Lemmens, H. Lindemann, M.F. Marshall, J.F. Merz, F.H. Miller, M.E. Mohrmann, H. Morreim, M. Nass, J.L. Nelson, J.H. Noble Jr., E. Reis, S.M. Reverby, A. Silvers, A.C. Sousa, R.G. Spece Jr., C. Strong, J.P. Swazey, L. Turner. 2013. The OHRP and SUPPORT: Another view, *New England Journal of Medicine*, 369(2): e3.

Magnus, D. and A.L. Caplan. 2013. Risk, consent, and SUPPORT, *New England Journal of Medicine*, 368(20): 1864–5.

McGuire, A.L. and L.M. Beskow. 2010. Informed consent in genomics and genetic research, *Annual Review of Genomics and Human Genetics*, 11: 361–81.

McNeil, P. 1997. Paying people to participate in research: Why not? A response to Wilkinson and Moore, *Bioethics*, 11: 390–6.

Merkatz, R.B., R. Temple, S. Sobel, K. Feiden, D.A. Kessler and the Working Group on Women in Clinical Trials. 1993. Women in clinical trials of new drugs -- A change in Food and Drug Administration policy, *New England Journal of Medicine*, 329: 292–6.

Merz, J.F. 2014. 'If the risk of death was not foreseeable...', Replies to Comparative Effectiveness Trials: Generic Misassumptions Underlying the SUPPORT Controversy. Online posting. Available: <http://pediatrics.aappublications.org/content/134/4/651/reply> (accessed November 18, 2014).

Meslin, E.M. and K.A. Quaid. 2004. Ethical issues in the collection, storage, and research use of human biological materials, *Journal of Laboratory and Clinical Medicine*, 144(5): 229–34.

Michener, L., J. Cook, S.M. Ahmed, M.A. Yonas, T. Coyne-Beasley and S. Aguilar-Gaxiola. 2012. Aligning the goals of community-engaged research: Why and how academic health centers can successfully engage with communities to improve health, *Academic Medicine*, 87(3): 285–91.

Miller, F.G. and H. Brody. 2003. A critique of clinical equipoise. Therapeutic misconception in the ethics of clinical trials, *Hastings Center Report*, 33: 19–28.

Millum, J. 2011. Post-trial access to antiretrovirals: Who owes what to whom?, *Bioethics*, 25(3): 145–54.

Moskop, J.C., C.A. Marco, G.L. Larkin, J.M. Geiderman and A.R. Derse. 2005. From Hippocrates to HIPAA: Privacy and confidentiality in emergency medicine – Part I: Conceptual, moral, and legal foundations, *Annals of Emergency Medicine*, 45(1): 53–9.

Münzel, T., S. Kurz, S. Rajagopalan, M. Thoenes, W.R. Berrington, J.A. Thompson, B.A. Freeman and D.G. Harrison. 1996. Hydralazine prevents nitroglycerin tolerance by inhibiting activation of a membrane-bound NADH oxidase: A new action for an old drug, *Journal of Clinical Investigation*, 98(6): 1465–70.

National Bioethics Advisory Commission. 1999. *Research involving human biological materials: Ethical issues and policy guidance*. Rockville, MD: National Bioethics Adivsory Commision.

National Commission for the Protection of Human Subjects of Biomedical and Behavioral Research. 1975. *Research on the fetus*. Washington, DC: U.S. Department of Health, Education, and Welfare.

National Commission for the Protection of Human Subjects of Biomedical and Behavioral Research. 1976. *Research involving prisoners*. Washington, DC: U. S. Department of Health, Education, and Welfare.

National Commission for the Protection of Human Subjects of Biomedical and Behavioral Research. 1977. *Research involving children*. Washington, DC: U.S. Department of Health, Education, and Welfare.

National Commission for the Protection of Human Subjects of Biomedical and Behavioral Research. 1979. *The Belmont Report: Ethical principles and guidelines for protection of human subjects of biomedical and behavioral research*. Washington, DC: U.S. Department of Health, Education, and Welfare.

National Institutes of Health. 1994. *H. Helicobacter pylori* in peptic ulcer disease, *NIH Consensus Statement*, 12(1): 1–23.

National Institutes of Health: Office of Extramural Research. 1994. NIH guidelines on the inclusion of women and minorities as subjects in clinical research, Online. Available: <http://grants.nih.gov/grants/funding/women_min/guidelines_amended_10_2001.htm> (accessed November 18, 2014).

National Research Act. 1974. Public Law. No. 93-348, 88 Stat. 342.

Nuremberg Code. In Nuremberg Military Tribunals. 1949–1953. *Trials of War Criminals before the Nuremberg Military Tribunals under Control Council Law No. 10, Nuremberg, October 1946–April 1949*. Washington, DC: United States Government Publishing Office.

Oberman, M. 1996. Minor rights and wrongs, *Journal of Law, Medicine & Ethics*, 24: 127–38.

Office for Human Research Protections. 2013a. Letter to the University of Alabama at Birmingham, Online. Available: <http://www.hhs.gov/ohrp/detrm_letrs/YR13/mar13a.pdf> (accessed September 26, 2014).

Office for Human Research Protections. 2013b. Letter to the University of Alabama at Birmingham, Online. Available: <http://www.hhs.gov/ohrp/detrm_letrs/YR13/jun13a.pdf> (accessed September 26, 2014).

Palmer, B.W., E.L. Cassidy, L.B. Dunn, A.P. Spira and J.I. Sheikh. 2008. Effective use of consent forms and interactive questions in the consent process, *Hastings Center Report*, 30(2): 8–12.

Participants in the 2006 Georgetown University Workshop on Ancillary-Care Obligations of Medical Researchers Working in Development Countries. 2008. The ancillary-care obligations of medical researchers working in developing countries, *PloS Medicine*, 5(5): e90.

Pratt, C.M. and L.A. Moye. 1990. The cardiac arrhythmia trial: Background, interim results and implications, *American Journal of Cardiology*, 65: 20B–29B.

Pratt, C.M. and L.A. Moye. 1995. The cardiac arrhythmia suppression trial: Casting suppression in a different light, *Circulation*, 91: 245–7.

Ravitsky, V. and B.S. Wilfond. 2006. Disclosing individual genetic results to research participants, *American Journal of Bioethics*, 6(6): 8–17.

Reame, N.K. 2001. Treating research subjects as unskilled wage earners: A risky business, *American Journal of Bioethics*, 1: 53–4.

Reingold, S.C., H.F. McFarland and A.J. Petkau. 2011. The growing need for alternative clinical trial designs for multiple sclerosis in J.A. Cohen (ed.) *Multiple sclerosis therapeutics*, 4th ed. Cambridge: Cambridge University Press.

Reverby, S.M. 2008. Special treatment: BiDil, Tuskegee, and the logic of race, *Journal of Law, Medicine & Ethics*, 36(3): 478–84.

Richardson, H.S. 2004. The ancillary-care responsibilities of medical researchers: An ethical framework for thinking about the clinical care that researchers owe their subjects, *Hastings Center Report*, 34(1): 25–33.

Richardson, H.S. 2008. Incidental findings and ancillary-care obligations, *Journal of Law, Medicine and Ethics*, 36(2): 255–270.

Rochon, P.A., J.P. Clark, M.A. Binns, V. Patel and J.H. Gurwitz. 1998. Reporting of gender-related information in clinical trials of drug therapy for myocardial infarction, *Canadian Medical Association Journal*, 159: 321–7.

Rosenthal, M.S., G.I. Lucas, B. Tinney, C. Mangione, M.A. Schuster, K. Wells, M. Wong, D. Schwarz, L.W. Tuton, J.D. Howell and M. Heisler. 2009. Teaching community-based participatory research principles to physicians enrolled in a health services research fellowship, *Academic Medicine*, 84(4): 478–84.

Ross, L.F., A. Loup, R.M. Nelson, J.R. Botkin, R. Kost, G.R. Smith Jr. and S. Gehlert. 2010. Human subjects protections in community-engaged research: A research ethics framework, *Journal of Empirical Research on Human Research Ethics*, 5(1): 5–17.

Sah, S. 2012. Conflicts of interest and your physician: Psychological processes that cause unexpected changes in behavior, *Journal of Law, Medicine & Ethics*, 40(3): 482–7.

Sankar, P. and J. Kahn 2005. BiDil: Race medicine or race marketing?, *Health Affairs*, W5: 455–63.

Saul, S. 2005. Maker of heart drug intended for Blacks bases price on patients' wealth, *New York Times*, July 8:business. Located at: <http://nytimes.com/2005/07/08/business/maker-of-heart-drug-intended-for-blacks-bases-prices-on-patients.html?_r=0> (accessed January 7, 2017).

Savulescu, J. 2001. The fiction of "undue inducement": Why researchers should be allowed to pay participants any amount of money for any reasonable research project *American Journal of Bioethics*, 1: 1a–3a.

Savulescu, J. and M. Spriggs. 2002. The hexamethonium asthma study and the death of a normal volunteer in research, *Journal of Medical Ethics*, 28: 3–4.

Schneider, C.E. 2010. The hydra, *Hastings Center Report*, 40(4): 9–11.

Scott, C.T. and D. Magnus. 2014. Wrongful termination: Lessons from the Geron clinical trial, *Stem Cells Translational Medicine*, 3(12): 1398–401.

Shah, S., W. Whittle, B. Wilfond, G. Gensler and D. Wendler. 2004. How do institutional review boards apply the federal risk and benefit standards for pediatric research?, *Journal of the American Medical Association*, 291(4): 476–82.

Simon, V. 2005. Wanted: Women in clinical trials, *Science*, 308: 1517.

Society for Adolescent Medicine. 2003. Guidelines for adolescent health research: A position paper of the society for adolescent medicine, *Journal of Adolescent Health*, 33: 396–409.

Solomon, M. and A.C. Bonham. 2013. Ethical oversight of research on patient care, *Hastings Center Report*, 43(S1): S2–3.

Stark, A.R., J.E. Tyson and P.L. Hibberd. 2010. Variation among institutional review boards in evaluating the design of a multicenter randomized trial, *Journal of Perinatology*, 30(3): 163–9.

Steinberg, L. 2013. Does recent research on adolescent brain development inform the mature minor doctrine?, *Journal of Medicine and Philosophy*, 38: 256–67.

Stunkel, L., M. Benson, L. McLellan, N. Sinaii, G. Bedarida, E. Emanuel and C. Grady. 2010. Comprehension and informed consent: Assessing the effect of a short consent form, *IRB: Ethics & Human Research*, 32(4): 1–9.

SUPPORT Study Group of the Eunice Kennedy Shriver NICHD Neonatal Research Network. 2010. Target ranges of oxygen saturation in extremely preterm infants, *New England Journal of Medicine*, 362(21): 1959–69.

Tait, R.C., J.T. Chibnall, A.S. Iltis, A. Wall and T.L. Deshields. 2011. Assessment of consent capability in psychiatric and medical studies, *Journal of Empirical Research on Human Research Ethics*, 6(1): 39–50.

Taylor, A.L., S. Ziesche, C. Yancy, P. Carson, R. D'Agostino Jr., K. Ferdinand, M. Taylor, K. Adams, M. Sabolinski, M. Worcel and J. Cohn for the African-American Heart Failure Trial Investigators. 2004. Combination of isosorbide dinitrate and hydralazine in Blacks with heart failure, *New England Journal of Medicine*, 351(20): 2049–57.

Taylor, H.A., M.W. Merritt and L.C. Mullany. 2011. Ancillary care in public health intervention research in low-resource settings: Researchers' practices and decision-making, *Journal of Empirical Research on Human Research Ethics: An International Journal*, 6(3): 73–81.

Temple, R. and N.L. Stockbridge. 2007. BiDil for heart failure in black patients: The U.S. Food and Drug Administration perspective, *Annals of Internal Medicine*, 146(1): 57–62:

U.S. Food and Drug Administration. 2005. *Joint meeting of the arthritis advisory committee and the drug safety and risk management advisory committee.* Washington: FDA. Located at: <http://www.fda.gov/oc/advisory/accalendar/2005/cder12532ddd0216171805. html> (accessed March 4, 2016.)

Usharani, P. and S.M. Naqvi. 2013. Post-trial access, *Perspectives in Clinical Research*, 4(1): 58–60.

Warren, S. and L. Brandeis. 1890 The right to privacy, *Harvard Law Review*, 4: 193–220.

Wegner, D. 2003. *The illusion of conscious will.* Cambridge: MIT Press.

Weijer, C. and P.B. Miller. 2004. When are research risks reasonable in relation to anticipated benefits?, *Nature Medicine*, 10(6): 570–3.

Weithorn, L. 1983. Children's capacities to decide about participation in research, *Hastings Center Report*, 5: 1–5.

Weithorn, L. and S. Campbell. 1982. The competence of children and adolescents to make informed treatment decisions, *Child Development'*, 53: 1589–98.

Wendler, D. and F.G. Miller. 2007. Assessing research risks systemically: The net risks test, *Journal of Medicine & Ethics*, 33: 481–6.

Whitney, S. and C. Schneider. 2011. A method to estimate the cost in lives of ethics board review of biomedical research, *Journal of Internal Medicine*, 269: 392–406.

Wilfond, B.S., D. Magnus, A.H. Antommaria, P. Appelbaum, J. Aschner, K.J. Barrington, T. Beauchamp, R.D. Boss, W. Burke, A.L. Caplan, A.M. Capron, M. Cho, E.W. Clayton, F.S. Cole, B.A. Darlow, D. Diekema, R.R. Faden, C. Feudtner, J.J. Fins, N.C. Fost, J. Frader, D.M. Hester, A. Janvier, S. Joffe, J. Kahn, N.E. Kass, E. Kodish, J.D. Lantos, L. McCullough, R. McKinney Jr., W. Meadow, P.P. O'Rourke, K.E. Powderly, D.M. Pursely, L.F. Ross, S. Sayeed, R.R. Sharp, J. Sugarman, W.O. Tarnow-Mordi, H. Taylor, T. Tomlinson, R.D. Truog, R.D. Unguru, K.L. Weise, D. Woodrum and S. Youngner. 2013. The OHRP and SUPPORT, *New England Journal of Medicine*, 368(25): e36.

Wilson, R.F. 2010. The death of Jesse Gelsinger: New evidence of the influence of money and prestige in human research, *American Journal of Law & Medicine*, 36: 295–325.

Wolf, S.M. 2012. The past, present, and future of the debate over return of research results and incidental findings, *Genetics in Medicine*, 14(4): 355–7.

Wolf, S.M., F.P. Lawrenz, C.A. Nelson, J.P. Kahn, M.K. Cho, E.W. Clayton, J.G. Fletcher, M.K. Georgieff, D. Hammerschmidt, K. Hudson, J. Illes, V. Japur, M.A. Keane, B.A. Koenig, B.S. Leroy, E.G. McFarland, J. Paradise, L.S. Parker, S.F. Terry, B. Van Ness and B.S. Wilfond. 2008. Managing incidental findings in human subjects research: Analysis and recommendations, *Journal of Law Medicine & Ethics*, 36(2): 219–48.

Wolford, B. 2014. Big pharma plays hide-the-ball with data, *Newsweek*.

Yoder, L.H., T.J. O'Rourke, et al. 1997. Expectations and experiences of patients with cancer participating in phase I clinical trials, *Oncol Nurs Forum*, 24(5): 891–6.

Yu, J., S. Goering and S.M. Fullerton. 2009. Race-based medicine and justice as recognition: Exploring the phenomenon of BiDil, *Cambridge Quarterly of Healthcare Ethics*, 18: 57–67.

Zink, S. 2001. Maybe we should pay them more, *American Journal of Bioethics*, 1: 88.

Zong, Z. 2008 Should post-trial provision of beneficial experimental interventions be mandatory in developing countries?, *Journal of Medical Ethics*, 34(3): 188–92.

14 Early Termination of Cardiovascular Research Protocols

Teresa Lynne Caples and Emily E. Anderson

I Introduction

An increasing number of randomized controlled trials (RCTs) are terminated early before they have completed enrollment and follow-up of all patients (Montori et al., 2005, p. 2203). In medical research, it is ethically imperative that researchers protect the safety and well-being of participants (National Commission for the Protection of Human Subjects of Biomedical and Behavioral Research, 2014). Society must also be protected from overzealous premature claims of treatment benefit (Pocock, 1992, p. 239). There can be tension between these two ethical obligations in situations where researchers, due to new information or circumstances, are faced with the question of whether or not a research study should continue. Regardless of which consideration is given ethical primacy, guidance is needed to help researchers, sponsors, and members of institutional review boards (IRBs) and data safety monitoring boards (DSMBs) evaluate whether or not it is appropriate to stop a trial early.

Reasons for stopping clinical trials early vary, and some reasons may be more ethically acceptable than others. In this chapter, we will review the primary reasons that trials are stopped early and evaluate the ethics of doing so, providing examples from different areas of cardiovascular research. In our overview, we will focus on trials that are stopped early for apparent benefit or for commercial reasons, as these are the most ethically complex and troubling, respectively. We will discuss the potential impact that stopping trials early may have on research participants, patients, and future research as well as the implications for clinical decision-making. We will conclude with some recommendations.

II Reasons for Stopping Trials Early

Major reasons for stopping trials early include safety concerns, determinations of futility, the availability of new information from other studies, apparent benefit for the population, or commercial reasons. These will be the focus of this chapter. Other factors that may influence early termination but will not be discussed include natural or catastrophic disasters (e.g., fire), the loss of key study personnel,

DOI: 10.4324/9781003240273-20

or highly problematic scenarios such as rushing to publish before a competing trial or for academic promotion (Friedman et al., 2010, pp. 301–302).

Decisions to stop a trial early may be initiated by research sponsors, investigators, and/or data safety monitoring boards (DSMBs) (also known as data safety monitoring committees (DSMCs)). DSMBs are independent review groups that monitor participant safety and the overall integrity of clinical trials, usually through periodic review of preliminary data. They can recommend that a study be stopped if there are concerns about safety or efficacy or if the trial does not appear to be meeting scientific objectives (National Institutes of Health, 2013). However, there is evidence that DSMB members are relatively inexperienced and lack appropriate training, and, therefore, that many committees may not be functioning properly (Goodman, 2007, p. 886).

Ideally, a randomized controlled trial protocol will include predetermined, statistically-calculated stopping rules, which are established by reviewing previous trial study designs and outcomes. If, at interim analysis (after a sufficient number of events has occurred) data fall outside the upper or lower boundaries of the stopping rules, the research team must review the risks and benefits to participants, as well as overall safety and efficacy of the trial and predictive probabilities that the trial will continue as intended. However, applying previous outcomes to new research may be challenging, and it is often difficult for a DSMB to determine conclusively when stopping boundaries have been crossed. These uncertainties emphasize the importance of interim oversight and transparency in the decision-making process so DSMBs can make the best possible determination (Montori et al., 2005; Slutsky and Lavery, 2004, p. 1146).

Researchers and sponsors may also decide to stop a trial for reasons beyond DSMB recommendations. Sponsors may want to stop early to minimize costs and appease shareholders. Pharmaceutical companies may also get favorable publicity and the opportunity to reduce research expenses when a drug shows promise and is available for sale sooner. Other stakeholders may also influence decisions to stop trials early. For example, journals want to publish exciting new results that encourage readership. Patients, patient advocates, and clinicians want to speed the delivery of promising interventions into clinical practice (Bassler et al., 2008, p. 243).

III Trials Stopped Early for Safety Reasons

The decision to stop a trial early due to concerns about participant safety is generally not ethically controversial (Bassler et al., 2008, p. 241). If serious adverse events occur during a trial or preliminary data analysis suggests that a particular intervention is doing more harm than good, the trial can and should be terminated in order to protect the research participants. The MOXonidine CONgestive Heart Failure trial (MOXCON) is an example of a cardiovascular clinical trial that was appropriately stopped early due to safety concerns. MOXCON was a placebo-controlled randomized trial comparing moxonidine (a central sympathetic nervous system inhibitor) against placebos in patients with chronic heart failure. The study planned to follow participants over two years and assess all-cause mortality. Although previous trials of monoxidine raised no safety concerns, the DSMB planned for interim analyses at least every six months. Early on, the DSMB observed a trend of almost twice as many deaths in the monoxidine arm than in the placebo arm, far exceeding the pre-determined stopping rule. The trial was stopped after 10 months given that the observed negative trend in mortality suggested a true reduction in mortality due to monoxidine was highly unlikely to be present and detectable with more data (Pocock et al., 2004, pp. 1975–1978). To continue collecting data given the evidence of harm was not worth the risk to participants.

IV Trials Stopped Early for Reasons of Futility

It may be ethical to stop a clinical trial for unforeseen reasons of futility. For example, interim analysis may suggest that differences between intervention and control groups are so insignificant that the money, time and effort cannot be justified (Bassler et al., 2008, p. 241). With no potential for meaningful results, the risks to participants are not balanced by any potential benefit of knowledge gained. Trials stopped appropriately for reasons of futility should not be confused with trials that must be stopped due to poor planning, insufficient oversight or leadership, or insufficient resources (Friedman et al., 2010, pp. 301–302). In these cases, lack of potential scientific worth is foreseen and, therefore, such trials should not be initiated.

However, some trials simply do not go as expected, which is why oversight is so critical. For example, the AleCardio study aimed to investigate aleglitazar in patients with diabetes. The drug had been shown to reduce cardiovascular risks, but had not been tested in patients with diabetes. After only 55% of projected participant enrollment, an unplanned DSMB analysis was recommended due to the high incidence of adverse events in the aleglitazar group. The DSMB's review of cardiovascular criteria suggested there was no benefit from the intervention and that no benefit could be shown even if the trial was carried through to completion, so the trial was terminated early (Lincoff et al., 2014, p. 1517).

V Trials Stopped Early Due to New Information From Other Related Studies

New information may be published that makes current trial outcomes obsolete and, therefore, to continue the research would be unethical given any lack of potential benefit gained from new knowledge. For example, the Canadian Atrial Fibrillation Anticoagulation trial was a 3.5-year, placebo-controlled, randomized controlled trial designed to evaluate the efficacy of warfarin to prevent strokes. At the same time, there were six other studies with similar study designs evaluating the effects of warfarin. Shortly after the Canadian Atrial Fibrillation Anticoagulation trial began, data from two of the other studies were published, confirming the benefits of warfarin with fewer embolic and major bleeding events. Given this new information, the Canadian Atrial Fibrillation Anticoagulation trial investigators determined it would be unethical to randomize participants into the placebo arm of the trial, knowing the benefits of warfarin from these other trials (Laupacis and Sullivan, 1996, p. 1672).

VI Trials Stopped Early for Apparent Benefit

The three reasons for stopping trials early that have been discussed so far are fairly straightforward, presenting situations where the risk–benefit balance to research participants is clear. However, when preliminary analysis suggests that individuals in one study arm benefit significantly compared to those in other arms, decisions become a bit more complicated. In some cases, obvious benefits within a trial suggest overwhelming benefits to the population, and the ethical response is to end the trial and make the drug available to the population for the greater good (Bassler et al., 2008, p. 244). In fact, between 1990 and 2007, the number of randomized trials reported in the literature that were stopped early because of apparent benefit has doubled, and these outcomes are being published more frequently in high impact journals (Montori et al., 2005, p. 2207).

Care is needed when stopping early for benefit, because misinterpreting interim analysis can lead to overestimation of treatment effects. The Candesartan in Heart Failure Assessment of Reduction in Mortality and Morbidity (CHARM) study provides an example of a study in which stopping early was considered, but ultimately the trial continued (see Pocock et al., 2005). CHARM involved three separate randomized trials comparing candesartan with placebo in patients with chronic heart failure. At several interim analyses, significant differences in all-cause mortality were observed. At the fourth interim analysis, the DSMB observed a 24% risk reduction in the candesartan compared to the placebo group, which met their stopping boundary. However, the study aimed to collect proof beyond a reasonable doubt that would influence clinical practice rather than strict reliance on a statistical stopping guideline (Pocock, 2005, p. 2229) and the DSMB recommended continuing. Ultimately, candesartan was found to be insignificant in reducing cardiovascular risks and subsequent analyses showed a much less significant difference in mortality (Pfeffer et al., 2003, p. 759).

The Anglo-Scandinavian Cardiac Outcomes Trial (ASCOT) study compared atorvastatin with placebo in patients with hypertension who were not dyslipidemic, challenging the traditional standard of care for prevention of cardiovascular disease in these patients (Dahlof et al., 2005, p. 895). Early interim analyses showed a highly significant reduction of coronary heart disease-related events (the primary outcome) and a significant reduction of stroke in participants taking atorvastatin (Sever et al., 2003, p. 1151). The decision to stop the trial was supported by evidence from other related trials and, therefore, generally judged to be appropriate (Pocock, 2005, p. 2229).

The Study of Trial Policy of Interim Truncation (STOPIT) used a systematic strategic review to identify problematic areas of bias across a wide spectrum of trials that were stopped early for benefit. Study investigators compared reported treatment effects with a pooled estimate of randomized trials addressing similar questions to study the magnitude and determinants of bias introduced by stopping early (Bassler et al., 2010, pp. 1180–1181).

Initially, STOPIT investigators had difficulty identifying when a reported trial had been truncated, as this is not always explicitly stated in trial abstracts or methods. The quality of the STOPIT review is directly related to the quality of data published by investigators, and publication bias may exclude some trials from being published at all. Reviewers observed that investigators, journal editors, and clinical investigators "remain mostly unaware of the problematic inferences that may arise from truncated RCTs" (Briel et al., 2009). Despite these limitations, STOPIT provides evidence to suggest that published outcomes from trials stopped early for apparent benefit are biased and therefore bias meta-analyses and provide misinformation to clinicians and patients (Briel et al., 2009).

VII Trials Stopped Early for Commercial Reasons

Due to anticipated profits from a drug or device, a company may want to terminate a trial early in order to benefit financially from product distribution on the quarterly returns (Psaty and Rennie, 2003, p. 2128). In other cases, changing market priorities may suggest there is little profit to be made if a drug is brought to market, and sponsors may decide they are not willing to invest in long-term research and end the trial early to avoid financial loss. These business decisions to discontinue the trial may be made with little regard for participant welfare or other ethical considerations. From an ethical perspective, an interim analysis of the trial would need to determine if the benefit to the population, or the risk to the participants, is great enough to warrant early termination of the study (Bassler et al., 2008, p. 244).

Ana Iltis suggests that early termination is unethical if there is still important scientific information to be gained and enrolled participants have already been exposed to some risk. In such a case, stopping a trial early not only retrospectively changes the risk–benefit ratio (participants are exposed to risk without the prospect of societal benefit), it violates the basic principles of informed consent. Essentially, the study is not the same study for which participants provided informed consent (Iltis, 2005, pp. 412–413).

For example, Controlled Onset Verapamil Investigation of Cardiovascular Endpoints (CONVINCE) was a large trial to assess the equivalence of the calcium channel blocker verapamil to standard therapy (atenolol or hydrochlorothiazide) in preventing cardiac events among patients with hypertension. The trial was scheduled to last five years but was stopped two years early for "commercial reasons" (Black et al., 2003, p. 2074) and "business considerations" (Psaty and Rennie, 2003, p. 2128), even though results were inconclusive and the DSMB had recommended the trial continue. While the sponsor never gave investigators a specific rationale for the decision, this case was unique in that investigators still published their findings (Psaty and Rennie, 2003, p. 2128;

Black et al., 2003, p. 2074). The truncated study did not demonstrate equivalence of verapamil compared with diuretic or beta blocker, in large part because it was underpowered. As one commentary argued, "The participants in CONVINCE were not only deprived of personal benefit from the completed trial but also the social benefit of genuine scientific contributions from an adequately powered study" (Psaty and Rennie, 2003, p. 2129). Under such circumstances, termination is not due to unforeseen circumstances but a "willful, informed" decision of the sponsor, who fully anticipated that the proposed research could lose money (or might not be financially beneficial) as this is a risk of all research by the definition of equipoise (Iltis, 2005, p. 413).

There may be exceptional instances in which discontinuing a trial due to financial reasons may be ethically acceptable, but in such cases financial hardship must be due to unforeseen circumstances, not poor planning. In some cases, if financial resources are significantly lacking, it may be dangerous to continue the trial. If there are difficulties in recruiting a sufficient number of participants, it may be ethical to stop in order to prevent exposure of already enrolled participants to risk, given that the scientific aims of the study will not be able to be met without full enrollment. In the case of a trial stopped early for apparent benefit, in which financial considerations may come into play, a DSMB may determine there is sufficient benefit to individual participants that may compensate for risk exposure, and in such a case it may be permissible to end a trial early (Iltis, 2005, pp. 413–414).

VIII Potential Impact on Medical Research

If a trial is terminated early for apparent benefit, the results are likely to be highly publicized as part of the marketing strategy, with potentially questionable analysis available for media and public interpretation. Once a trial has been terminated early, any results that may have come about from the fully completed trial are lost to science. Researchers or sponsors often do not wish to publish negative results, or they cannot find journals that will publish them. However, it is an ethical imperative that all clinical trial results – negative or positive – are made known to other scientists so that future research can build upon what has been established. Further, publishing negative outcomes will limit exposure of future research participants to unnecessary risks. Unfortunately, there is troubling evidence to suggest that not all truncated clinical trials are reported, or if they are, information is lacking in substance and transparency (Montori et al., 2005, p. 2207).

Imagine the following case: Dr. M would like to design a clinical trial to investigate the potential benefits of using a certain non-steroidal anti-inflammatory drug (NSAID) in patients with cardiovascular disease. In reviewing clinicaltrials.gov (a "registry and results database of publicly and privately supported clinical studies of human participants conducted around the world" (ClinicalTrials.gov, 2014)), Dr. M finds three industry-sponsored trials investigating the cardiovascular risks of this specific NSAID, yet it appears all three were terminated early without listing any trial outcomes or reason for early termination. He has contacted the principal investigators and funding sponsors, but he cannot get any information about the trials. Based on other research, Dr. M hypothesizes that there could be a benefit for patients with cardiovascular disease, but he is unsure if he should proceed without full knowledge of what has already been studied.

Repeated, unnecessary trials are unethical because they expose participants to risks needlessly without any potential benefit to society. Currently, there are international movements underway to promote the registry of all clinical trials and reporting of all data results, so that all may benefit from knowledge of the outcomes – positive, negative, or incomplete (see "All trials registered - All results reported", 2013; Anderson, Sprott, and Olsen, 2013; Sprott, 2013). Increasing transparency in this manner could also reduce overall costs by reducing repeated research and supporting scientists to build upon established research.

IX Potential Impact on Patient Care and Clinical Decision-Making

Regardless of the reasons, stopping a clinical trial earlier than participants anticipated may negatively affect trust. Consider the following case: Mr. L, 45 years old, recently experienced an acute myocardial infarction (MI). He has not responded to standard treatments. Electrocardiograms revealed significant heart rate variability. His cardiologist suggested he enroll in a clinical trial testing the effectiveness of anti-arrhythmic drugs to reduce the risk of future arrhythmic death in post-myocardial infarction patients. Mr. L enrolled, but after only two months into the two-year study, he received a phone call informing him that the DSMB has recommended that the study be discontinued because an interim analysis determined the drug had increased the risk of death from a heart attack. Mr. L is confused because his own heart rate variability had improved while taking the new drug, and he did not feel he was at greater risk from a heart attack. His cardiologist would not prescribe the anti-arrhythmic drug that he had been taking during the trial because it had been determined to be unsafe, yet Mr. L felt he was at a greater risk for a heart attack without the trial drug. He feels somewhat betrayed by the research team who offered him a drug that was reducing his heart rate variability, which he thought reduced his risk of future heart attacks, but had now taken this drug away.

Mr. L may have been suffering from the therapeutic misconception, or the misguided perception that the research was intended to benefit him, rather than provide empirical knowledge to add to medical science (Henderson et al., 2007, p. 1735). Regardless, this case highlights the need for the informed consent process to include information regarding the potential for a trial to be stopped, as well as a plan for effectively communicating the reasons for stopping to all participants. Otherwise, stopping trials early may result in loss of public trust in the research enterprise and have a negative impact on the physician–patient relationship (Iltis, 2005, pp. 411–412). Not only might patients, like Mr. L, be concerned that a beneficial intervention has been taken away, they may also fear that they will suffer additional harm from a dangerous drug. For example, in the AleCardio study, there were concerns that suddenly and completely stopping use of aleglitazar might negatively impact participants' ability to control their diabetes, because of the drug's known side-effects relating to glucose reduction. Therefore, investigators sent participants letters which relayed safety concerns, suggested proper stopping procedures, and explained the ultimate futility of continuing the study (Nainggolan, 2013).

When trials are stopped early for apparent benefit, this can also impact patient care, as demonstrated by the Justification for the Use of Statins in Primary Prevention: An Intervention Trial Evaluating Rosuvastatin (JUPITER). JUPITER hypothesized that statin therapy would be effective in preventing first-ever cardiovascular events in patients at risk for vascular disease due to elevated high-sensitivity C-reactive Protein (hsCRP) levels, but who were not traditional candidates for statin therapy due to low cholesterol levels of low-density lipoprotein (LDL). The DSMBs interim analysis observed a 44% reduction in all vascular events, a 54% reduction in MI, a 48% reduction in stroke, and a 20% reduction in all-cause mortality. Additionally, all groups showed benefit from rosuvastatin, including those previously considered to be at low risk (e.g., women, those with normal body mass index, etc.). The trial was stopped early when rigorous pre-specified stopping rules were met (Ridker, 2009, p. 279). However, the trial has received criticism, namely that commercial interests biased the study's leading investigators to overlook the fact that there were not significant differences between groups on the most objective criteria: *mortality* from stroke and myocardial infarction (de Lorgeril et al., 2010, p. 1032). As a result of this "statistical-tug-of-war" between the risks and benefits of statins in primary prevention (Curtiss and Fairman, 2010, p. 420), clinicians have been cautious about prescribing drugs from data analysis that seemed overly optimistic or biased by commercial motivations. In balance, this clinical trial revealed how lifestyle modifications, such as diet, exercise and weight loss, are superior to pharmacological interventions for primary prevention measures (Kaul, Morrissey, and Diamond, 2010, 1076).

X Guidelines for Clinical Decision Analysis to Stop a Trial Early

From our literature search, the primary rules regarding the decision to stop a clinical trial early are: (1) a trial needs independent monitoring; (2) stopping rules should use a high p-value; (3) there should be no interim analysis until a minimum number of events have occurred that would allow for a valid analysis that detects potential harms and adverse events (Bassler et al., 2008, p. 243; Mueller et al., 2007, p. 880); (4) journals should require any trials stopped early to provide sufficient justification for their decisions (Mueller et al., 2007, p. 880); and (5) some new treatments, chronic conditions, or trials seeking regulatory approval should not allow early stopping of any kind to ensure long-term evidence of efficacy and safety (Pocock, 2005, p. 2228).

Understanding the methods of predicting future trial outcomes can be particularly confusing for oversight committees. Goodman recommends a Bayesian approach to interpreting interim results, which incorporates prior trial evidence and "formalizes the notion that surprising effects are probably overestimated and provides a more tempered estimate of the true difference" (Goodman, 2007, p. 885). In short, this is a formal method of incorporating "evidence-based skepticism." Some have argued more conservatively that DSMBs should focus on harm and not review effectiveness of the data while the trial is ongoing (Montori et al., 2005, p. 2208).

Superiority trials aim to detect the clinically relevant difference between two treatments, while equivalence trials aim to determine that the new treatment is neither worse nor better than an established treatment, and non-inferiority trials aim only to show whether the new treatment is not inferior to the established treatment. There is greater potential for misinterpretation of results during interim analysis in non-inferiority and equivalence trials as compared with a superiority trial. Regulatory guidelines often use vague terms such as "clinically acceptable" or "justified clinically" to dictate how large the difference between groups should be (a pre-defined irrelevance margin, or delta), leaving much up to the investigator, statistician, and sponsor. Normally, the study sponsor determines what this difference will be and outlines this in the protocol. Not surprisingly, current methodologies suggest a bias in favor of the trial aim or intervention. A more standardized approach is needed to ensure the comparative validity of results, particularly if the results are used to justify stopping a trial early (Lange and Freitag, 2005, pp. 12, 13, 22).

CONsolidated Standards Of Reporting Trials (CONSORT) were developed by an international group of clinical trial specialists, statisticians, epidemiologists, and biomedical journal editors to improve the complete and transparent reporting of randomized control trial outcomes (Moher et al., 2012; Turner et al., 2012). The details in CONSORT could assist in identifying trials that were stopped early and provide justification for stopping. CONSORT guidelines have only been around for a few years and have not yet gained wide acceptance; therefore, their current impact is marginal (Montori et al., 2005, p. 2207). The CONSORT checklist is reprinted here (Table 14.1) to assist readers in evaluating the reporting of research studies.

XI Conclusion

While much is expected from medical research, there is an "acceptable speed of medical progress" (Goodman, 2007, p. 886). That is, in all research, risks to individual participants must be appropriately balanced against the potential risks and benefits to future patients (National Commission for the Protection of Human Subjects of Biomedical and Behavioral Research. 2014; "Trials of war criminals before the Nuremberg military tribunals under control council law no. 10", 1949). While often conceived of as a primarily scientific issue, stopping a clinical trial early — whether for reasons of safety, apparent benefit, futility, or money — has significant ethical implications.

Table 14.1 CONSORT 2010 Checklist of Information to Include When Reporting a Randomized Trial

Section/Topic	Item No.	Checklist Item
Title and abstract		
	1a	Identification as a randomized trial in the title
	1b	Structured summary of trial design, methods, results, and conclusions (for specific guidance see CONSORT for abstracts)
Introduction		
Background and objectives	2a	Scientific background and explanation of rationale
	2b	Specific objectives or hypotheses
Methods		
Trial design	3a	Description of trial design (such as parallel, factorial) including allocation ratio
	3b	Important changes to methods after trial commencement (such as eligibility criteria), with reasons
Participants	4a	Eligibility criteria for participants
	4b	Settings and locations where the data were collected
Interventions	5	The interventions for each group with sufficient details to allow replication, including how and when they were actually administered
Outcomes	6a	Completely defined pre-specified primary and secondary outcome measures, including how and when they were assessed
	6b	Any changes to trial outcomes after the trial commenced, with reasons
Sample size	7a	How sample size was determined
	7b	When applicable, explanation of any interim analyses and stopping guidelines
Randomization:		
	8a	Method used to generate the random allocation sequence
	8b	Type of randomization; details of any restriction (such as blocking and block size)
Allocation	9	Mechanism used to implement the random allocation concealment mechanism sequence (such as sequentially numbered containers), describing any steps taken to conceal the sequence until interventions were assigned
Implementation	10	Who generated the random allocation sequence, who enrolled participants, and who assigned participants to interventions

(Continued)

Table 14.1 (Continued)

Section/Topic	Item No.	Checklist Item
Blinding	11a	If done, who was blinded after assignment to interventions (for example, participants, care providers, those assessing outcomes) and how
	11b	If relevant, description of the similarity of interventions
Statistical methods	12a	Statistical methods used to compare groups for primary and secondary outcomes
	12b	Methods for additional analyses, such as subgroup analyses and adjusted analyses
Results		
Participant flow	13a	For each group, the numbers of participants who were (a diagram is randomly assigned, received intended treatment strongly recommended) and were analysed for the primary outcome
	13b	For each group, losses and exclusions after randomization, together with reasons
Recruitment	14a	Dates defining the periods of recruitment and follow-up
	14b	Why the trial ended or was stopped
Baseline data	15	A table showing baseline demographic and clinical
Numbers analysed	16	For each group, number of participants (denominator) included in each analysis and whether the analysis was by original assigned groups
Outcomes and estimation	17a	For each primary and secondary outcome, results for each group, and the estimated effect size and its precision (such as 95% confidence interval)
	17b	For binary outcomes, presentation of both absolute and relative effect sizes is recommended
Ancillary analyses	18	Results of any other analyses performed, including subgroup analyses and adjusted analyses, distinguishing pre-specified from exploratory
Harms	19	All-important harms or unintended effects in each group (for specific guidance see CONSORT for harms
Discussion		
Limitations,	20	Trial limitations, addressing sources of potential bias, imprecision, and, if relevant, multiplicity of analyses
Generalizability	21	Generalizability (external validity, applicability) of the trial findings
Interpretation	22	Interpretation consistent with results, balancing benefits and harms, and considering other relevant evidence
Other information		
Registration	23	Registration number and name of trial registry
Protocol	24	Where the full trial protocol can be accessed, if available
Funding	25	Sources of funding and other support (such as supply of drugs), role of funders

Source: Moher et al. (2012).

DSMBs play a critical role in determining whether or not it is ethical and scientifically appropriate to continue a trial and, therefore, more resources must be invested in training and supporting DSMB members in the important work they do. In addition, the complexities of oversight are compounded since it is not possible to create standardized methods to evaluate the unknowns in emerging research, which are often unpredictable. Each research project presents its own challenges. DSMBs and sponsors must be as transparent as possible when justifying their decision for early termination or continuation of a trial. This transparency may extend to a full public disclosure of their rationale, including relevant risks to participants, to maximize the scientific and clinical value of the trial (Slutsky and Lavery, 2004, p. 1146).

Although there has been substantial discussion in the literature regarding the problems encountered by stopping trials early, it appears that researchers, journal editors, and clinicians are largely unaware of the problems that may arise from truncated clinical trials (Briel et al., 2009). Journal editors and publishers play a major role in encouraging more transparency and accountability in the research process. We recommend that journals mandate the use of the CONSORT checklist. And, of course, when reviewing the medical literature, physicians should review all trials, but truncated trials in particular, with a healthy skepticism.

References

All trials registered - All results reported. 2013. http://www.alltrials.net/find-out-more/all-trials/ (Accessed June 22, 2014).

Anderson, G., H. Sprott, and B.R. Olsen. 2013. *Publish negative results; Non-confirmatory or "negative" results are not worthless.* http://www.the-scientist.com/?articles.view/articleNo/33968/title/Opinion--Publish-Negative-Results/ (Accessed June 22, 2014).

Bassler, D., M. Briel, V.M. Montori, M. Lane, P. Glasziou, Q. Zhou, D. Heels-Ansdell, S.D. Walter, G.H. Guyatt, D.N. Flynn, M.B. Elamin, M.H. Murad, N.O. Abu Elnour, J.F. Lampropulos, A. Sood, R.J. Mullan, P.J. Erwin, C.R. Bankhead, R. Perera, C.C. Ruiz, J.J. You, S.M. Mulla, J. Kaur, K.A. Nerenberg, H. Schunemann, D.J. Cook, K. Lutz, C.M. Ribic, N. Vale, G. Malaga, E.A. Akl, I. Ferreira-Gonzalez, P. Alonso-Coello, G. Urrutia, R. Kunz, H.C. Bucher, A.J. Nordmann, H. Raatz, S.A. da Silva, F. Tuche, B. Strahm, B. Djulbegovic, N.K. Adhikari, E.J. Mills, F. Gwadry-Sridhar, H. Kirpalani, H.P. Soares, P.J. Karanicolas, K.E. Burns, P.O. Vandvik, F. Coto-Yglesias, P.P. Chrispim, and T. Ramsay. 2010. Stopping randomized trials early for benefit and estimation of treatment effects: Systematic review and meta-regression analysis, *JAMA* 303 (12): 1180–1187.

Bassler, D., V.M. Montori, M. Briel, P. Glasziou, and G. Guyatt. 2008. Early stopping of randomized clinical trials for overt efficacy is problematic, *Journal of Clinical Epidemiology* 61 (3): 241–246.

Black, H.R., W.J. Elliott, G. Grandits, P. Grambsch, T. Lucente, W.B. White, J. D. Neaton, R.H. Grimm Jr., L. Hansson, Y. Lacourciere, J. Muller, P. Sleight, M.A. Weber, G. Williams, J. Wittes, A. Zanchetti, and R.J. Anders. 2003. Principal results of the Controlled Onset Verapamil Investigation of Cardiovascular End Points (CONVINCE) trial, *JAMA* 289 (16): 2073–2082.

Briel, M., M. Lane, V.M. Montori, D. Bassler, P. Glasziou, G. Malaga, E.A. Akl, I. Ferreira-Gonzalez, P. Alonso-Coello, G. Urrutia, R. Kunz, C.R. Culebro, S.A. da Silva, D.N. Flynn, M.B. Elamin, B. Strahm, M.H. Murad, B. Djulbegovic, N.K. Adhikari, E.J. Mills, F. Gwadry-Sridhar, H. Kirpalani, H.P. Soares, N.O. Abu Elnour, J.J. You, P.J. Karanicolas, H.C. Bucher, J.F. Lampropulos, A.J. Nordmann, K.E. Burns, S.M. Mulla, H. Raatz, A. Sood, J. Kaur, C.R. Bankhead, R.J. Mullan, K.A. Nerenberg., P.O. Vandvik, F. Coto-Yglesias, H. Schunemann, F. Tuche, P.P. Chrispim, D.J. Cook, K. Lutz, C.M. Ribic, N. Vale, P.J. Erwin, R. Perera, Q. Zhou, D. Heels-Ansdell, T. Ramsay, S.D. Walter, and G.H. Guyatt. 2009. Stopping randomized trials early for benefit: A protocol of the Study Of Trial Policy Of Interim Truncation-2 (STOPIT-2), *Trials* 10: 49.

ClinicalTrials.gov. 2014. Washington, D.C.: National Institutes of Health. Available from http://clinicaltrials.gov/ct2/home (Accessed June 22, 2014).

Curtiss, F.R., and K.A. Fairman. 2010. Tough questions about the value of statin therapy for primary prevention: Did JUPITER miss the moon? *Journal of Managed Care Pharmacy* 16 (6): 417–423.

Dahlof, B., P.S. Sever, N.R. Poulter, H. Wedel, D.G. Beevers, M. Caulfield, R. Collins, S.E. Kjeldsen, A. Kristinsson, G.T. McInnes, J. Mehlsen, M. Nieminen, E. O'Brien, and J. Ostergren. 2005. Prevention of cardiovascular events with an antihypertensive regimen of amlodipine adding perindopril as required versus atenolol adding bendroflumethiazide as required, in the Anglo-Scandinavian Cardiac Outcomes Trial-Blood Pressure Lowering Arm (ASCOT-BPLA): A multicentre randomised controlled trial, *Lancet* 366 (9489): 895–906.

de Lorgeril, L.M., P. Salen, J. Abramson, S. Dodin, T. Hamazaki, W. Kostucki, H. Okuyama, B. Pavy, and M. Rabaeus. 2010. Cholesterol lowering, cardiovascular diseases, and the rosuvastatin-JUPITER controversy: A critical reappraisal, *Archives of Internal Medicine* 170 (12): 1032–1036.

Friedman, L.M., C.D. Furberg, and D.L. DeMets. 2010. *Fundamentals of clinical trials*. New York: Springer.

Glossary of common site terms. 2013. Washington D.C.: National Institutes of Health. Available http://clinicaltrials.gov/ct2/about-studies/glossary (Accessed June 22, 2014).

Goodman, S.N. 2007. Stopping at nothing? Some dilemmas of data monitoring in clinical trials, *Annals of Internal Medicine* 146 (12): 882–887.

Henderson, G.E., L.R. Churchill, A.M. Davis, M.M. Easter, C. Grady, S. Joffe, N. Kass, N. King, C.W. Lidz, F.G. Miller, D.K. Nelson, J. Peppercorn, B.B. Rothschild, P. Sankar, B.S. Wilfond, and C.R. Zimmer. 2007. Clinical trials and medical care: Defining the therapeutic misconception, *PLoS Med* 4 (11): e324.

Iltis, A.S. 2005. Stopping trials early for commercial reasons: The risk-benefit relationship as a moral compass. *Journal of Medical Ethics* 31 (7): 410–414.

Kaul, S., R.P. Morrissey, and G.A. Diamond. 2010. By Jove! What is a clinician to make of JUPITER? *Archives of Internal Medicine* 170 (12): 1073–1077.

Lange, S., and G. Freitag. 2005. Choice of delta: requirements and reality — Results of a systematic review, *Biometrical Journal* 47 (1): 12–27.

Laupacis, A., and K. Sullivan. 1996. Canadian atrial fibrillation anticoagulation study: Were the patients subsequently treated with warfarin? Canadian Atrial Fibrillation Anticoagulation Study Group, *Canadian Medical Association Journal* 154 (11): 1669–1674.

Lincoff, A.M., J.C. Tardif, G.G. Schwartz, S.J. Nicholls, L. Ryden, B. Neal, K. Malmberg, H. Wedel, J.B. Buse, R.R. Henry, A. Weichert, R. Cannata, A. Svensson, D. Volz, and D.E. Grobbee. 2014. Effect of aleglitazar on cardiovascular outcomes after acute coronary syndrome in patients with type 2 diabetes mellitus: The AleCardio randomized clinical trial, *JAMA* 311 (15): 1515–1525.

Moher, D., S. Hopewell, K.F. Schulz, V. Montori, P.C. Gotzsche, P.J. Devereaux, D. Elbourne, M. Egger, and D.G. Altman. 2012. CONSORT 2010 explanation and elaboration: Updated guidelines for reporting parallel group randomised trials, *International Journal of Surgery* 10 (1): 28–55.

Montori, V.M., P.J. Devereaux, N.K. Adhikari, K.E. Burns, C.H. Eggert, M. Briel, C. Lacchetti, T.W. Leung, E. Darling, D.M. Bryant, H.C. Bucher, H.J. Schunemann, M.O. Meade, D.J. Cook, P.J. Erwin, A. Sood, R. Sood, B. Lo, C.A. Thompson, Q. Zhou, E. Mills, and G.H. Guyatt. 2005. Randomized trials stopped early for benefit: A systematic review, *JAMA* 294 (17): 2203–2209.

Mueller, P.S., V.M. Montori, D. Bassler, B.A. Koenig, and G.H. Guyatt. 2007. Ethical issues in stopping randomized trials early because of apparent benefit, *Annals of Internal Medicine* 146 (12): 878–881.

Nainggolan, L. 2013. *All trials of diabetes drug Aleglitazar are abandoned.* 2014. Available from http://www.medscape.com/viewarticle/807585 (Accessed June 22, 2014).

National Commission for the Protection of Human Subjects of Biomedical and Behavioral Research. 2014. The Belmont Report. Washington D.C.: Department of Health, Education, and Welfare. Available from http://www.hhs.gov/ohrp/policy/belmont.html (Accessed June 22, 2014).

Pfeffer, M.A., K. Swedberg, C.B. Granger, P. Held, J.J. McMurray, E.L. Michelson, B. Olofsson, J. Ostergren, S. Yusuf, and S. Pocock. 2003. Effects of candesartan on mortality and morbidity in patients with chronic heart failure: The CHARM-Overall programme, *Lancet* 362 (9386): 759–766.

Pocock, S.J. 1992. When to stop a clinical trial, *BMJ* 305 (6847): 235–240.

Pocock, S., L. Wilhelmsen, K. Dickstein, G. Francis, and J. Wittes. 2004. The data monitoring experience in the MOXCON trial, *European Heart Journal* 25 (22): 1974–1978.

Pocock, S.J. 2005. When (not) to stop a clinical trial for benefit, *JAMA* 294 (17): 2228–2230.

Pocock, S., D. Wang, L. Wilhelmsen, and C.H. Hennekens. 2005. The data monitoring experience in the Candesartan in Heart Failure Assessment of Reduction in Mortality and morbidity (CHARM) program, *American Heart Journal* 149 (5): 939–943.

Psaty, B.M., and D. Rennie. 2003. Stopping medical research to save money: A broken pact with researchers and patients. *JAMA* 289 (16): 2128–2131.

Ridker, P.M. 2009. The JUPITER trial: Results, controversies, and implications for prevention. *Circulation, Cardiovascular Quality and Outcomes* 2 (3): 279–285.

Sever, P.S., B. Dahlof, N.R. Poulter, H. Wedel, G. Beevers, M. Caulfield, R. Collins, S.E. Kjeldsen, A. Kristinsson, G.T. McInnes, J. Mehlsen, M. Nieminen, E. O'Brien, and J. Ostergren. 2003. Prevention of coronary and stroke events with atorvastatin in hypertensive patients who have average or lower-than-average cholesterol concentrations, in the Anglo-Scandinavian Cardiac Outcomes Trial—Lipid Lowering Arm (ASCOT-LLA): A multicentre randomised controlled trial, *Lancet* 361 (9364): 1149–1158.

Slutsky, A.S., and J.V. Lavery. 2004. Data safety and monitoring boards. *New England Journal of Medicine* 350 (11): 1143–1147.

Sprott, H. 2013. *Why publish your negative results? 2013.* Available from http://blogs.biomedcentral.com/bmcblog/2012/08/28/why-publish-your-negative-results-2/ (Accessed June 22, 2014).

Trials of war criminals before the Nuremberg military tribunals under control council law no. 10, vol. 2 1949. (181–182). Washington, DC: US Government Printing Office. Available at http://www.hhs.gov/ohrp/archive/nurcode.html (Accessed June 22, 2014).

Turner, L., L. Shamseer, D.G. Altman, L. Weeks, J. Peters, T. Kober, S. Dias, K.F. Schulz, A.C. Plint, and D. Moher. 2012. Consolidated standards of reporting trials (CONSORT) and the completeness of reporting of randomised controlled trials (RCTs) published in medical journals. *Cochrane Database Sysem Review* 11, MR000030.

Index

For Product Safety Concerns and Information please contact our EU
representative GPSR@taylorandfrancis.com
Taylor & Francis Verlag GmbH, Kaufingerstraße 24, 80331 München, Germany